RISK MANAGEMENT HANDBOOK

FOR HEALTH CARE FACILITIES

American Society for Healthcare Risk Management
Linda Marie Harpster, J.D., and Margaret S. Veach, Editors

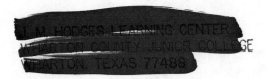

AHA books are published by American Hospital Publishing, Inc.,
an American Hospital Association company

The views expressed in this publication are strictly those of the authors and do not necessarily represent official positions of the American Hospital Association.

Library of Congress Cataloging-in-Publication Data

Risk management handbook for health care facilities / American Society
 for Healthcare Risk Management ; Linda Marie Harpster and Margaret
 S. Veach, editors.
     p.   cm.
  Includes bibliographical references.
  Includes index.
  ISBN 1-55648-054-7 (paper)
  1. Health facilities—Risk management. I. Harpster, Linda Marie.
II. Veach, Margaret S. III. American Society for Healthcare Risk
Management.
  [DNLM: 1. Health Facilities—economics. 2. Health
Facilities—organization & administration. 3. Risk Management.
WX 157 R5953]
RA971.38R58   1990
362.1'1'068—dc20
DNLM/DLC
for Library of Congress   90-1087
                                               CIP

Catalog no. 178157

©1990 by American Hospital Publishing, Inc.,
an American Hospital Association company

Printed in the USA

AHA is a service mark of the American Hospital Association used under license by American Hospital Publishing, Inc.
Text set in Palacio
4M—9/90—0223
1.5M—5/93—0350
1M—7/95—0422
Audrey Kaufman, Project Editor
Linda Conheady, Manuscript Editor
Sophie Yarborough, Editorial Assistant
Marcia Bottoms, Managing Editor
Peggy DuMais, Production Coordinator
Marcia Vecchione, Designer
Brian Schenk, Books Division Director

Table of Contents

List of Figures

List of Tables

Contributors

Megan A. Adams is director of risk management/quality assurance at Hahnemann University in Philadelphia. She was past president and is current treasurer of the Delaware Valley Health Care Risk Management Association and is a member of the Delaware Valley Ethics Committee Network.

Gregory E. Alvarez, J.D., is an attorney with the law firm of Matthews & Branscomb in San Antonio. Mr. Alvarez is a member of the San Antonio Young Lawyer's Association and the San Antonio chapter of the Mexican–American bar association. He is also a member of the American and San Antonio bar associations and the State Bar of Texas.

Ellen L. Barton, C.P.C.U., J.D., is director of corporate risk management at the Franciscan Health System, Aston, Pennsylvania, and president of Neumann Insurance Company in Chadds Ford, Pennsylvania. She is currently the president-elect of the American Society for Healthcare Risk Management. Ms. Barton sits on the boards of directors of several insurance organizations. From 1985 to 1987 she was the director of risk management at the University of Pennsylvania. From 1981 to 1985 she held positions as associate director and director of risk management at the University of Cincinnati. She also holds the distinction of Chartered Property and Casualty Underwriter. She has conducted national and regional seminars on risk management issues and has published articles in related areas, including a series of articles in *Nursing Economic$*. She served as the contributing author of the second edition of *Commercial Liability Risk Management and Insurance* (CPCU 4), published by the American Institute for Property and Liability Underwriters. She is admitted to the Bars of Ohio, Maryland, and Pennsylvania and is a member of numerous organizations of legal, insurance, and health care professionals.

Sanford M. Bragman is assistant vice-president of risk management services at the Daughters of Charity National Health System in St. Louis, which supports health care activities in seventeen states and the District of Columbia. He has served as president of the American Society for Healthcare Risk Management and the Michigan Society of Hospital Risk Management and has participated in numerous AHA presentations and publications.

Susan N. Chernoff, J.D., is a senior associate with the Chicago-based law firm of Gardner, Carton & Douglas, specializing in health and hospital law. She is coauthor, with William H. Roach, Jr., and Carole L. Esley, of *Medical Records and the Law,* published by Aspen Publishers in 1985. She also has been a contributing author to *Topics in Health Record Management, Journal of the American Medical Record Association,* and *Computers in Healthcare.* She is a member of the American Academy of Hospital Attorneys, the American Society of Law & Medicine, and the Chicago Bar Association.

John C. Dronsfield is vice-president of risk management for MMI Companies, Inc., Bannockburn, Illinois. He participated in the development of and is on the advisory board for the Healthcare Risk Management Certificate Program (HRM) developed jointly by MMI and the University of Health Sciences. Previously he was director of risk management and quality assurance at North Kansas City Hospital, North Kansas City, Missouri, and director of risk management for the Illinois Hospital Association.

Guy Fragala, Ph.D., is director of environmental health and safety at the University of Massachusetts Medical Center in Worcester, Massachusetts. He also is a member of the National Safety Council's Healthcare Section Executive Committee and a former member of the board of directors for the American Society for Hospital Risk Management. Dr. Fragala is a certified safety professional, a certified health care safety professional, and a faculty member of the Joint Commission on Accreditation of Healthcare Organizations Educational Programs.

Mary Elizabeth Giblin, J.D., is an associate in the health care group at Reed Smith Shaw & McClay, a Washington, D.C., law firm.

Trudy A. Goldman is director of the American Society for Healthcare Risk Management in Chicago. She previously was risk manager at the University of Illinois at Chicago and was president of the Healthcare Risk Management Society of Metropolitan Chicago in 1987.

Paul A. Greve, Jr., J.D., is vice-president and general counsel of St. Luke's Hospital in Cleveland. He began his health care career with the Cleveland Clinic Foundation in 1973, serving as an administrative coordinator until 1978. From 1978 to 1979, he was a claims representative for the Ohio Joint Underwriting Association. He spent seven years at Columbus Children's Hospital as director of risk management and director of legal services before becoming assistant vice-president and associate general counsel for University Hospitals of Cleveland in 1986. He is past president of the Ohio Society of Hospital Risk Managers and has published, lectured, and consulted on risk management and medical–legal topics.

Sheila R. Hagg, M.H.A., M.B.A., J.D., is director of risk management and health care services at Sisters of Charity Health Care Systems, Inc., and Novare Services, Inc., Cincinnati. She is responsible for development and monitoring of clinical and medical staff risk management programs for a system of 23 Catholic hospitals as well as risk management consulting services. She previously was associate vice-president of Memorial Hospital in Belleville, Illinois.

Linda Marie Harpster, M.A., J.D., is in the private practice of law in Cincinnati, Ohio. During the preparation of this book, she was vice-president and general counsel for Lutheran Hospital of Indiana, Fort Wayne, Indiana, a 589-bed regional referral center serving northeast Indiana, northwest Ohio, and southern Michigan. Previously, she served for three years as director of legal services for Sisters of Charity Health Care Systems, Inc., Cincinnati, and she also contributes "Case Law Update" to *Perspectives in Health Care Risk Management* and serves on the editorial advisory board of *Perspectives.* Ms. Harpster was also past president of the Ohio Society of Hospital Risk Managers and is a member of the American College of Health Care Executives.

Ann Helm, R.N., M.S., J.D., is associate professor at the School of Medicine at the Department of Public Health and Preventive Medicine, Oregon Health Sciences University, Portland, Oregon, and consultant on quality assurance to the United States Air Force Surgeon General. She also is director of quality assurance and risk management, Department of Veteran Affairs, VA Medical Center, Portland, Oregon, and a major in the United States Air Force Reserves, 40th Aeromedical Evacuation Squadron, McChord Air Force Base, Tacoma. She has been a United Nations intern and a fellow of the W. K. Kellogg Foundation. She has had an HEW internship on bioethics, and has written extensively on bioethics, legal issues, quality assurance, and risk management. She is a member of the Communications and Resources Committee at the American Society for Healthcare Risk Management and serves on the board of directors of the American Association for World Health and Public Health International.

Virginia P. Johnson, R.N., M.S.N., is director of quality assurance and risk management at the General Hospital Center at Passaic, New Jersey. She previously was nurse supervisor at the psychiatric unit of St. Joseph's Hospital and Medical Center in Paterson, New Jersey.

Leilani Kicklighter, R.N., M.B.A, is vice-president and director of risk management services for the National Health Care Division of Alexander & Alexander, Inc., in St. Louis. Her past experience includes infection control and quality assurance. She has over 13 years of experience in health care risk management in a variety of settings, including a university and teaching hospital, a medium-sized community hospital, a large multispecialty physician clinic, an HMO, and a multihospital, multistate health care system. She has been active in state and local health care risk management organizations and in the American Society for Healthcare Risk Management, serving on committees, on the board of directors, and as president-elect. Ms. Kicklighter has achieved the Associate in Risk Management (A.R.M.) designation and holds the distinction of diplomate in the American Society for Healthcare Risk Management.

James H. Kizziar, Jr., J.D., is a partner with the law firm of Matthews & Branscomb in San Antonio, where he represents management in labor relations and employment law. A substantial segment of his labor practice consists of health care institutions throughout the United States. Mr. Kizziar has 14 years of experience in representing management in labor issues. He is board certified in labor law by the Texas Board of Legal Specialization. He is a frequent lecturer and author on labor and employment law issues for health care institutions.

Frances Kurdwanowski, R.N., is risk manager at St. Joseph's Hospital and Medical Center, Paterson, New Jersey, a 701-bed regional medical center that includes a 136-bed long-term care facility and two satellite clinics. She has served in clinical and administrative positions in nursing for over 20 years at St. Joseph's Hospital and Medical Center. She has been a member of the American Society for Healthcare Risk Management's Communications and Resources Committee since 1987, serving as chairperson for the past two years.

Stephan E. Lawton, J.D., is a partner in the health care group at Reed Smith Shaw & McClay, a Washington, D.C., law firm. From 1971 to 1979 he was chief counsel of the Subcommittee on Health and the Environment, U.S. House of Representatives.

Melissa J. Long, M.S.H.H.A., J.D., was most recently an attorney at Wyatt, Tarrant & Combs in Louisville, Kentucky, where she worked primarily in health care law. She has six years of experience in health care administration and health care risk management at Methodist Hospitals of Memphis, Baptist Memorial Health Care Development Corporation in Memphis, and Baylor University Medical Center in Dallas. She is currently a member of the Kentucky and Tennessee Bar Associations, the American Bar Association, and the Memphis Bar Association.

Jonathan T. Lord, M.D., is medical quality assurance director at the Anne Arundel Medical Center in Annapolis, Maryland, and a consultant surveyor at the Joint Commission on Accreditation of Healthcare Organizations in Chicago. Dr. Lord previously was director of quality assurance for the Department of the Navy, Office of the Navy Surgeon General, and is a coauthor of *Integrated Quality Assessment: A Model for Concurrent Review,* published by American Hospital Publishing, Inc., in 1989.

Joan S. MacDonald, M.S., is risk manager at Colchester Regional Hospital, Truro, Nova Scotia, and a board member of Community and Hospital Infection Control-Canada (CHICA Canada). Ms. MacDonald also is a consultant at LEFAR Health Associates, Inc., a health care consulting firm with offices in Halifax, Nova Scotia, and Providence, Rhode Island.

Peggy Berry Martin, M.S., is director of education at the Risk Management Foundation (RMF) of the Harvard Medical Institutions, Cambridge, Massachusetts. She has been a member of the American Society for Healthcare Risk Management for 10 years, has served on the nominating committee, chaired the education committee in 1987 and 1990, and currently serves on the board of directors. In addition, she was a charter member and first president of the Massachusetts Society for Healthcare Risk Management. She came to RMF in 1978 as their first loss control director, went to Children's Hospital in Boston as director of risk management and quality assurance from 1982 to 1987, and returned to RMF in 1987 in her present position. She has published a number of articles in the *RMF Forum.*

Jane C. McConnell, R.N., J.D., is vice-president of risk management at FOJP Service Corporation in New York City, a not-for-profit corporation providing risk management, insurance, and litigation support services to eight major medical centers, eight nursing homes, and over 100 community and social service agencies affiliated with the Federation of Jewish Philanthropies of New York. She is a member of the Ad Hoc Committee on Medical Malpractice of the Association of the Bar of the City of New York, a member of the New York State Bar Association, and past president and board member of the Association of Hospital Risk Management of New York, Inc. In 1989 she was chair of the Education Committee of the American Society for Healthcare Risk Management, and in 1988 a member of its legislative committee.

Brad R. Norrick is vice-president of Johnson & Higgins of Oregon, Inc., in Portland. Mr. Norrick is a frequent speaker at risk management and health care organization meetings and is a member of the American Society for Healthcare Risk Management's Risk Financing Committee.

James E. Orlikoff is president of Orlikoff & Associates, a Chicago consulting firm specializing in health care leadership, quality, and risk management. He was formerly the director of the American Hospital Association's Division of Hospital Governance and director of the Institute on Quality of Care and Patterns of Practice of the AHA's Hospital Research and Educational Trust. Mr. Orlikoff has been involved in quality, leadership, and risk management issues for over 10 years. He has designed and implemented hospital quality assurance and risk management programs in four countries, and since 1985 has worked with hospital governing boards to strengthen their oversight of quality assurance and medical staff credentialing. He has authored four books and over 40 articles and currently serves on hospital and civic boards. He is the primary author of the best-selling book *Malpractice Prevention and Liability Control for Hospitals* (American Hospital Publishing, 1988), now in its second edition.

Andrea M. Praeger, M.P.H., J.D., is associate general counsel at FOJP Service Corporation in New York City, a not-for-profit corporation providing risk management, insurance, and litigation support services to eight major medical centers, eight nursing homes, and over 100 community and social service agencies affiliated with the Federation of Jewish Philanthropies of New York.

Fay A. Rozovsky, M.P.H., J.D., is president of LEFAR Health Associates, Inc., a Rhode Island and Nova Scotia health care consulting firm specializing in quality assurance, risk management, staff privileges issues, and related matters. She is a visiting lecturer in health law at Harvard University, and a member of the Massachusetts and Florida bars. Ms. Rozovsky is the author of *Consent to Treatment: A Practical Guide,* 2nd edition, published in 1990 by Little, Brown & Company in Boston. Rozovsky acts as a consultant for hospitals, nursing homes, home care agencies, and government on health care law and risk management issues.

Patricia Scully, R.N., M.S., J.D., is director of risk management at Tucson Medical Center. Her past experience includes clinical nursing in intensive/coronary care units, private law practice, and community college teaching. She has presented numerous educational programs on health care law, and her work has been published in *Nursing Life* and *Perspectives in Healthcare Risk Management.*

Myra C. Selby, J.D., is a partner at the Indianapolis, Indiana, law firm of Ice Miller Donadio & Ryan, where she practices in the area of health care law. She is a frequent lecturer and the author on health law topics. She coauthored the 1988 Case Law Update for the Annual Meeting of the National Health Lawyers Association.

Michael D. Smith, J.D., is an associate in the health care group at Reed Smith Shaw & McClay, a Washington, D.C., law firm.

Audrone M. Vanagunas, M.P.H., has served since 1980 as the director of risk management services for the Chicago Hospital Risk Pooling Program (CHRPP), which provides professional and comprehensive general liability coverage for several Chicago-area hospitals. Before joining CHRPP, she was project manager of education program development for the Joint Commission on Accreditation of Hospitals, Chicago, and is past president of the American Society for Healthcare Risk Management. With James Orlikoff, Ms. Vanagunas wrote *Malpractice Prevention and Liability Control for Hospitals* (2nd ed.), published in 1988 by American Hospital Publishing, Inc.

Margaret S. Veach is staff specialist for the American Society for Healthcare Risk Management of the American Hospital Association, as well as editor of *Perspectives in Healthcare Risk Management.* She was previously editor with the Editorial Services Department of the American Hospital Association and before joining AHA did freelance editorial work for Care Communications in Chicago. Ms. Veach also wrote "Minimizing the Hospital's Risk of Liability Exposure: The Trustee's Role," which appeared in the June 1987 issue of *Trustee.*

Edgar A. Zingman, J.D., of Wyatt, Tarrant & Combs in Louisville, Kentucky, is counsel to the Kentucky Hospital Association and numerous hospitals in Kentucky and other locations. Mr. Zingman was past president of the American Academy of Hospital Attorneys and past president of the Kentucky Academy of Hospital Attorneys. He also has been a member of the House of Delegates of the American Hospital Association.

How to Use This Book

This book has been organized into six parts to facilitate an understanding of the various responsibilities and issues important to risk managers. Beginning risk managers will find the first three sections helpful in understanding how the elements of a risk management program fit together. Part One provides background and highlights legislative and regulatory concerns, Part Two explores how risk managers interact with the board of trustees, the medical staff, the nursing staff, and others within and external to the health care setting, and Part Three describes key functions, such as safety, that affect risk management.

Experienced risk managers may wish to concentrate on the last three parts, which deal with more specific risk management areas. Part Four covers many different high-risk areas, Part Five describes how to identify and control risk from various perspectives, and Part Six focuses on contract review, employment issues, and record management.

Three useful appendixes supplement the text. They include documents that are essential to the practice of risk management—the risk management standards of the Joint Commission on Accreditation of Healthcare Organizations, the federal Health Care Quality Improvement Act (HCQIA), and the regulations implementing HCQIA, which established the National Practitioner Data Bank. The standards are those for 1990 and may change from year to year. Risk managers must refer to the most recent Joint Commission *Accreditation Manual for Hospitals* for updates.

As this book is written, the National Practitioner Data Bank created by the HCQIA is not yet operational. The forms for reporting and accessing data are not included because they are in draft form only. There are many other statutes and regulations important to risk managers, which are discussed in Part One, but space does not permit publication of them all. Sources for copies of other legislation include the institution's attorney, the public library, the local or state hospital association, and the American Hospital Association.

Acknowledgments

We would be remiss if we did not acknowledge the many individuals who contributed their support, suggestions, criticism, and advice throughout the course of this project.

Before a book of this nature is begun, it takes the unflagging enthusiasm of key people to make the idea come alive. Those who supplied that enthusiasm were Trudy Goldman, director, American Society for Healthcare Risk Management (ASHRM), and the members of the 1988 ASHRM board of directors: Sanford Bragman, Roberta Carroll, John Cossa, M.D., Lawrence Herron, Leilani Kicklighter, LeAna Osterman, Stephen Trosty, and Audrone Vanagunas.

Invaluable to the quality of this book were the suggestions and criticism of those individuals who served as initial reviewers: Karen Arcidiacono, Jane Bryant, Aileen Evans, Sheila Hagg, Judy Hart, Ann Helm, James Holzer, James Jensen, Eric Joseph, Frances Kurdwanowski, Clifford Roe, Fay Rozovsky, Steven Salman, and Audrone Vanagunas. They supplied us with careful, reasoned, thoughtful reviews under sometimes nearly impossible deadline demands.

We acknowledge the uncomplaining assistance of Cherrell Jackson, ASHRM administrative assistant, who performed essential tasks of keeping us to our deadlines, inputting and formatting manuscripts, and conducting voluminous correspondence with the authors. The staff at AHPI—particularly Audrey Kaufman, product line manager, Linda Conheady, assistant managing editor, and Sophie Yarborough, editorial assistant—are thanked for the editorial review of the chapters, copyediting of the manuscript, and production of the book.

Part One

Background

How risk management is performed in health care settings is determined by the needs of each particular health care institution and the qualifications of the personnel performing the risk management functions. However, risk management programs have a common structure that is determined by the goals of risk management—to reduce the risk of financial loss to the institution—and by the regulatory environment of health care. The chapters in this section will describe these fundamentals and the major pieces of federal legislation that affect health care risk management.

Chapter 1

Introduction

Linda Marie Harpster

The people who wrote this book are, for the most part, health care risk managers who have been in the field at least five years; some have been in it much longer. Most of them taught themselves how to be health care risk managers. When they began their careers, there were no books explaining the principles or how-to's of risk management; there were no seminars on managing risk in health care settings; the American Society for Healthcare Risk Management (ASHRM) had not yet been organized, nor had the state societies; and the chief executive officers or boards of directors who hired them did not really know what risk management was but knew only that the hospital's insurance carrier encouraged risk management. The things they have learned by setting up and running risk management programs for hospitals are shared in this book.

☐ A Brief History of Health Care Risk Management

The impetus to establish risk management in hospitals came from the insurance crisis in the mid-1970s, when the number of malpractice claims against hospitals and physicians rose dramatically and the amount required for settlements and judgments seemed to skyrocket. Some malpractice carriers withdrew from the market, leaving the hospitals they had insured without coverage. Many states took action by establishing underwriting funds for health care providers.

Hospitals came together to fund hospital-owned insurance companies. Many of those, as well as the insurance companies that remained in the market, offered reduced premiums to hospitals that set up risk management programs. They perceived that risk management programs were the answer to bringing the cost of malpractice claims under control. Also, Medicare conditions of participation required those hospitals with their own trust to have risk management programs.

Fifteen years later, hospitals have survived still another "insurance crisis," and health care risk management has matured as a discipline to become an integral part of the operations of most health care institutions. Beginning risk managers now have a multitude of resources on which to draw for direction.

☐ The History of This Handbook

In the 1980s, the American Society for Healthcare Risk Management realized that there was no single source that explained the fundamentals of risk management—there was no primer from which someone undertaking the risk management job could learn the principles upon which risk management programs are built. Therefore, the 1987–1988 Communication and Resources Committee of ASHRM gave itself the ambitious task of creating such a primer. Because the committee membership changes each year and because the project would take more than one year, the 1987–1988 Communication and Resources Committee, which envisioned the project, constituted itself as a task force to develop the manuscript. The task force comprised the following members: Linda Marie Harpster, Ann Helm, Frances Kurdwanowski, Fay Rozovsky, and Audrone Vanagunas.

The task force first developed a detailed outline of what the book should cover. It then identified ASHRM members and supporters who had expertise in each area covered by the outline and asked them to write those parts of the book. Once the authors had submitted their manuscripts, the task force reviewed the submissions for inclusiveness, accuracy, consistency of style, and readability. Above all, the committee wanted the book to be a practical guide with as many examples as possible so that new risk managers could put the principles discussed into the context of the problems they faced each day.

All committee members and all authors were volunteers on this project. The hundreds of hours of work that they put in were in addition to their regular responsibilities and without monetary reward. They provide this book so that risk managers undertaking the job for the first time do not have to teach themselves and so that experienced risk managers will have a reference tool. Readers who find a particular section helpful can provide a well-deserved reward by letting the author of that section know.

☐ Emphasis on General Principles

Because legislation affecting health care practitioners and health care institutions changes rapidly and because health care business practices change in response, some of the information in this book may become quickly outdated. The authors and editors made an effort not to include issues that were sure to change by the publication date. The authors have emphasized general principles and have used examples that provide general guidance to beginning risk managers. For advice on issues specific to the institution, the risk manager should continue to rely on the institution's attorneys, insurance brokers, and other consultants.

☐ Organizational Differences

The purpose of risk management programs—to identify the risk of loss, determine the most effective way to manage the risks identified, and monitor the effectiveness of the programs—is the same in every institution. Regardless of the particular tasks assigned in the job description, the methods by which the tasks are accomplished are the same. These include educating health care personnel on topics important to risk management, anticipating losses and providing a method to handle them, responding to losses quickly to minimize them, putting systems in place to deal with problems that repeat themselves, protecting patient safety, and maintaining confidentiality of documents.

Despite the similarity in goals and methodology, however, risk management programs are organized differently in each institution. First, they differ in the areas that risk managers are expected to handle. Some assign oversight of the workers' compensation system, or even the entire employee benefits section, to risk management, but most do not. Some institutions want the risk manager to manage only the facility's safety program.

Some put the quality assurance function under risk management; some put the risk management function under quality assurance; and some separate quality assurance and risk management entirely.

Institutions provide varying resources to the risk management program. Many large institutions have one person functioning as both in-house counsel and risk manager. The smaller community hospital across town may have a department of risk management with several employees responsible for safety, loss prevention, legal services, claims management, and workers' compensation. Many hospitals do not have a position they call "risk manager," but they have someone who performs the functions that make up risk management. In those institutions without a risk manager, the risk management tasks are usually done by a number of different people, from the director of safety and security to the chief financial officer to the patient representative. Each hospital puts together those functions that belong together for that institution and devotes the resources to risk management that seem appropriate.

☐ Tips for Beginning Risk Managers

Despite the lack of consistency in job descriptions and organization of risk management programs, there are common problems that, because of the nature of the job, almost every beginning risk manager encounters. The following suggestions may assist beginning risk managers to avoid some natural pitfalls.

Priority Setting

Doing the job that risk managers expect of themselves requires both an omniscience and an omnipresence not usually possessed by mortals. The risk manager's tasks include:

- Controlling losses to the institution from medical malpractice
- Managing claims
- Reviewing contracts
- Overseeing the hospital safety program
- Reviewing hospital policies to minimize loss exposures
- Ensuring the adequacy of disaster plans
- Keeping management informed of new legislation affecting operations
- Identifying potential loss exposures from medical staff credentialing
- Setting up risk management programs in outpatient care settings
- Conducting ongoing orientation and inservice programs on risk management issues
- Serving on hospital committees that discuss loss prevention and risk management issues
- Reporting regularly to management and the board on the effectiveness of the risk management program
- Facilitating resolution of crisis situations in patient care areas
- Managing the institution's insurance program
- Complying with the Joint Commission's standards related to risk management and safety

In addition, employees in other departments are busy creating other exposures that the risk manager should know about.

In short, risk managers become involved in every facet of the health care organization's business. A person assuming the job for the first time will be overwhelmed not only by issues identified by fellow employees, but also by those issues the risk manager himself or herself sees as important. There is a great danger that the risk manager's energy and attention will be diffused to the extent that a little bit of everything gets done, but not enough of anything to make much difference.

One of the most difficult risk management tasks is to decide where risk management attention will be most effective for the institution. The risk manager who rushes from crisis to crisis in response to the demands of line managers will not be as effective as the risk manager who makes time to analyze those areas of greatest exposure to the institution, makes those areas the focus of the program, establishes a plan to manage them, and then sticks to the plan despite the incessant demands on risk management time that others may make.

Furthermore, the medical treatment of the hospital's patients, which is the area where the financial impact of a loss may be the greatest, is the hardest to manage. It is much easier for the risk manager to spend time analyzing data on patient falls or lost patient valuables than alerting hospital management that a physician who admits many patients to the hospital does not have the medical skills to manage those patients successfully. However, the cost to the hospital of one anesthesia mishap may far exceed the cost of all patient falls for an entire year. Both areas require attention, but risk management time must be given where it will have the greatest impact.

Visibility

To be effective, the risk manager must maintain high visibility and be easily accessible to others. That means the risk manager will spend a lot of time visiting departments, making presentations, seeking information, providing guidance, answering questions, investigating, talking by telephone, and serving on committees. The volume of paperwork required, including responding to interrogatories, completing insurance applications, and drafting policies, must be sandwiched in between meetings, visits to departments, and phone calls, or done after everyone else has gone home.

Patient care personnel, including physicians, must be confident that if they call the risk manager for assistance, the response will be prompt and helpful. If it is not, they will not seek risk management assistance when it will be most beneficial. Problems that are brought to the risk manager's attention by the people caring for patients are excellent sources of information about what is going on in the institution.

Even though serving on committees takes a lot of time, committee service provides excellent visibility. It also provides opportunities for the risk manager to seek information and provide guidance before decisions are made, which can prevent problems from developing after action has been taken. Most committees in health care institutions will benefit from risk management expertise, but because of time limitations, the risk manager, with the direction of management and the board, must select only those committees that will most benefit the institution.

Visibility generates business—more business than there is time to handle. The risk manager's ability to set priorities will be sorely tested, and the ability to communicate the goals of the risk management program may become his or her most valuable skill.

Communication

The axiom that anything that can go wrong will go wrong is well accepted and has particular relevance to risk management. The risk manager who recognizes and accepts with equanimity the fact that many losses suffered by the hospital may result from exposures that risk management has not dealt with, either because of lack of time or because the exposure is unanticipated, understands the nature of risk management. To avert such crises, the risk manager must have the support of senior management, which requires that there be a risk management plan with priorities that are well thought out, communicated in easily understood terms, and approved by senior management and the board.

As important as it is for the risk manager to be an advocate to get support from senior management and the board, it is equally important that he or she be an advocate for risk management principles among the physicians and staff of the hospital. Risk managers do not *do* risk management as much as they *teach* risk management principles to those who provide patient care, either directly or indirectly. The more persuasive the risk manager can be in teaching risk management principles and getting other people to incorporate them in their daily tasks, the more successful the risk management program will be. In effect, every employee becomes a risk manager. The key to getting other people to employ risk management techniques is the risk manager's skill in showing people that those techniques make a difference in patient, employee, and visitor safety.

Recognition

Risk managers spend most of their time helping line managers do a better job. If loss prevention is given the proper attention, risk management help will always be welcomed, but it may not always be publicly acknowledged. The better the job the risk manager does, the more credit that will go to the line manager who follows risk management advice.

Another dilemma for the risk manager is that preventing a multimillion-dollar malpractice suit does not provide as much recognition as managing one. It is difficult to demonstrate the results of a well-run program, because the emphasis of risk management is on preventing catastrophe. Also, the risk management function is always vulnerable to budget cuts because risk managers do not produce revenue for the institution. Furthermore, the job that risk managers do is not as visible or dramatic as that of the trauma nurse, for example.

Because the results of the risk management program may not be as self-evident as those of other programs, the risk manager must devise ways to demonstrate what the program achieves. There are no objective criteria that the risk manager can use to quantify the success of the hospital's loss prevention activities. Some risk managers write an annual report that emphasizes the year's achievements. Some compare the amounts spent on judgments, settlements, and costs of defending claims from year to year. Others simply count risk management contacts and activities to show that the risk management program affects every facet of the institution's operation.

Regardless of the difficulty of creating an effective evaluation tool, the risk manager must provide an assessment of the program at least annually and make the results available to the senior management staff. Even if the report does not provide a complete picture of the effectiveness of the risk management program, it will remind the staff of the institution's risk management objectives.

Resources

When people in the hospital call the risk manager to ask a question, they expect that the answer will be simple and that the risk manager will be able to provide it quickly. Because other people expect easy answers, risk managers expect themselves to be able to provide them. It takes several years of being a risk manager not to feel a momentary panic when questions are asked and to know that few answers are simple and quickly apparent.

There are a number of inexpensive resources available to the skillful risk manager who wants to find answers to tough questions. The most obvious is to ask colleagues who may have dealt with similar issues and who are glad to share their expertise.

Many health care professionals belong to professional and trade associations that provide members with information on risk management issues. If the question comes from a nurse in the operating room, for example, the Association of Operating Room Nurses may provide information on the topic, particularly if the question has to do with a standard of practice. The resources section at the end of the book lists many professional organizations that provide information on risk management issues.

Risk managers should develop working relationships with risk management, safety, or other related professionals at their state or local hospital association who can serve as resources. State departments of health, state industrial commissions, and other departments of state and local government provide not only information but also some services to hospitals. For example, the state industrial commission may do air sampling within the hospital to test for unacceptable levels of noxious gases.

The hospital's insurance broker, especially one who has worked with health care institutions for many years, may have a wealth of experience on which the risk manager can draw for insight into tough issues. In addition, the broker provides a variety of services, such as contract review, for which there may be no additional charge to the hospital. The best risk managers are those who know how to draw on other people's experiences; this book is designed to help risk managers to do just that.

Chapter 2

The Legislative/Regulatory Setting for Risk Management

Patricia Scully

Health care is one of the most highly regulated industries. There are many levels of regulation by which health care organizations are bound. Some are mandatory, such as federal and state law; others, such as the requirements of the Joint Commission, are voluntary. The role of the courts is to interpret statutes and regulations as they apply to particular situations.

This chapter will provide an overview of legislative and regulatory schemes at the federal, state, and local levels. Selected federal statutes with significant impact on the professional practice of risk managers will be discussed. Elements of state statutes and local rules that are common to many jurisdictions also will be discussed.

Risk managers assist their institutions in complying with federal, state, and local law, call attention to new legislation affecting health care operations, and assist in interpreting laws and regulations as they affect the operations of their institutions. The new risk manager is advised to develop and maintain an effective working relationship with the employer's in-house or outside counsel and with any specialty counsel that the employer may use. Those resources are invaluable in interpreting regulatory requirements and in assisting with the development of institutional policies and procedures to comply with those requirements. In addition, the chapter endnotes provide leads to other sources of information and support.

☐ Federal Legislation and Regulation

The following discussion of federal legislation and regulation includes the Health Care Quality Improvement Act (out of which comes the National Practitioner Data Bank), regulations that protect human research subjects, rules published by the Nuclear Regulatory Commission to protect the public health and safety, Medicare regulations for long-term care facilities, the Consolidated Omnibus Budget Reconciliation Act, which deals with the issue of patient dumping, and hazardous materials management, including regulation of hazardous and infectious waste.

Health Care Quality Improvement Act

On November 14, 1986, Public Law 99-660, or the Health Care Quality Improvement Act (HCQIA),[1] became effective. In its statement of findings, Congress noted the nationwide increase in medical malpractice, a need to improve the quality of care, and a method of accomplishing such improvement—that is, effective professional peer review. Congress further noted the impediments to effective peer review, such as the threat of litigation, including that under the federal antitrust laws. Noting that the problem is national in scope, Congress decided that a uniform system of protection of physicians conducting peer review would be more effective than leaving the task to state legislatures. Hospitals with procedures that provide due process to physicians adversely affected by credentialing decisions and comply with the requirements of the act are not liable in damages under federal or state law.

Due Process

Section 11112 of the act outlines the process of a peer review proceeding. Qualified immunity from liability in civil actions will attach to those engaged in peer review if the professional review action is taken:

- To further high-quality health care
- After reasonable effort to ascertain the facts
- After notice and fair hearing opportunities are afforded to physicians (includes M.D.s, D.O.s, and dentists)
- In the reasonable belief that the action is supported by the facts

Physicians' due process rights are detailed in this section of the act. The notice of a proposed professional review action must include the reasons for such review, the time frame within which a physician may request a hearing (not less than 30 days), and a summary of fair hearing rights.

The physician has the right to the following:

- Notice of the time, place, and date of hearing (not less than 30 days after the date of notice)
- The list of witnesses appearing for the reviewer
- Representation by counsel
- A written record of the proceedings
- Examination and cross-examination of witnesses
- Presentation of relevant evidence
- Submission of a written closing statement
- The written recommendations/rationale of the reviewer
- The written decision/rationale of the health care entity

Notwithstanding these specific protections afforded to the physician, the institution may suspend or restrict privileges for 14 days, during which an investigation may be conducted to determine the need for a professional review action. In addition, the institution may summarily suspend privileges, subject to subsequent notice and hearing, if the failure to take such action would jeopardize the health of any individual.

The National Practitioner Data Bank

In addition to providing protection for the peer review process, the HCQIA created a National Practitioner Data Bank. This bank's function is to collect information on health care practitioners, primarily physicians and dentists, who have been defendants in malpractice claims that have been concluded either with a judgment against the practitioner or a settlement. The bank also collects information about practitioners against whom adverse action has been taken against their hospital membership or privileges or their licenses to practice. The information is collected from insurance companies, self-insurance trusts, and state licensing boards (who get the information from the health care entity taking the action), who are required to report all such judgments, settlements, privileges, or licensure actions.

The public law, as further delineated by the regulations (45 C.F.R. Part 60), describes the reporting requirements of the National Practitioner Data Bank. The time lines are as follows:

- Information on malpractice payments is due within 30 days of the date of payment.
- Information on adverse actions on medical staff membership or clinical privileges must be reported by the entity to the board of medical examiners within 15 days; that board must then forward the information to the data bank and other applicable licensing boards within 10 days.
- Licensure actions must be reported within 30 days of the date the action was taken.

Malpractice payments must be reported by the payer, either an insurance carrier or self-insurer. The regulations specify the information that the reporting bodies must include about the physicians, in addition to the claims and financial data. The regulations provide for civil money penalties up to $10,000 per violation for failure to make a required report. A report must be made regardless of amount if any money is paid in response to a written demand; however, administrative adjustment to a patient's bill is not a reportable event. The regulations do not provide for allocating fault in a settlement involving several defendants, an issue that may cause difficulty in those insurance programs that feature risk pooling among physicians and hospitals.

Boards of medical examiners must report to the data bank any action taken against the licenses of physicians or dentists. Health care entities must report to the board of medical examiners (1) any action taken that adversely affects a practitioner's medical staff membership or clinical privileges for a period exceeding 30 days, and (2) the voluntary relinquishing of membership privileges by a physician to avoid disciplinary action.

Hospitals must request information from the data bank about a new physician at the time he or she makes an initial application for membership and clinical privileges. Information on current members of the staff must be requested at a minimum of every two years. Unlike the sanctions for failure to report, there is no provision for civil money penalties for entities that fail to request information. Instead, the hospital is presumed to have knowledge of the information on file in the data bank. In addition, a plaintiff's attorney bringing a medical malpractice action against the hospital will be given access to the information presumed to have been given to the hospital if the attorney provides evidence that the hospital did not request the information. The data bank must disclose information about a practitioner to the practitioner upon request at no charge. All other requests are subject to a fee schedule. Practitioners may dispute the accuracy of the data by simultaneously filing with the reporter and the data bank a written notice of dispute. The data will then be reported as "disputed" until the issue is resolved. Other requesters, specifically researchers, will have access to anonymous aggregate data.

It would be prudent for risk managers to confer with facility administration and reach a consensus on procedures for reporting to the data bank. The facility's board of trustees, as final arbiter in physician credentialing matters and with knowledge of the sensitivities involved in hospital–physician relations, may deem it appropriate to vest the reporting responsibility within the executive suite. To achieve maximum protection for the facility under the new law, facility counsel should be involved in reconciling the medical staff bylaws with these new federal requirements.

Protection of Human Research Subjects

Risk managers working in facilities that conduct research or treat patients who are enrolled in research protocols or whose physicians conduct clinical trials of experimental drugs and devices need to become familiar with the federal regulations that protect human research subjects. Risk managers may be asked to serve on committees that function as institutional review boards (IRBs). Members of IRBs need a working knowledge of the requirements for patient informed consent and the requirements for research-related record keeping. If a patient is injured while participating in a research project, the risk manager will need access to the appropriate information in order to create a claim file.

There are two sets of federal rules governing research on human subjects. The first set, promulgated in 1980, consists of those rules applicable to clinical investigations regulated by the Food and Drug Administration (FDA) under selected sections of the federal Food, Drug and Cosmetic Act.[2]

The other is a set of regulations for the protection of human subjects, most recently amended in 1983, that applies to research conducted or funded by the Department of Health and Human Services (HHS).[3] For a detailed summary of the FDA rules and HHS regulations, see chapter 23, "Institutional Review Boards and Human Research Issues."

Nuclear Regulatory Commission

For the purpose of protecting the public health and safety, the federal Nuclear Regulatory Commission (NRC) has published rules for the handling, storage, and use of radioactive substances ("byproduct material") in the health care environment.[4] Risk managers who work in a clinical environment where radioactive substances are used need to know the federal regulations applicable to those substances.

The NRC issues licenses for five-year periods to qualified medical institutions or individuals who file the appropriate forms, pay the required fees, and observe the federally prescribed safety standards. The institution must file licensure amendments for approval by the agency when it makes a material change, such as adding authorized users, changing the designated radiation safety officer, or changing the address where radioactive substances are used.

Each licensee must develop and implement a written radiation protection program, which must include the following:

- Mandatory participation by institution management, the radiation safety officer, and all authorized users (licensed physicians, dentists, or podiatrists)
- Notice to workers about the types and amounts of byproduct materials used, doses, safety procedures, continuing education, and training
- Provisions for keeping doses as low as reasonably achievable (known as ALARA levels)

Licensees must appoint a radiation safety officer who is responsible for implementing the radiation safety program. As of October 1, 1986, a person listed as a radiation safety officer on a commission license must comply with the specific education and training requirements of section 35.900 of the NRC rules. The responsibilities of the radiation safety officer include:

- Developing and implementing written policies and procedures for the purchase, storage, inventory, use, and disposal of byproduct material
- Training of personnel
- Investigating accidents, misadministrations, and other deviations from approved radiation safety practice

- Assisting the institutional radiation safety committee in its oversight role for the radiation safety program
- Maintaining appropriate records

The rules state that the minimum retention period for records is two years.

Each institutional licensee must establish a radiation safety committee to oversee the use of byproduct material. The rules require that the committee meet at least quarterly and keep minutes that conform with requirements specified in the rules. The responsibilities of the committee include (1) approval or disapproval of authorized users and the radiation safety officer; (2) review and approval of minor changes in operating procedures; (3) review of personnel radiation dose records; (4) review of incidents; and (5) the annual program review.

The occurrence of a therapeutic or diagnostic misadministration (defined specifically in the rules) triggers certain reporting obligations. Errors involving therapy must be reported by phone within 24 hours to the regional NRC office. During the same time interval, the patient's referring physician must be informed. The patient or a responsible relative must also be advised; this notification, or the decision to defer patient notice, may be made by the physician. Errors involving diagnostic procedures are investigated and documented by the radiation safety officer. In some circumstances, additional information must be provided to the physician and the NRC within 15 days.

The rules outline minimum requirements for the safety instruction of patients and health care workers. Safety instructions and precautions are specified for three categories of therapeutic intervention: radiopharmaceuticals, sealed sources or implants, and teletherapy. Basic principles to be included in the teaching of health care workers for all classes of patients are visitor control, contamination and waste control, and notification of the radiation safety officer in the event of a medical emergency or death of the patient.

As always, it is prudent to check state and local health department sources for any additional regulatory requirements for the treatment of patients with radioactive substances.

Medicare Regulations for Nursing Homes

In 1983, the Health Care Financing Administration (HCFA) of HHS contracted with the Institute of Medicine to study the long-term care regulatory system. The institute's report, available in 1986, recommended that new regulations be promulgated to shift the focus of care from a process to an outcome, or quality orientation. The Health Care Financing Administration published proposed rules on October 16, 1987, and invited public comment. More than 5,500 comments were generated in response to the proposed rule, and HCFA issued its final rule (with additional comment period) with most provisions effective August 1, 1989.[5]

Two months after HCFA published its proposed regulations for nursing homes, Congress enacted the Omnibus Budget Reconciliation Act (COBRA) of 1987, which included extensive revisions to the Medicare and Medicaid statutory requirements for nursing facilities. The OBRA revisions are effective October 1, 1990. Both effective dates have been incorporated into the regulations.

The purpose of the rules is to consolidate the requirements for participation in both Medicare and Medicaid programs by facilities furnishing long-term care. Such facilities include skilled nursing facilities (SNFs) under Medicare, and SNFs and intermediate care facilities (ICFs) under Medicaid. After October 1, 1990, those facilities that participate in Medicaid will be known collectively as nursing facilities (NFs). The regulations do not apply to facilities treating patients with mental disorders or retardation.

The rules emphasize residents' rights, including the requirement for notice to the residents and their written acknowledgment of those rights. The rules attempt to promote the dignity of residents, their self-determination, and open communication between resident and provider. The term "resident" was selected in lieu of "patient" to emphasize the homelike living arrangement. Residents are entitled to:

- Information about their physical condition
- Access to a physician
- Copies of their medical records
- The right to refuse treatment
- Freedom from physical restraints and psychoactive drugs that are not required as part of the medical plan of care

Residents also are entitled to information on medical benefits and associated costs. The protection of financial assets, including a requirement to pay interest on funds in excess of $50 handled by the facility after October 1, 1990, also is required. Residents may file formal complaints about infractions of any rights.

Facilities have certain obligations to meet. Facilities that have more than 120 beds must have a full-time social worker and a therapeutic recreation specialist to coordinate the activities program. A comprehensive resident assessment is required within four days of admission (effective October 1, 1990), and every 12 months thereafter, to include a nursing care plan. With certain specific exceptions, facilities are mandated to provide coverage by registered nurses for eight hours each day, seven days per week. A licensed nurse must be on duty at all times. Physician coverage is also prescribed. Physicians, who may alternate visits with a physician's assistant or nurse practitioner, are required to see each resident every 30 days for three successive 30-day periods, then once every two months as long as the resident remains in the facility. In an ICF, the ongoing physician visitation schedule is lengthened to once every three months. Nursing assistants must have training. Finally, the facility must have a quality assurance committee with representation by the director of nursing, a physician, and three staff members. The committee must meet at least quarterly.

The most significant impact of these regulations is expected to be the staffing requirements, especially for registered nurses.

COBRA

Any facility with an emergency department undoubtedly has become familiar with a small section of the federal legislation known as COBRA, or the Consolidated Omnibus Budget Reconciliation Act of 1985.[6] Although COBRA is primarily tax legislation, it includes a section that attempts to halt what the law calls patient "dumping," or the inappropriate transfer of patients from hospital emergency departments. Congress perceived that these inappropriate transfers usually were economically based, that is, they moved indigent, uninsured patients from private to county facilities.

The COBRA provisions, amended again in late 1989,[7] apply to hospitals, specifically including rural primary care hospitals, with a Medicare provider agreement covering emergency department services. They require that any individual who appears at a hospital emergency department for treatment be provided a medical screening examination to determine whether that individual has an emergency medical condition. The term *emergency medical condition* has been redefined to include women in labor. If the individual has not been "stabilized" (also defined in the statute), that person may not be transferred to another medical facility unless the individual requests transfer after (s)he is informed of the hospital's obligation and the risks of transfer; and the transferring physician certifies in writing that the benefits of transfer outweigh the risks.

In addition, the receiving facility must agree to accept the transfer; and the transferring facility must provide copies of all emergency department medical records, including copies of the individual's informed consent or the physician's certification. Appropriate transport, with qualified personnel, is also mandated.

The 1989 COBRA amendments, effective July 1, 1990, imposed several new requirements upon hospitals. These are:

1. Mandatory adoption and enforcement of a COBRA policy
2. Maintenance of medical records related to patient transfers for a period of five years
3. Maintenance of lists of on-call physicians
4. Mandatory acceptance of appropriate transfers by regional referral centers or hospitals with specialized capabilities
5. Examination and stabilization of individuals who present for care, prior to an inquiry on insurance status
6. Posting of signs in the emergency department advising patients of their rights under COBRA and whether the hospital participates in a Medicaid program under a state plan approved under Title XIX.

The amendments also feature a "whistleblower" provision that protects physicians from adverse actions by hospitals when the physician refuses to transfer an unstable patient.

Those who violate COBRA provisions are subject to more stringent sanctions. Civil money penalties up to $50,000 per violation may be imposed upon hospitals, emergency department physicians, and on-call physicians who refuse or fail to appear within a reasonable time to provide necessary stabilizing treatment. Transferring facilities must report to receiving facilities the names and addresses of such noncompliant on-call physicians.

Sanctions may be imposed for negligent as well as intentional acts. The facility's Medicare provider agreement may be terminated or suspended; physicians may be excluded from participation in Medicare and state health care programs. In addition, the statute creates a cause of action for individuals who have been harmed by inappropriate transfers and a cause of action for receiving facilities that may be economically disadvantaged as a result of a "dumping" episode.

Hazardous Materials Management

Nowhere is the excursion into the alphabet soup of government acronyms more complex than in the area of hazardous waste. There's the EPA, CERCLA, RCRA, MWTA—and all the regulations associated with them. Perhaps the most helpful information for the new risk manager is to know to whom questions may be posed about these very confusing requirements. At the federal level, the Environmental Protection Agency (EPA) has a regional office in each of 10 regions of the country. A map of the regions and directory information on each can be found in appendix A of the EPA's handbook on rules for the small-quantity generator.[8] There is also a toll-free federal hotline: 1-800/424-9346. In the same EPA handbook, there is a list of the state hazardous waste management agencies. Every state is included, as well as American Samoa, the District of Columbia, Guam, the Mariana and Virgin islands, and Puerto Rico. It is also advisable to check with the city and county offices to determine whether there are local regulations that may be applicable.

Some important tasks for risk managers to consider are the following:

- Inventorying and quantifying the hazardous and infectious materials generated by the facility to determine what regulations apply
- Developing and implementing a hazardous materials policy and procedure
- Developing and implementing an infectious waste policy and procedure
- Providing for orientation and continuing education for staff on hazardous and infectious waste
- Saving all insurance policies (old policies may be occurrence forms with coverage available for pollution exposures; policies with exclusions may, nevertheless,

respond to losses because the courts construe policy language in favor of the insured)

- Putting all insurance carriers on notice whenever there is reason to suspect a pollution claim
- Using the resources available to respond to questions and concerns
- Soliciting administrative support for the appropriate response to regulations; soliciting funding for consultants as needed
- Knowing the location of any underground storage tanks
- Keeping records diligently
- Using approved transporters who use RCRA-approved dump sites
- Contracting carefully, requesting indemnity agreements and proof of insurance from transporters and other contractors
- Implementing and maintaining a close working relationship among departments of risk management, safety, employee health, and infection control to ensure compliance with these complex regulations

Hazardous Waste

In 1976, Congress passed the Resource Conservation and Recovery Act, known as RCRA. The purpose of the law is to encourage industry to minimize or recycle waste that would otherwise be hazardous. The EPA was required to define hazardous waste and license all those who generate, transport, treat, store, or dispose of hazardous waste. In 1984, Congress amended RCRA to require the EPA to regulate previously exempt generators. Effective September 22, 1986, there are three categories of hazardous waste generators:

- Those producing less than 100 kg of hazardous waste per month (still virtually exempt from regulation)
- Those producing in excess of 1,000 kg of hazardous waste per month (subject to all hazardous waste regulations)
- Those generating between 100 and 1,000 kg (previously exempt, but now categorized as "small-quantity generators" and subject to EPA regulation)

Under current law, regulated facilities are required to do the following:

- Identify the type and quantity of wastes generated by the facility
- Obtain an EPA identification number (submit EPA Form #8700-12: "Notification of Hazardous Waste Activity")
- Limit the storage of hazardous waste on site to 180 days (or 270 days if the waste must be transported more than 200 miles)
- Contract only with transporters and facilities with verified EPA identification numbers
- Comply with Department of Transportation shipping requirements
- Use a multipart hazardous waste manifest to accompany the shipment to its final destination (EPA Form #8700-22, "Uniform Hazardous Waste Manifest," may be used, or a state-mandated facsimile)
- Maintain copies of manifests for at least three years

The generator of hazardous waste is ultimately liable for any hazards the waste causes long after it is disposed of. It is an area of tremendous exposure and fertile ground for future litigation. The Comprehensive Environmental Response, Compensation, and Liability Act of 1980, or CERCLA (known as the "Superfund" law), imposes joint and several liability for cleanup operations of toxic dump sites on any person or entity that contributed waste to the site. The generator is strictly liable, regardless of fault, so long as the waste is able to contaminate.

Another hazardous waste issue that risk managers must be concerned about is pollution of groundwater as a result of leaking underground storage tanks. All underground storage tanks should be monitored, and, if they leak, they should either be repaired or removed from service.

Infectious Waste

Although there is currently no federal mandate to manage infectious waste, regulation is likely. In 1986, the EPA released the *EPA Guide for Infectious Waste Management*, which included technical advice on waste segregation, packaging, storage, transport, treatment, and disposal. The publication also recommended six categories of infectious waste. These categories were not the same as those described the previous year by the Centers for Disease Control (CDC). The CDC defined infectious waste more narrowly, leaving hospitals in a quandary because neither set of definitions represented formal federal policy. Some states developed infectious waste management plans of varying complexity and rigor.

In 1988, in response to the public outcry after medical waste was washed up on the shores of East Coast beaches, Congress amended RCRA with the Medical Waste Tracking Act (MWTA).[9] The act mandates a two-year demonstration project, which may become the national model for medical waste management. The 10 states originally targeted for the project were New York, New Jersey, Connecticut, and the states bordering the Great Lakes. The designated states were given the opportunity to opt out, and other states were given an opportunity to join.

Under interim final regulations,[10] the EPA has decided to track seven types of medical waste: cultures and stocks, pathological wastes, human blood and blood products, sharps, animal waste, isolation waste, and unused sharps. Generators of less than 50 pounds of medical waste per month need not file formal manifests but should maintain in-house records. Administration of the program is through state EPAs. Sanctions available include civil money penalties, criminal fines, and incarceration.

Although it is not likely that medical waste management will be formally regulated for at least two more years, it would be prudent for risk managers to scrutinize the proposed regulations and plan for the future.

☐ State Legislation and Regulation

The following sections provide an overview of tort reform, professional practice, peer review, and risk management statutes currently existing in 10 states.

Tort Reform

The system for compensating persons injured by health care providers has come under increasing scrutiny and attack. Insurers have been accused of being greedy for raising premiums for medical malpractice insurance and for paying "nuisance settlements" in cases of questionable merit. Attorneys have come under attack for charging "contingent" fees, which are paid only if the attorney wins the case. Under a contingent fee arrangement, plaintiffs have little risk, and successful plaintiffs' lawyers often get more of the claim dollar than the injured clients. The plaintiffs' bar has lobbied state legislatures to thwart any attempt to limit the ability of plaintiffs to seek legal assistance.

The courts have not escaped notice. Courts seldom mandate alternative dispute resolution, which would shorten the litigation process and save money. Courts have also found tort reform legislation unconstitutional. The medical profession itself has not escaped notice for its ineffective attempts at quality management.

Most tort reform has been and continues to be at the state level, because professional malpractice issues are creatures of state law. Some of the common methods employed by state legislatures to effect tort reform are discussed in the following sections.

Joint and Several Liability

The concept of joint and several liability is economically devastating to a defendant with minimal liability but deep pockets. Each defendant can be held responsible for the entire loss even if that defendant may have been only tangentially involved in the event. Plaintiffs' attorneys add as many defendants as possible to a lawsuit to ensure that there will be a solvent defendant from whom to collect a judgment. Some state legislatures have abolished joint and several liability so that culpable defendants are held responsible only for the portion of the loss their conduct caused.

Statutes of Limitations

One way to improve the position of malpractice defendants is to shorten the time frames within which plaintiffs may bring an action for damages, known as the "statutes of limitations." States may have statutes of limitations for negligence actions and separate statutes covering actions against health care providers. Risk managers need to know the provisions of their respective states' statutes.

Attorneys' Fees

Some states have statutorily limited the fees that attorneys may charge to represent injured plaintiffs in personal injury and medical malpractice cases. Those laws have been protested vigorously by members of the plaintiffs' bar. Usually the fees are awarded on a sliding scale as a percentage of the damage award. The theory is that injured clients, rather than attorneys, should get the maximum benefit from a significant award.

Caps on Damages

The amount of money that may be awarded to an injured claimant is capped by law in some states. One hurdle that may need to be overcome is a state's constitutional ban on limiting damage awards. Arizona has such a constitutional provision, which prevents legislative effort to cap damages.

Professional Practice Acts

Risk managers often investigate incidents in which the scope of professional practice is at issue. For example, a question may arise as to whether an insurer could deny coverage if a nurse performed an act that, under state statute, is defined as medical practice. The place to look for information about such issues is the individual state's professional practice acts. For each group of health care professionals licensed by the state there will be state laws that define the scope of practice and outline the powers and duties of the professional regulatory boards.

State professional practice statutes commonly begin with a definition section. For the practice of nursing, significant definitions are those for "registered" and "licensed practical/vocational" nurse. The scope of nursing practice, as well as the degree of interdependence with medical practitioners, may be deduced from the state legislature's definition of "nurse" and such other terms as "direction," "supervision," "collaboration," and "nursing diagnosis."

Professional practice regulatory boards are created by statute. The composition of the boards is outlined, and broad powers and duties are listed. The legislature delegates to the professional board the power to develop and implement rules and regulations that clarify the broad language of the statutes.

It is in the rules and regulations that specific requirements for professional practice may be found. The process of licensure will be detailed, including the state's requirement, if any, for mandatory continuing education. Elements of "unprofessional conduct" may be discussed, and the impact of that behavior upon licensure will be stated.

The unlawful use of controlled substances is listed in state statutes as being unprofessional conduct. Many states require a medical professional to report a colleague to the licensing board if there is a reasonable belief that the public welfare may be compromised as a result of the colleague's substance abuse.

Disciplinary and licensure matters are administrative proceedings, not court proceedings. However, licensure matters can be litigated by a practitioner who takes legal action to challenge an administrative decision.

Peer Review

The concept of physician peer review received national attention when the Oregon statute was scrutinized by the U.S. Supreme Court in *Patrick v. Burget*. Risk managers will be intimately involved in the peer review process as members of committees, advisors on the peer review process, and arbitrators of requests for data. Risk managers who know the provisions of state statutes will be able to develop reasoned responses to the questions raised by others in the organization.

The goal of peer review is the full and fair evaluation of medical practice to reduce morbidity and mortality. Absent significant statutory protections, physicians are understandably reluctant to admit professional errors in judgment that may have economic and career consequences. Most states have enacted statutes that both mandate peer review and provide protection from suit for the participants and protection from discovery for the documents that are generated by the process.

Protections may range from absolute or complete immunity to some form of qualified immunity, usually if action is taken in good faith. Absolute immunity, although preferred by peer reviewers, may result in abuses of the process and damage to professional reputations if documents and discussions become public.

The rules covering document production are articulated in peer review statutes. In many states, plaintiffs' attorneys do not have access to records created by peer review committees. The privilege usually does not include documents prepared for purposes other than peer review but used in peer review. On the other hand, there is a common exception to the nondisclosure rules that favors reviewed practitioners who are either protesting disciplinary action or being reviewed, in an administrative or licensure context, by state boards of medical examiners. Medical practice boards have broad authority to examine documents, including peer review materials.

The issue of confidentiality is particularly sensitive, requiring constant educational reminders to peer review participants. The urge to gossip is often overwhelming, but the integrity of the peer review process is of paramount importance and must be reinforced by risk management and quality assurance professionals.

Risk Management Statutes

Risk managers in 10 states have their professional practice regulated by specific risk management laws. Those states are Alaska, Colorado, Florida, Kansas, Maryland, Massachusetts, New York, North Carolina, Rhode Island, and Washington. Statutes in two states, New York and Washington, use the term "quality assurance" rather than "risk management." Two other states, Alaska and Rhode Island, have never implemented enabling regulations, with the result that incentives for implementing risk management programs are lacking in those states.

The 10 states differ in their approach to risk management. Some, such as Kansas and Florida, mandate reporting of specific incidents to the state. The Maryland law is the closest to the model risk management statute drafted by the American Society for Healthcare Risk Management (ASHRM). Although ASHRM does not endorse a state legislative scheme for health care risk management, its model prescribes the elements of an acceptable health care risk management program. Those elements include a system for identifying, evaluating, and handling of risk exposures; the employment of a qualified risk manager; data sharing and continuing education; and, most important, a commitment from the governing body to the risk management effort.

In addition, ASHRM developed sample statutory language for confidentiality of all risk management–related documents and immunity of participants in risk management activities. The Maryland and Florida risk management statutes have expanded those protections. Florida, the site of many liability insurance problems in recent years, has significantly augmented its tort reform activity, of which the risk management legislation is a part. Florida remains the only state to require certification of risk managers. Criteria for such certification are outlined in regulations available from the Florida Hospital Association in Tallahassee. More detailed information on risk management statutes has been published by the U.S. General Accounting Office[11] and by ASHRM in seminar manuals available through the American Hospital Association.[12,13]

☐ Local (City/County) Regulation

In addition to federal and state regulators, there are other rule-making bodies that affect the risk manager's professional practice. City and county codes may contain additional requirements; for example, the requirement that certain chemicals found in waste water may not exceed established thresholds. Local health departments may prescribe procedures such as reporting of positive results of tests for the human immunodeficiency virus.

The health care institution may have many volumes of rules and regulations developed by administration, nursing, and ancillary departments. Those in-house standards are often based on federal, state, and local laws. In addition, the standards articulated by nationally recognized accrediting bodies are frequently incorporated into policy and procedure manuals.

Such manuals are valuable resources for facility personnel and are evidence of compliance with regulatory requirements. Input from risk managers and legal counsel in creating these manuals is encouraged so that reasonable and achievable standards are developed. The standards of care in medical malpractice litigation are partially established by the facility's own policies and procedures.

☐ Case Law

Statutes passed by Congress, and statutes and regulations crafted by states, cannot cover every individual situation to which those laws apply. Statutes and regulations must be interpreted by judges when litigants take their particular disputes to court. When the judge, usually at the appellate level, renders a decision in the form of a written opinion, the opinion forms part of the body of the law to which future litigants look to build their cases.

☐ Conclusion

The regulatory milieu is one in which the risk manager must function effectively. All aspects of a risk manager's professional life are governed in some measure by some regulation. In addition to the sampling of statutes reviewed in this chapter, there are many other laws and cases that will affect a risk manager's job. Those who work in a clinical environment will have some involvement with issues of guardianship, termination of life support, living wills, powers of attorney, release of medical records, subpoenaes, workers' compensation, and many others. This is an area that provides risk management its unique appeal: an infinite variety of professional challenges.

References

1. 42 U.S.C. §§11101–52.

2. 21 C.F.R. Ch. 1 (April 1, 1988 ed.); Food and Drug Administration, HHS Part 50–Protection of Human Subjects, pp. 215–21, May 30, 1980, and Jan. 27, 1981; Part 56–Institutional Review Boards, pp. 221–29, Jan. 27, 1981.

3. 45 C.F.R. Subtitle A (Oct. 1, 1988 ed.); HHS Part 46–Protection of Human Subjects, §§46.101–46.409.

4. 10 C.F.R. Ch. 1 (January 1, 1988 ed.); Nuclear Regulatory Commission, Part 35–Medical Use of Byproduct Material, pp. 382–411, Oct. 16, 1986.

5. Medicare and Medicaid; requirements for long-term care facilities, HCFA. Part 483–Conditions of Participation and Requirements for Long-Term Care Facilities; Subpart B–Requirements for Long-Term Care Facilities. *Federal Register* 54(21):5316–73, Feb. 2, 1989.

6. Social Security Act, §1867; 42 U.S.C. §1395dd; Proposed Regulations. *Federal Register* 53:22513–27, June 16, 1988.

7. P.L. 101–239, §6018: Hospital Anti-Dumping Provisions, and §6211: Medicare Hospital Patient Protection Amendments.

8. U.S. Environmental Protection Agency. *Understanding the Small Quantity Generator Hazardous Waste Rules: A Handbook for Small Business. EPA/530SW-86-019.* Washington, DC: EPA Office of Solid Waste and Emergency Response, Sept. 1986.

9. Public Law 100-582.

10. Standards for the tracking and management of medical waste. 40 C.F.R. Parts 22 and 259. *Federal Register* 54(56):12326–95, Mar. 24, 1989.

11. U.S. General Accounting Office. *Health Care Initiatives in Hospital Risk Management.* GAO/HRD-88-79. Washington, DC: U.S. General Accounting Office, July 1989.

12. Scully, P. Risk management statutes. In: *Risk Management: The Widening Circle of Responsibility.* American Society for Healthcare Risk Management Third Annual Summer Symposium. Chicago, Aug. 1987.

13. Scully, P. Risk management legislation update. In: *Proceedings of the 10th Annual Meeting of the American Society for Healthcare Risk Management.* Chicago, Oct. 1988, pp. 204–10.

Chapter 3
Elements of a Risk Management Program

Sheila R. Hagg

□ Risk Management Program Structure

Although the exact structure of a given hospital's risk management program depends on the size of the facility and the scope of the patient care and other services it offers, several key structural components are necessary for any hospital risk management program to succeed. Whether a hospital is just beginning to organize its risk management efforts or is seeking to revamp an existing program, attention to those structural factors will help ensure that the program has a solid foundation.

Authority

The hospital's risk manager must command sufficient authority and respect to enact the changes in hospital practice, policy, and procedure and in employee and medical staff behavior necessary to fulfill the essential functions of the risk management program. Because the risk manager must deal on a daily basis with highly sensitive and confidential information that directly affects the hospital's public image and financial status, and because the risk manager is responsible for coordinating risk management activities with members of the hospital's medical staff as well as managers and employees at all levels, the risk manager's position must be relatively high in the organizational hierarchy. Ideally, the risk manager should report directly to the chief executive officer, or at least to another member of the senior administrative management team. Risk managers whose positions fall below the department manager level on the hospital's organizational chart will almost certainly face difficulty in dealing authoritatively with medical staff and nursing and department managers. They may also have difficulty gaining the attention of hospital administration and representing the hospital in its relations with insurers, attorneys, and other outside parties involved in the risk management process.

Visibility

The position of hospital risk manager should be a highly visible one. No one individual can perform every function of a comprehensive risk management program single-handedly, even in the smallest health care facility. It is therefore necessary for the hospital risk manager, through consciousness raising, education, and communication, to foster an awareness of risk management practices and techniques among medical staff members and hospital employees at all organizational levels. The risk manager's position must be structured so as to enhance opportunities for interaction through serving on hospital committees, participating in educational activities such as new-employee orientation and staff inservice offerings, and having access to hospitalwide communications mechanisms.

Coordination

Because of the wide range of risk management functions and the diversity of activities necessary for a successful risk management program, there should be both formal and informal mechanisms for coordination and information exchange between the risk management program and other hospital departments and functions. In order to adequately integrate and coordinate risk management with other hospital functions, the risk manager should establish reporting and communication relationships with the following individuals:

- *The chief executive officer,* who provides a vital link to the hospital's governing board and medical staff and sets the tone and provides necessary support for the risk management program. The CEO serves as the key decision maker for many activities crucial to the hospital's risk management program, such as authorizing the settlement of larger claims.
- *The quality assurance director,* who serves as an important source of information on adverse clinical events occurring within the hospital that may have serious risk management implications. The risk management standards promulgated by the Joint Commission on Accreditation of Healthcare Organizations emphasize the interdependence of risk management and quality assurance activities.[1] The quality assurance director may also be able to assist the risk manager who lacks clinical training in interpreting and analyzing information contained in the medical record.
- *The infection control nurse (or staff epidemiologist),* who provides information regarding hospital-acquired infections that may give rise to liability claims. He or she can assist the risk manager in understanding infection control protocols aimed at reducing the frequency and severity of nosocomial infections and in establishing guidelines for coping with acquired immunodeficiency syndrome (AIDS).
- *The safety officer,* who may assist the risk manager in performing fire safety, hazardous materials management, disaster planning, and employee safety activities in compliance with Joint Commission standards[2] or may have primary responsibility for those activities. He or she usually chairs the hospitalwide safety committee,[3] which serves as a vital source of risk management information and problem solving.
- *The patient representative (or ombudsman),* who relays information to the risk manager regarding patient complaints and dissatisfaction. Patient representatives, whether hospital employees or volunteers, must be trained to recognize and appropriately handle potential risk management concerns, as they are often in a position to deal directly with dissatisfied patients and thus resolve minor problems more effectively than the risk manager.
- *The employee health nurse (or workers' compensation coordinator or personnel director),* who manages the daily operational activities related to the hospital's employee safety and workers' compensation program and provides claims and injury information to the risk manager.
- *The medical records director,* who notifies the risk manager of requests from attorneys for medical records, which may signal the initiation of a professional liability

action. The risk manager must work with the medical records director to develop policies and procedures relating to the documentation of patient care activities and patient confidentiality and the release of information.

- *The medical director (or vice-president of medical affairs or chief of staff)*, who serves as a liaison between the hospital's risk management program and the medical staff and assists the risk manager in "selling" risk management to physicians. In addition, the risk manager must work with the medical director to ensure that the hospital's medical staff appointment, credentialing, privileging, and disciplinary procedures are conducted in accordance with sound risk management practices.
- *The patient accounts representative*, who works with the risk manager to identify patient complaints and concerns that surface during the billing and collections process. Those concerns may be based on perceived patient care problems and hold the potential for liability claims.
- *Nursing and departmental managers*, who offer the risk manager technical and clinical expertise necessary to identify and analyze potential risks and assist with the investigation of liability claims and incidents. Middle-management personnel play a crucial role in building and maintaining support for the hospital's risk management program and in educating and raising the risk management consciousness of employees within their areas.
- *The education director (or inservice program coordinator)*, who can assist the risk manager in identifying staff educational needs and in planning, organizing, and presenting inservice education programs pertaining to risk management.

Accountability

Just as the risk manager needs sufficient authority to perform assigned functions, he or she should be held accountable for that performance. Every hospital risk manager, including those in small institutions who have job duties in addition to risk management, must have a written job description that outlines key risk management responsibilities. Annual performance appraisals assessing the risk manager's achievement of specific, measurable risk management goals and objectives should be conducted in order to gauge and document the risk manager's effectiveness. The risk manager should prepare an annual report for administration and the governing board that summarizes claims, insurance, and risk management program activities.

☐ Risk Management Program Documentation

A hospital risk management program, like other integral hospital functions, requires certain documented plans, policies, and procedures in order to ensure program consistency and uniformity and to provide the framework for operating decisions. Plans, policies, and procedures should be in writing, approved and adopted in accordance with established hospital policy, and reviewed and revised as necessary at least annually.

Plans Related to Risk Management

Each hospital should adopt a comprehensive written risk management plan that states the goals of the hospital's risk management program, describes the program's organizational structure, and assigns responsibility for the various risk management functions. The plan should specify the flow of information and reporting relationships among various risk management components and the individuals responsible for risk management activities. Flowcharts and organizational charts depicting the structure of the risk management program may be helpful accompaniments to the plan.

When drafting a risk management plan, care must be taken to ensure consistency with other hospital documents, such as quality assurance plans, hospital and medical staff bylaws, and hospital policies and procedures, as well as current Joint Commission and state licensure requirements and local, state, and federal laws and regulations. In addition to the risk management plan, each hospital needs comprehensive written plans covering fire safety,[4] internal and external disaster preparedness,[5] and the interruption of essential utility services (such as water, electricity, telephone, and natural gas)[6] in accordance with Joint Commission standards.

Risk Management Policies

In order to document support and authority for the hospital's risk management program, policies or resolutions must be adopted by both the governing board and hospital administration (figures 3-1 and 3-2). Such policies or resolutions should be reviewed and revised as necessary on an annual basis.

Risk Management Procedures

In addition to plans and policies or resolutions, each hospital risk manager needs to develop a comprehensive set of risk management procedures that describe in detail how various risk management activities are carried out within the facility and by whom. Risk management procedures may be assembled in a single risk management manual, or they may be included in various other manuals, such as safety manuals or nursing service procedure manuals. Regardless of how such procedures are kept, it is important that a mechanism be devised to ensure that everyone within the hospital who is expected to follow a given procedure is apprised of its existence, is informed

Figure 3-1.   Board Resolution Regarding Risk Management

WHEREAS, the Board of Directors of _____ Hospital recognizes that the primary purpose of _____ Hospital is to provide for the safe and professional care of patients, visitors, and personnel;

THEREFORE, be it resolved by the Board of Directors of _____ Hospital concurring:

    That the Board of Directors shall hereby make a commitment to provide for the safe and professional care of all patients, visitors, and hospital personnel.

    That the Board of Directors hereby directs the Chief Executive Officer to take whatever action is necessary to implement a hospitalwide risk management program.

    That this Resolution shall go into full force and effect from the date of its passage.

Adopted by the Board of Directors
of _____ Hospital
Date: _____

_____
For Board of Directors

Source: Reprinted, with permission, from St. Elizabeth Community Hospital, Red Bluff, CA.

Figure 3-2. Administrative Policy Regarding Risk Management

```
SUBJECT: Risk Management
Adopted: _____ , 19 _____
Reviewed and Revised: _____ , 19 _____

POLICY:    It shall be the policy of _____ Hospital, in accordance with a Resolution of
           its Board of Directors, to develop, implement, support, monitor, and evaluate a comprehen-
           sive hospitalwide risk management program aimed at:

                1. Eliminating or reducing the risk of loss or injury to the facility, its patients,
                   employees, and visitors, and
                2. Eliminating or reducing the risk of liability losses due to such injuries.

RESPONSIBILITY:  The Chief Executive Officer, through the hospital's designated Risk Manager,
                 shall be responsible for the development, implementation, support, monitoring,
                 and evaluation of the risk management program.
```

of any changes in the procedure, and knows where a copy of the procedure is kept for reference.

The following is a list of some procedures that should be included in a hospitalwide risk management program:

- *Incident reporting procedure,* including where incident report forms are kept, when and by whom they are to be completed, where completed reports are to be sent, and whether copies are to be made or retained
- *Patient complaint resolution procedure,* including to whom patient complaints are to be channeled and any forms to be completed
- *Attorney contact procedure* instructing employees as to how to handle contacts or requests for information from attorneys representing current or former patients
- *Patient confidentiality/release of information procedure* regarding the release of patient information to the media, third-party payers, and others
- *Informed consent procedure,* including parties responsible for securing an informed consent to medical or surgical treatment and who may grant such consent under various circumstances
- *Sponge and needle count procedure* for ensuring that such items are accounted for prior to wound closure in the surgical suite
- *Visitor injury procedure* indicating what should be done, who should be called, and what forms should be completed when an employee encounters an injured visitor
- *Employee injury procedure* indicating actions to be taken and forms to be completed in the event of an employee injury
- *Body mechanics procedure* describing techniques for the safe lifting and moving of patients, objects, and equipment
- *Sharps safety and disposal procedure,* including a prohibition on needle recapping and instructions for the disposal of used syringes
- *Preventive maintenance procedure* for ensuring scheduled preventive maintenance of hospital equipment and documenting maintenance activities
- *Loaner equipment procedure* covering lending equipment to and borrowing equipment from other facilities
- *Defective equipment procedure* for sequestering defective equipment and notifying appropriate parties to arrange for testing and repair
- *Product and device recall procedure* assigning responsibility for and prescribing forms to be completed when a product or medical device is recalled

Other specific procedures will be included in the hospital's fire plan, safety manual, disaster plans, and hazardous materials plan. Although the foregoing list is by no means exhaustive, it reinforces the need for the risk manager to think in broad terms when developing a comprehensive risk management program.

☐ Claims Management

In addition to the loss prevention duties outlined, the risk manager is primarily responsible for the hospital's claims management activities. Such activities include notifying the hospital's liability insurance carrier and/or defense counsel of potential claims and lawsuits, assisting with the defense of claims by scheduling employees for deposition, providing documents in response to requests for production, and supplying answers to written interrogatories. Often the risk manager has authority to settle small claims (such as for reimbursement for lost or damaged patient valuables) and to write off hospital bills up to a designated dollar amount. In conjunction with defense counsel, the risk manager may recommend to hospital administration the settlement of larger claims.

☐ Risk Management Strategies

In order to approach the process of health care risk management systematically, it is helpful to think in terms of the following four-step generic model for risk management:[7]

1. The identification of risk
2. The analysis of the risks identified
3. The treatment of risk
4. The evaluation of risk treatment strategies

This model will assist the beginning risk manager in setting priorities for his or her activities and, in conjunction with a vigorous claims management program, ensure a comprehensive risk management effort.

Risk Identification

Risk identification is the process through which the risk manager becomes aware of risks in the health care environment that constitute potential loss exposures for the institution. Such exposures can include not only losses of the facility's financial assets through liability judgments and out-of-court settlements, but also casualty losses to its physical plant and property, human losses through death or injury, and less tangible losses to the institution's public image and reputation.

The risk manager can use many information sources to identify potential risks. Incident reporting, in which hospital employees report accidents and occurrences not consistent with normal hospital routine, is the cornerstone of most risk identification systems. In addition, the following provide valuable information to assist the risk manager in identifying risks:

- Generic occurrence screening often performed as part of the hospital's quality assurance programs
- Patient complaints and satisfaction-survey results tallied by patient representatives (or community relations or marketing departments)
- Prior professional liability, property and casualty, and workers' compensation claims
- Surveys by the Joint Commission,[8] liability insurers, or risk management consultants
- State licensure surveys

Contracts, leases, and other agreements entered into by the health care facility often reveal additional risk exposures, as does information generated through the hospital's infection control and quality assurance functions, which the risk manager should routinely review to the extent permitted by law. (Some concerns have been expressed that free access to medical staff quality assurance peer review information by the hospital risk manager for use in preparing a defense for professional liability claims may waive statutory protections provided under state peer review protection statutes. The reader is advised to seek the counsel of an attorney when developing a mechanism for reviewing such information.) Finally, informal discussions with line managers and other staff members are excellent sources of information for the beginning risk manager about potential risks.

Risk Analysis

Risk analysis is the process of determining the potential severity of the loss associated with an identified risk and the probability that such a loss will occur. Those factors taken together establish the seriousness of a risk and guide the risk manager's selection of an appropriate risk treatment strategy. Risk managers need to give priority to areas that hold the greatest potential risk of financial loss, such as anesthesia or obstetrical mishaps, even though claims in these areas may occur infrequently; they should give less emphasis to small claims that may occur more frequently.

Although risk analysis is in part an art—a judgment call based upon the training, experience, and instincts of the risk manager—there are sources of information that may prove helpful. In particular, closed claims data, which reveal the frequency of occurrence and financial consequences of prior risks, should be reviewed to gain insight into the analysis of current risks. The hospital's legal counsel and liability insurance carrier may also be consulted for additional information.

Risk Treatment

Risk treatment refers to the range of choices available to the risk manager in handling a given risk. Risk treatment strategies include the following:

- Risk acceptance
- Risk avoidance
- Risk reduction or minimization
- Risk transfer

In addition to exploring these risk treatment strategies individually, the risk manager can fashion the combination of strategies that is best suited to managing a given risk exposure.

Risk Acceptance

One strategy for managing an identified risk is risk acceptance. Risk acceptance involves assuming the potential losses associated with a given risk and making plans to cover any financial consequences of such losses, either through access to the general assets of the institution or by creating a special set-aside fund or self-insurance mechanism.

Risk acceptance is most appropriate for managing (1) those risks that cannot be otherwise reduced, transferred, or avoided; and (2) those for which the probability of loss is not great and the potential consequences are not beyond the institution's ability to self-fund.

For the purposes of illustration, let us assume that a hospital risk manager has identified a risk of birth trauma injuries associated with the facility's obstetrical services. Because the hospital's governing board and administration may have identified obstetrical services as central to both its mission and market-positioning strategy, the hospital may be unwilling to forgo providing such services as a means of eliminating the risk. The hospital may then choose to self-insure for losses associated with birth trauma injuries, or perhaps to purchase an insurance policy to cover such losses (a risk transfer strategy), but with a self-funded deductible as a means of risk acceptance.

Risk Avoidance

Risk avoidance represents another risk treatment strategy. When a given risk poses a particularly serious threat that cannot be effectively reduced or transferred, the conduct or service giving rise to the risk may perhaps be avoided.

In our obstetrical example, the hospital might elect not to provide obstetrical services, thus avoiding the risk of a birth trauma claim. Although that strategy may be very effective in terms of controlling risk exposure, it may come at the high cost of a loss of hospital mission effectiveness, market share and revenues, patient satisfaction, and medical staff relations, which could well outweigh its benefits.

Risk Reduction or Minimization

Risk reduction or minimization involves various loss control strategies aimed at limiting the potential consequences or frequency of a given risk without totally accepting or avoiding the risk. Risk reduction or minimization efforts are at the heart of most hospital risk management programs and include such activities as staff education, policy and procedure revision, and other interventions aimed at controlling adverse occurrences without completely eschewing potentially risky activities.

In the obstetrical example, risk reduction strategies may include mandating specific training for obstetricians and obstetrical nursing staff, eliminating high-risk obstetrical services, and providing for adequate staff and equipment to cope with obstetrical emergencies.

Risk Transfer

Risk transfer techniques involve shifting the risk of loss to another entity, either through contract or by purchasing insurance. Through risk transfer, an institution can continue to engage in a risk-producing activity while, for a price, transferring the risk of loss. In the obstetrical example, the hospital may purchase a professional liability policy to pay for any losses associated with an adverse obstetrical occurrence or may contract with another facility to provide such services as methods of risk transfer.

It should be clear from the preceding discussion that, for most identified risks, the health care facility may employ a combination of risk treatment strategies to best manage a given situation. In the obstetrical example, a hospital would likely accept a certain amount of risk through an insurance deductible or self-insured retention, avoid some of the potential risk (perhaps by not offering high-risk obstetrical services), seek to reduce risk through inservice education and appropriate staffing and privileging, and transfer some of the risk by purchasing insurance.

Risk Management Evaluation

The final step in the risk management process is risk management evaluation, whereby the effectiveness of the techniques employed to identify, analyze, and treat risks is gauged and assessed. Risk evaluation involves not only the risk manager, but also hospital administration, the medical staff and governing board, insurers, claims managers, and legal counsel. This multidisciplinary approach to evaluating the effectiveness of a risk management program ensures that the impact of various risk management activities is measured accurately and that additional risk management opportunities are fully explored. To facilitate the risk management evaluation process, the risk manager needs to prepare a comprehensive annual report of risk management activities that highlights significant claims activity, new program developments, changes in insurance coverage, and contractual modifications.

☐ Functional Components of a Risk Management Program

Although many risk managers tend to focus on the professional liability aspects of health care risk management, the discipline extends into many other areas that are equally important to the survival of the modern hospital. Defined broadly, health care risk management is concerned with a tremendous variety of issues and situations that hold the potential for liability or casualty losses for an institution. In order to be truly comprehensive, a risk management program must address the full scope of the following categories of risk.

Patient-Related Risks

Throughout much of the late 1970s and early 1980s, U.S. health care institutions and practitioners experienced a "malpractice crisis" evidenced by escalating numbers of professional liability claims, as well as by rising settlement amounts, jury verdicts, and insurance premiums.[9,10] As many state legislatures debated tort reform proposals aimed at slowing the trend[11] and some states enacted statutes mandating specific health care risk management programs,[12] increasing national attention was focused on the patient care aspects of health care risk management.

Therefore, it is not surprising that many hospital risk management efforts begin with patient care–related issues. Patient care or clinical risk management, including information gathering, loss prevention efforts, professional liability risk financing, and claims management activities, form the core of hospital risk management programs.

Although most patient-related risk management focuses on direct clinical patient care activities and the consequences of inappropriate or incorrectly performed medical treatments, other important patient-related issues also confront the hospital risk manager, including the following:

- Confidentiality and appropriate release of patient medical information
- Protection of patients from abuse and neglect and from assault by other patients, visitors, or hospital staff
- The securing of appropriate informed patient consent to medical treatment
- Nondiscriminatory treatment of patients, regardless of race, religion, national origin, or payment status
- Protection of patient valuables from loss or damage

Medical Staff-Related Risks

Closely aligned with the patient care–related management issues that a hospital deals with are those experienced by the hospital's medical staff. Many, if not most, of the potentially serious occurrences related to the delivery of clinical patient care also involve the facility's medical staff. It is therefore imperative that the health care risk manager include the hospital's medical staff in clinical loss prevention and claims management programs and elicit the staff's support of overall risk management activities.

Risk management concerns stemming from the unique relationship between the hospital and its medical staff merit the health care risk manager's particular attention. Of particular importance to the hospital risk manager are:

- Medical staff peer review and quality assurance activities
- The confidentiality and protection of the data generated

- The medical staff credentialing, appointment, and privileging processes
- Medical staff disciplinary proceedings and related issues of due process, antitrust, and restraint of trade

In this era of expanding legal theories of hospital corporate liability and broadened notions of vicarious liability, the activities of the medical staff are often deemed the activities of the hospital. It has become increasingly difficult for defense attorneys to persuade judges and juries to distinguish between the institution and its physicians. Thus, the hospital risk manager must actively assist the hospital in managing the quality of medical care provided by the hospital's physicians and in overseeing the fairness of the appointment and credentialing process.

Employee-Related Risks

Several issues relating to the employment of hospital personnel deserve the health care risk manager's attention. Of obvious importance are maintaining a safe work environment for employees, reducing the risk of occupational illnesses and injury, and providing for the treatment and compensation of workers who suffer on-the-job injuries and work-related illnesses. In this regard, it is important that the risk manager maintain a working knowledge of relevant state workers' compensation law as well as federal regulations promulgated by the Occupational Safety and Health Administration in order to work effectively with the health care facility's human resources department.

Posing particularly serious problems for today's hospital are issues involving allegations of discrimination in recruitment, hiring, and promotion based on age, race, sex, national origin, or handicap; wrongful termination; and claims filed with the Equal Employment Opportunity Commission. The risk manager must work with the facility's human resources director in minimizing such claims exposures.

Other Risks

There are, of course, other areas of potential interest for the hospital risk manager. Among those are the wide variety of property safety issues, including mechanisms to prevent and reduce the risk of losses associated with fire, flood, earthquake, and severe weather phenomena such as strong winds and hail; boiler and heating, ventilation, and air-conditioning system malfunction; and losses involving hospital-owned and nonhospital-owned vehicles such as automobiles, ambulances, and helicopters. Through disaster planning and simulated disaster drills, the risk manager must be concerned both with protecting hospital patients and employees from injuries stemming from such occurrences and with minimizing resulting property and liability damages. Risk financing, through both insurance and self-insurance, often proves to be a central focus of risk management activity in this regard.

Hazardous materials management is yet another area of risk management that has gained much recent attention. Ensuring that appropriate protocols are in place for the safe storage, use, and disposal of a myriad of toxic chemicals and radioactive materials is a highly regulated[13] and increasingly important risk management activity. It has implications for hospital patients and employees as well as for the community at large should such materials find their way into the environment. Infectious biological waste generated by hospitals came under increased public scrutiny after contaminated syringes and other medical waste products washed up on eastern U.S. beaches in 1988,[14] making the assurance of proper disposal procedures all the more important.

Special issues involving auxilians and other volunteers who provide services at the hospital, and students involved in clinical training experiences, all of whom may sustain injury in the course of their duties or may inflict harm on others, also merit the risk manager's attention. Because neither volunteers nor students are typically hospital employees, the hospital may not be able to purchase insurance coverage for such occurrences at a reasonable cost, and therefore some other risk management strategy must be developed.

References

1. Joint Commission on Accreditation of Healthcare Organizations. *Accreditation Manual for Hospitals.* Chicago: JCAHO, 1988.

2. Joint Commission on Accreditation of Healthcare Organizations, pp. 23, 59, 121, 135, 205–8, 255.

3. Joint Commission on Accreditation of Healthcare Organizations, pp. 203–4.

4. Joint Commission on Accreditation of Healthcare Organizations, p. 207.

5. Joint Commission on Accreditation of Healthcare Organizations, p. 205.

6. Joint Commission on Accreditation of Healthcare Organizations, p. 209.

7. Troyer, G., and Salman, S. L. *Handbook of Health Care Risk Management.* Rockville, MD: Aspen Publishers, 1986, p. 153.

8. Joint Commission on Accreditation of Healthcare Organizations. 1 Renaissance Blvd., Oakbrook Terrace, IL 60181.

9. DiPaulo, S. Spiraling premiums predicted. *Modern Healthcare* 9(12):56, Dec. 1979.

10. The crisis in Missouri. Case study Medical Malpractice Insurance. Jefferson City, MO: Missouri Hospital Association, 1985, p. 6.

11. Professional liability legislation: looking to '86. *Medical Staff* 14:2, Oct. 1985.

12. Nelson, S. States adopt risk-management regulations. *Hospitals* 62(6):56, Jan. 20, 1988.

13. Hazard Communication Standard. Final Rule. Occupational Safety and Health Administration. 29 C.F.R. 1910.1200, Aug. 24, 1987.

14. Holthaus, D. States seek tighter rules on infectious waste. *Hospitals* 62(17):70, Sept. 5, 1988.

☐ Bibliography

Brown, B. L. *Risk Management for Hospitals: A Practical Approach.* Rockville, MD: Aspen Publishers, 1979.

Jessee, W. F. *Quality of Care Issues for the Hospital Trustee: A Practical Guide to Fulfilling Trustee Responsibilities.* Chicago: Hospital Research and Educational Trust, 1984.

Kraus, G. P. *Health Care Risk Management: Organization and Claims Administration.* Owings Mills, MD: National Health Publishing Co., 1986.

Monagle, J. F. *Risk Management: A Guide for Health Care Professionals.* Rockville, MD: Aspen Publishers, 1985.

Orlikoff, J., and Vanagunas, A. *Malpractice Prevention and Liability Control for Hospitals.* 2nd ed. Chicago: American Hospital Publishing, 1988.

Richard, E. P., and Rathburn, K. C. *Medical Risk Management: Preventive Legal Strategies for Health Care Providers.* Rockville, MD: Aspen Publishers, 1983.

Troyer, G., and Salman, S. L. *Handbook of Health Care Risk Management.* Rockville, MD: Aspen Publishers, 1986.

Wade, R. D. *Risk Management Hospital Professional Liability Primer.* Columbus, OH: Ohio Hospital Insurance Co., 1983.

Part Two

Roles

The effective risk manager interacts with every other function within the health care setting. Although no one function is more important in the care of patients than any other, the risk manager primarily serves the board of trustees, the medical staff, and the nursing and patient care staff in facilitating the safe care of patients. The first chapter in this section describes the various responsibilities risk managers may have and discusses qualifications for risk managers. The following chapters explain how risk management principles are integrated into these functions and how the risk manager coordinates with the hospital's insurers, attorneys, and federal and local safety officials to accomplish risk management goals.

Chapter 4
The Risk Manager

Trudy A. Goldman

The risk manager's role in a health care organization, as in any organization, is strategic to its survival. In view of the degree of responsibility vested in this position, the individual who holds it must be academically and experientially prepared for a continuous flow of challenges. This chapter explores how the risk manager fits into the framework of the health care organization and how he or she can be effective in this demanding role.

☐ Qualifications

The sample job descriptions in figures 4-1 through 4-3 illustrate the range of responsibilities the risk manager is expected to assume in various organizations. The degree of responsibility assigned to the position in figure 4-1 is limited, focusing on the process of risk identification and evaluation. Figure 4-2 (pp. 41–43) describes an expanded position that requires the risk manager to become more involved in risk financing and claims management activities. Figure 4-3 (pp. 44–46) illustrates broader expectations for the risk management role, demanding that the candidate be capable of developing and implementing a more comprehensive program that includes management of the risk financing and claims programs.

Because the responsibilities of the position can be so diverse, it is difficult to develop a profile of qualifications for a risk manager. In 1983, the American Society for Healthcare Risk Management (ASHRM) conducted a survey to obtain an overview of risk management responsibilities and salaries. The resulting product provided insight into the activities of a risk manager. Table 4-1 (p. 47) illustrates the wide range of components of a risk management program and the percentage of respondents surveyed who are responsible for those functions. The greatest concentration of responsibilities of those who responded was in the area of risk control, labeled as risk identification/evaluation, loss prevention, and safety administration. Fewer respondents indicated involvement in risk financing activities.

The diversity of activity that a risk manager may have responsibility for suggests that a variety of academic and experiential backgrounds may be suitable for that role.

Figure 4-1. Risk Manager Position Description, Level 1

Position Summary

The risk manager is responsible for the facility's risk management activities, which include coordinating insurance coverage and risk financing, managing claims against the facility, interfacing with defense legal counsel, administering the risk management program on a day-to-day basis, managing and analyzing risk management data, conducting risk management educational programs, and complying with the Joint Commission's risk management standards, all with the objective of controlling and minimizing loss to protect the assets of the facility. The level 1 risk manager performs these functions at the direction of first-level management. This individual participates in formulating policy or organizational changes but must seek advice and approval from higher authority for same.

Insurance/Risk Financing

Overview

The level 1 risk manager has general knowledge of and is familiar with the facility's insurance coverage against liability and casualty loss, including self-insurance funding and budgeting for payment of deductibles, risk retentions, and coinsurance. Participates in management reviews of insurance coverage and related issues. May prepare summaries of facility's insurance program for information of management and staff.

Specific Activities

- Notifies the liability insurance carrier of all actual and potential claims, including primary and excess carriers as necessary.
- May verify that each voluntary physician provides proof of adequate professional liability insurance.
- Acts as liaison with the insurance carrier. Completes insurance applications and responds to surveys. Prepares materials necessary for renewal of primary and excess insurance policies.
- Provides insurance information to outside agencies. Assists in compliance with state insurance reporting requirements.

Claims Management and Incident Reporting

Overview

The level 1 risk manager receives complaints and claims related to professional liability and transmits that information to the insurance carrier or legal counsel. At the request of management, legal counsel, or the adjuster, participates in responding to the complaint or claim to obtain information and facilitate settlement at an early stage. Works in coordination with patient ombudsman or acts as same to resolve complaints before they develop into professional liability claims. Receives incident reports and other information regarding untoward occurrences in the facility, such as quality assurance outliers or variations, and collates such information systematically to permit analysis pursuant to risk management policy and procedure. Reviews collated data to identify trends regarding accidents or occurrences, and recommends corrective action to management if appropriate. Prepares reports to management regarding data systems and findings. Recommends electronic data-programming initiation and improvement, working with data-processing professionals.

Specific Activities

- Designs, implements, and maintains a direct referral system for hospital staff to report potential claims against the hospital through such input sources as medical records, business office, patient advocate, nursing, medical staff, quality assurance, etc.
- Designs, implements, and maintains a hospitalwide incident reporting system.
- Investigates and analyzes actual and potential risks in the institution. Assesses liability and probability of legal action for potential notification of insurance carriers.
- Receives and investigates reports of product problems to determine appropriate response (in-house recalls, independent evaluations, etc.).
- Participates on selected committees related to assessment of patient care.
- Directly refers to administration those incidents with claims potential. Reports to higher authority any serious event involving actual or potential injury to patients, visitors, or employees.

Figure 4-1. (Continued)

- Takes steps to ascertain that risks are minimized through follow-up and actions on all regulatory/insurance survey report recommendations/deficiencies.
- Assists in processing summonses and complaints served on present and previous employees. Assists defendants in completing necessary documents.
- With director of patient representatives, reviews patient complaints that may be the source of potential legal action. Discusses and offers solutions when possible to resolve with patient and/or family any grievances against the hospital that are perceived as potential liability claims.
- Participates in evaluating claims for settlement. Negotiates settlement of small claims within administrative authority. Advises collection department of appropriate action for unpaid accounts involved in litigation. Approves payment for or replacement of lost property after evaluating claims.
- Reviews national and local claims data. Analyzes prior claims, lawsuits, and complaints against the hospital.
- May have on-call responsibility.

Program Administration

Overview

The level 1 risk manager has specific responsibilities regarding gathering and analyzing data and preparing reports to management and outside agencies as required (the latter is subject to final approval by facility management). Responsible for keeping management advised of developments in professional liability, which entails ongoing review of applicable literature. May recommend budget items to management.

Specific Activities

- Develops, coordinates, and administers hospitalwide systems for risk identification, investigation, and reduction. Maintains a hospitalwide network of informational sources and experts. Performs risk surveys and inspects patient care areas. Reviews facility and equipment to assess loss potential.
- Maintains risk management statistics and files in compliance with the Joint Commission and state and federal agencies. Ensures maximum confidentiality of and access to such information. Ensures that the following information is accurate, available, and secure: medical records, patient billing records, policies and procedures, incident reports, medical examiner's reports (if available), and any other data pertinent to a particular claim.
- Collects, evaluates, and distributes relevant data concerning patient injuries: aggregate data summaries, monthly trend analyses of incidents, claims profiles, and workers' compensation trends. Provides aggregate analysis of risk data. Maintains statistical trending of losses and other risk management data.
- Informs directors of service and department heads regarding occurrences, issues, findings, and risk management suggestions. Provides feedback to directors at all levels in the effort to eliminate risks. Assists clinical chairmen and department heads in designing risk management programs within their departments.
- Advises security on procedures to prevent or minimize loss of property or assets.
- Provides assistance to departments in complying with Joint Commission risk management and related standards.
- Recommends appropriate revisions to new or existing policies and procedures to prevent future occurrences. Recommends ways to eliminate risks through organization, equipment, or other changes. Reviews and revises hospital policies as appropriate to maintain adherence to current standards and requirements.

Legal Interface

Overview

On request of legal counsel, the level 1 risk manager may provide assistance in gathering information regarding individual claims or claims history. Seeks approval from management before requesting legal opinions or advice.

Specific Activities

- Works with hospital legal counsel to coordinate the investigation, processing, and defense of

(continued on next page)

Figure 4-1.   (Continued)

---

claims against the hospital. Records, collects, documents, maintains, and provides to hospital attorneys any requested information and documents necessary to prepare testimony in pending litigation.
- Responds to professional liability and hospital liability questions posed by hospital physicians, nurses, and other personnel.
- Maintains awareness of legislative and regulatory activities related to health care risk management.

Education/Inservices

Overview

The level 1 risk manager presents periodic inservices and routine orientation for facility employees and medical staff members regarding health care risk management and related subjects. May be authorized to obtain outside speakers and faculty for such programs, subject to the approval of hospital management, and may coordinate such efforts with the facility's education department.

Specific Activities

- Provides inservice training to medical center personnel to enhance their awareness of their role in reducing liability exposures.
- Disseminates information on claim patterns and risk control, as well as on legislative and regulatory changes.
- Maintains a risk management education calendar.

In table 4-2 (p. 48), respondents indicated which academic qualifications they pursued in preparation for their careers. Table 4-3 (p. 48) demonstrates the disciplines in which ASHRM survey respondents indicated their professional experience had been concentrated. Both tables illustrate that the greatest number of respondents devoted their career preparation and prior work history to business or management.

A successful risk management program often can demonstrate the existence of top management support. This support is most apparent when the risk manager reports to an individual at or near the top of the organization. Table 4-4 (p. 49) lists the ASHRM survey findings concerning the titles of those professionals to whom the individual with responsibility for risk management reports. This table indicates that almost 75 percent of the respondents report to the CEO, president of the organization, or a vice-president.

To conduct a health care risk management program limited to loss prevention and risk control, the candidate may be well qualified with a background in a health care profession. However, a candidate seeking a corporate position, a risk management leadership role in a multihospital system, or control of a comprehensive risk management program for any organization must have:

- Strong management skills, in order to effectively plan and coordinate activities to be accomplished by others.
- Knowledge of the functioning of a health care facility.
- Familiarity with law pertaining to medical malpractice liability, in order to maintain a meaningful position in the claims management process.
- Ability to assume responsibility for both risk financing and risk control. This requires insurance expertise to control or participate in all the components of a complete risk management program.
- Excellent writing and speaking skills, in order to effectively carry out key education and communication functions.

Figure 4-2.   Risk Manager Position Description, Level 2

Position Summary

The risk manager is responsible for the facility's risk management activities, which include coordinating insurance coverage and risk financing, managing claims against the facility, interfacing with defense legal counsel, administering the risk management program on a day-to-day basis, managing and analyzing risk management data, conducting risk management educational programs, and complying with the Joint Commission's risk management standards, all with the objective of controlling and minimizing loss to protect the assets of the facility. The level 2 risk manager performs these functions and reports to management at the vice-president level. This individual is responsible for reviewing and formulating policy or organizational changes and making recommendations for final approval by the vice-president, chief executive officer, and governing body.

Insurance/Risk Financing

Overview

The level 2 risk manager performs or coordinates the functions outlined under level 1 and, in addition, participates in negotiating coverage issues with carriers or trust administrators, including levels of coverage, scope of coverage, and premiums. Participates in formulating recommendations for purchase of coverage or funding of self-insurance for submission to management for final approval. Participates in preparing other financial analyses of facility's insurance program for the information of management and the governing body.

Specific Activities

- Reviews and maintains insurance policies. Analyzes existing policies for coverage and exclusion clauses. Anticipates and deals with policy expirations in a timely manner.
- Participates in managing the hospital's insurance programs and financing by preparing statistical data to support the continuation or the reduction of premiums paid or reserves.
- Participates in negotiating of policy provisions.
- May assess appropriate reserve funding levels, both insured and self-insured, in conjunction with an actuary.

Claims Management and Incident Reporting

Overview

The level 2 risk manager performs the functions outlined under level 1 and, in addition, works actively with legal counsel or the adjuster in investigating claims, developing defense strategy, and evaluating the monetary value of the claim. Participates as a team member in negotiating settlements for management approval. In litigated claims, assists legal counsel in accessing facility records and personnel and may act as a corporate representative during pretrial and trial. Recommends defense strategies for approval by chief executive officer, governing board, and legal counsel. Provides advice to senior management or the chief financial officer regarding reasonableness of expenses for claims defense.

Specific Activities

- Oversees investigation of all incidents/accidents/events that could lead to financial loss, including professional liability, general liability, and workers' compensation.
- Ensures investigation of all risks involving actual or potential injury to patients, visitors, and employees. Ensures collection of all information necessary to prepare for the defense of claims.
- Serves as liaison to brokers and insurance company representatives in negotiating and settling specific general liability claims. Directs conferences with claimants, attorneys, and insurance carriers, when applicable.
- Interacts with hospital legal counsel, insurance carrier, and patients and their families to effect quick settlement.
- Provides direction and advice to medical staff as necessary in connection with malpractice litigation and medicolegal matters.
- Coordinates reporting of patient care;edrelated incidents to the Department of Health as required by law. Directs investigation and development of corrective plans. Submits required reports to state and federal agencies.

(continued on next page)

Figure 4-2. (Continued)

Program Administration

Overview

The level 2 risk manager performs the functions outlined under level 1 and, in addition, manages a facility department or office of risk management. Is responsible for data management, claims management, and the education components of the facility's risk management program. Develops department budget for management approval.

Specific Activities

- Has full responsibility for all operations of the risk management program.
- Directs loss control/loss prevention activities.
- Supervises the statistical trending of losses and analyzes patterns.
- Designs and implements risk management surveys and studies. Conducts surveys, studies, and special projects to assist in long-term planning and changes to hospital policies and systems that will reduce risk and losses.
- Designs and/or administers safety systems and procedures to prevent or minimize loss from employee casualties and ensures compliance with OSHA regulations.
- Analyzes the risk of loss versus cost of reducing risk.
- Supervises accumulation of risk management cost data for budgetary and historical purposes. Prepares budgets for departmental operations.
- Develops and maintains risk management profiles on individual physicians and ensures integration of that information into the credentialing process in compliance with requirements of state and federal agencies, the Joint Commission, and the institution.
- Submits recommendations for changes in the existing risk control and risk financing procedures based on changes in properties, operations, or activities.

Legal Interface

Overview

The level 2 risk manager performs the functions outlined under level 1 and, in addition, works directly with legal counsel as a team member in the defense of claims. Has ongoing access to hospital liability defense counsel to consult regarding preventive as well as corrective measures to be taken in situations having legal connotation. On request, may provide information to facility management concerning reasonableness of cost and quality of legal services.

Specific Activities

- Evaluates correspondence from attorneys, patients, and other outside sources and formulates responses as necessary.
- Records, collects, documents, maintains, and communicates to insurance carrier and/or hospital attorney any information necessary to prepare testimony in pending litigation.
- Directs and coordinates release of records and information in response to subpoenas, court orders, attorney requests, state and federal agency investigations, OHM investigations, IPRO investigations, and other inquiries from outside sources.
- Maintains all legal case files and ensures maximum protection from discoverability of all such files.
- Approves defense postures or settlement values at lower levels routinely.
- Answers medicolegal inquiries from physicians, nurses, and administrators regarding emergent patient care issues and loss control.
- Is available to resolve treatment issues, including patient refusal of treatment, consent issues, and issues involving AMAs (against medical advice). Initiates court orders as appropriate via in-house and outside legal counsel.
- Reviews relevant contracts for risk exposure and insurance purposes before approval, including affiliation agreements, leases, construction agreements, and purchase orders, as appropriate.
- Maintains awareness of legislative activities that may affect risk management programs and participates in the legislative process.

Figure 4-2. (Continued)

Education/Inservices

Overview

The level 2 risk manager performs the functions outlined under level 1 and, in addition, organizes and manages facilitywide educational programs on health care risk management and related subjects for health care practitioners. Presents such programs in conjunction with the facility's education department or other organizations.

Develops a budget for health care risk management educational activities, or recommends risk management educational items in facility education budget for management's final approval.

Specific Activities

- Plans, develops, and presents educational material to administration, the medical staff, nursing personnel, and other department personnel on topics related to risk management as they affect hospital personnel.
- Develops and implements educational programs to reduce or eliminate potential safety hazards throughout the facility.

☐ Types of Certification

Risk managers are assigned a high level of responsibility, and their credentials enhance and support the credibility they need to carry out that responsibility. Although there are a growing number of colleges and universities that offer or are developing programs leading to a baccalaureate or master's degree in risk management, several other avenues exist for the certification of achievement in risk management.

The American Society for Healthcare Risk Management's Professional Recognition Program

Through its Professional Recognition Program, ASHRM formally acknowledges individual achievement and professional excellence in the health care risk management field. Risk management achievement is recognized through the award of designations at two levels: Fellow of the American Society for Healthcare Risk Management (FASHRM) for superior achievement, and Diplomate of the American Society for Healthcare Risk Management (DASHRM) for outstanding achievement.

Risk managers with a minimum of five years of active membership in ASHRM must satisfy prescribed criteria to receive these designations. Requirements for these awards must be satisfied in the following areas: academic credentials, continuing education, employment experience, and contributions to the field. Complete details for each requirement can be obtained by contacting ASHRM, 840 North Lake Shore Drive, Chicago, Illinois 60611.

The Associate in Risk Management Program

The Associate in Risk Management Program, known as ARM, is offered by the Insurance Institute of America. It consists of three courses that introduce the student to a decision-making process for identifying and analyzing all types of losses faced by any organization. The student learns techniques to treat those exposures and then practices risk control by focusing on the selection and application of appropriate methods for

Figure 4-3.   Risk Manager Position Description, Level 3

Position Summary

The risk manager is responsible for the facility's risk management activities, which include coordinating insurance coverage and risk financing, managing claims against the facility, interfacing with defense legal counsel, administering the risk management program on a day-to-day basis, managing and analyzing risk management data, conducting risk management educational programs, and complying with the Joint Commission's risk management standards, all with the objective of controlling and minimizing loss to protect the assets of the facility. The level 3 risk manager performs the functions described in levels 1 and 2, reporting directly to the chief executive officer or governing body. This position reviews, formulates, and implements policy and organizational changes, working within general programmatic authority delegated by the chief executive officer or governing body.

Insurance/Risk Financing

Overview

The level 3 risk manager performs or coordinates the functions outlined under levels 1 and 2 and, in addition, manages the facility's or system's insurance or self-insurance program within broad guidelines established by the chief executive officer or governing body. This position has authority to finalize selection and retention of carriers or self-funding mechanisms in conjunction with the chief financial officer. Sees to the preparation of loss experience reports and summaries for the information of the chief executive officer, chief financial officer, and governing body.

Specific Activities

- Evaluates property exposures, including new construction and renovation programs, to ensure coverage and minimize risk.
- Develops familiarity with insurance markets through frequent market contact and attendance at meetings and market symposiums.
- Plans, coordinates, and administers a broad comprehensive insurance program involving such activities as insurance purchasing, insurance consulting, administering self-insured coverages, and coordinating claims handling for all insurance lines.
- Directs and coordinates all aspects of insurance management for the institution, including developing alternatives such as self-insurance, excess insurance, and other risk financing mechanisms.
- Develops and manages the overall risk management program, involving risks of all types, which may include using deductibles, self-insurance, captive insurance companies, financial plans, commercial insurance, and insurance/reinsurance programs.
- For property insurance, boiler and machinery insurance, crime insurance, student health insurance, automobile insurance, and all other purchased insurance coverages, analyzes values and ensures that exposures are adequately insured. In the event of a loss, prepares data required by brokers and carriers and manages process through to settlement of claim.
- Develops familiarity with insurance markets through frequent market contact.
- Prepares specifications for competitive bidding. Negotiates with brokers, agents, or companies on insurance coverage, premiums, and services.
- Establishes and administers self-insurance trust funds for various types of insurance needs.

Claims Management and Incident Reporting

Overview

The level 3 risk manager performs the functions outlined in levels 1 and 2 and, in addition, has authority within broad guidelines established by the chief executive officer or governing body to approve settlement of all claims against the facility or system. Has authority to direct legal counsel and other personnel involved in claims management and give final approval to defense strategies. Approves payment of fees of defense counsel and payment of other expenses of claims defense.

Specific Activities

- Manages the claims program, which contains the following components:
  — Reporting procedures
  — System maintenance
  — Detailed claim investigations

Figure 4-3. (Continued)

- Establishment of reserves
- Selection and monitoring of legal counsel, as indicated
- Direct conferring with claimants, attorneys, physicians, employees, brokers, consultants, and carriers
- Settlement of claims
- Selection and utilization of actuarial firms, as needed and/or required
- Compliance with Medicare/Medicaid regulations
- Recommendations to senior management for funding requirements and necessary limits of coverage
- Reporting claims information to senior management
- Directs activities of investigators.
- Directs all claims-handling and defense-preparation activities of the insurance company and defense counsel.
- Is responsible for administering claims initiated in boiler/machinery, fire, and other loss areas.
- Procures outside loss prevention services.
- Projects future costs of losses, services, insurance, and other risk management devices.

Program Administration

Overview

The level 3 risk manager performs the functions outlined under levels 1 and 2 and, in addition, oversees all aspects of data management and analysis for the organization's loss control program. Establishes budget for data management and analysis aspects of loss control. Works within broad guidelines established by the chief executive officer or governing body regarding the use and integration of loss control data with other types of organizational data systems for audit and accountability purposes on a facilitywide or systemwide basis.

Specific Activities

- Conducts systems analyses to uncover and identify patterns that could result in compensable events.
- Assists clinical chairmen and department heads in designing risk management programs within their departments.
- Researches, writes, and implements departmental and hospital policies and procedures that affect liability exposures.
- Ensures that risks are minimized by following up and acting on all regulatory/insurance survey report recommendations/deficiencies.
- Selects and utilizes consulting services, brokers, carriers, etc.
- Provides quarterly board summary reports on incidents, claims, reserves, claim payments, etc.
- Develops and maintains risk management profiles on individual physicians and ensures integration of that information into the credentialing process in compliance with requirements of state and federal agencies, the Joint Commission, and the institution.

Legal Interface

Overview

The level 3 risk manager performs functions outlined in levels 1 and 2 and, in addition, has authority to retain, direct, and approve compensation of defense counsel.

Specific Activities

- Ensures compliance with various codes, laws, rules, and regulations concerning patient care, including those mandated by state and federal agencies, and incident reporting and investigational activities of federal, state, and local enforcement authorities.
- Implements relevant statutes and regulations, including mandated mechanisms of physician monitoring with feedback to medical staff office, reappointment process, etc.
- Assumes responsibility for contract compliance within appropriate guidelines and legal concepts. In preparing contracts for board approval, provides advice on contract language necessary to fulfill insurance and risk management requirements. Evaluates each contract negotiated by the hospital

(continued on next page)

Figure 4-3. (Continued)

to ensure that insurance and liability issues are adequately addressed and that risk is transferred to the other party if feasible. Establishes insurance requirements for all projects and contracts. Where appropriate, negotiates changes in contracts with other parties. Ensures that affiliated institutions have adequate insurance coverage.

- Reviews and approves all plans and specifications for new construction, alterations, and installation of equipment.

Education/Inservices

Overview

The level 3 risk manager performs the functions outlined under levels 1 and 2 and, in addition, develops loss control educational programs for the organization's use. This position establishes the education budget, subject to approval of the chief executive officer, chief financial officer, or governing body. May develop educational programs relative to health care risk management utilizing well-known experts in the field for national or regional representation. May develop risk management educational programs with broad appeal for marketing to other organizations.

Specific Activities

- Plans and implements a facilitywide program for both loss prevention and loss control and a comprehensive orientation program. Those programs will be directed to all current and future employees of the board, physicians at the hospital, and hospital employees to advise them of their responsibilities, obligations, and part in the board's risk management program.
- Directs and conducts educational sessions for medical staff and hospital staff on risk management topics.

identified hazards. This decision-making process is also applied in choosing the appropriate risk financing techniques, with attention given to retention, commercial insurance, and captives.

Although the program is generic to risk management in all industries, it offers significant benefits to the health care risk manager. The health care risk manager needs to look beyond medical malpractice and general liability risks to control or finance the risk of loss of property, net income, and personnel. Of greatest benefit may be the opportunity to study risk financing techniques, which enable the health care risk manager to better administer or assist in the institution's risk financing program.

The ARM designation is awarded after the successful completion of three examinations. Preparation for those examinations may be accomplished through self-study or classroom education. More information can be obtained from the Insurance Institute of America, Providence and Sugartown Roads, Malvern, Pennsylvania 19355.

The Certified Property Casualty Underwriter Program

The designation CPCU, for Certified Property Casualty Underwriter, awarded by the American Institute for Property and Liability Underwriters after completion of a program that focuses on the insurance business and its impact upon the economic, social, and legal environment.

Although the CPCU program has a greater insurance orientation than the ARM program, it will benefit health care risk managers who aspire to greater involvement in their institution's risk financing function. Successful completion of the required courses broadens the risk manager's knowledge of risk management techniques, provides a greater understanding of insurance contracts and functions, and enables risk managers to apply loss control and risk financing techniques to their institutions.

Table 4-1. Percentage of Respondents with Responsibility for Handling Individual Components of a Comprehensive Risk Management Program

Program Component	Percentage of Respondents with Responsibility (Number)	Percentage of Individuals Whose Authority Is:			Average Percentage of Respondent's Time Spent
		Complete	Shared	Consulting	
Risk identification/evaluation	94.3 (2,864)	39.5	55.9	4.6	12.6
Loss prevention	87.8 (2,665)	33.2	61.0	5.8	7.9
Safety administration	73.7 (2,239)	34.4	53.5	12.1	6.1
Handling patient complaints	65.9 (2,001)	24.3	66.1	9.6	4.3
Property/casualty claims	65.5 (1,989)	40.6	52.2	7.2	4.8
Product liability claims	52.9 (1,607)	38.1	51.3	10.6	1.8
Security	51.2 (1,554)	39.8	43.5	16.7	3.2
Workers' compensation claims	45.2 (1,373)	40.7	45.0	14.3	2.7
Conducting patient satisfaction surveys	40.6 (1,234)	27.3	58.2	14.5	1.6
Other employee benefits design/administration	31.2 (949)	29.5	54.4	16.1	1.3
Premium forecasting/budgeting	30.2 (916)	35.8	49.2	15.0	.9
Group insurance plan design/administration	29.2 (888)	31.0	53.0	16.0	1.3
Group insurance benefit claims	28.6 (868)	39.5	46.7	13.8	.1
Insurance accounting	27.0 (821)	33.4	52.1	14.5	1.0
Management of department personnel (2+)	25.6 (778)	66.6	28.4	5.0	3.4
Pension/retirement income payments	21.8 (663)	39.5	45.0	15.5	.6
Family counseling	20.3 (616)	22.9	55.3	21.8	.9

Source: American Society for Healthcare Risk Management, 1983.

N = 3,037.

Table 4-2. Subject Areas in Which Respondents Hold Academic Qualifications/Degrees

Subject	Number	Percentage
Health care administration	674	22.2
Business administration	577	19.0
Nursing and nursing administration	385	12.7
Social sciences	141	4.6
Law	107	3.5
Allied health care (except nursing)	106	3.5
Accounting	98	3.2
Medical records	91	3.0
Public administration	73	2.4
Education	66	2.2
Humanities	58	1.9
Biological and health sciences	54	1.8
Medicine (M.D.)	48	1.6
Personnel management	41	1.4
Physical sciences	26	.9
Engineering	24	.8
Risk management	13	.4
Health care education	8	.3
Industrial psychology	6	.2
Other	241	7.9
Missing responses	200	6.5
Total	3,037	100.0

Source: American Society for Healthcare Risk Management, 1983.

Table 4-3. Discipline in Which Respondent's Professional Experience Has Been Concentrated

Discipline	Number	Percentage
Hospital administration	1,385	45.6
Health care	577	19.0
Personnel management	209	6.9
Medical records administration	134	4.4
Accounting	106	3.5
Law	99	3.3
Business	87	2.9
Insurance	61	2.0
Engineering	50	1.6
Claims handling	49	1.6
Other[a]	240	7.9
Missing responses	40	1.3
Total	3,037	100.0

Source: American Society for Healthcare Risk Management, 1983.

[a] A 25 percent random sample suggests that this category includes approximately 153 safety, security, and criminal justice professionals; 28 quality assurance professionals; 14 food service management personnel; 10 health planners; 10 public relations specialists; 10 program analysts/evaluation specialists; 10 biomedical engineers; and 5 patient representatives.

Table 4-4. Generic Titles of Risk Management Professionals' Supervisors

Type of Professional	Number	Percentage
Chief executive officer/president	1,347	44.4
Senior officer/vice-president	917	30.2
Board of trustees member/president	140	4.6
Financial officer	93	3.1
Chief medical officer	63	2.1
Nursing administrator/director	63	2.1
Personnel officer	35	1.2
Chief of engineering or safety/security	31	1.0
Quality assurance coordinator/director	31	1.0
Operations officer	22	.7
Administrative asst. to CEO/senior officer	20	.7
Legal services officer	15	.5
Director of risk management & quality assurance	9	.3
Risk management coordinator/director	7	.2
Medical records manager/director	5	.2
Marketing/public relations officer	1	.0
Other	18	.5
Missing responses	220	7.2
Total	3,037	100.0

Source: American Society for Healthcare Risk Management, 1983.

The CPCU program consists of 10 courses that address personal and commercial risk management and insurance, law, management, economics, and accounting. To receive the CPCU designation, students must matriculate with the American Institute for Property and Liability Underwriters before taking the examinations. There also are ethics and experience requirements that must be satisfied before this designation is conferred.

Candidates with an ARM designation have an advantage in seeking the CPCU designation: for them, part 1 of the CPCU examination is waived.

For more information, contact the American Institute for Property and Liability Underwriters, 720 Providence Road, Malvern, Pennsylvania 19355.

☐ Responsibilities of the Risk Manager

The risk manager's duties include conducting staff orientation and inservice education programs, having access to formal and informal reporting systems within the institution, and establishing a risk management committee.

Staff Orientation and Inservice Education

The risk manager can guide and motivate the risk management practice of others in the organization by providing education. By conducting staff orientation and periodic inservice programs, the risk manager can train health care staff to practice more effective loss control techniques and employ risk management procedures. Often, little is known about the risk management function; therefore, members of the organization who wish to clarify their role in this process may be a captive audience for this type of educational program.

A risk management orientation should present general risk management techniques together with specific risk control information tailored to the clinical area being addressed. The following outline suggests an orientation program the risk manager can deliver to health care staff.

I. General Risk Management Information

- Generic definition of risk management
- Functions of the risk management office
- Overview of the professional liability program
  - Who is insured in the organization
  - Description of coverage provided
  - Discussion of whether employees need to obtain additional private professional liability coverage
- Reasons why risk management practice is critical to the survival of the organization, and the health care staff's obligation to support risk management
  - The significance of early reporting of potentially compensable events
  - Criteria to be used to identify a claim
  - How trending data are used in the organization's loss control efforts
- The flow of risk management information, including linkage with quality assurance

II. General Risk Control Methods

- The importance of good medical records documentation
- The practicing of informed consent
  - Description of the difference between obtaining a signature on a consent form prior to a procedure and the educational process of informed consent
  - Discussion of how documentation of informed consent can be of benefit in the event of a claim
- Patient relations and techniques for communicating with the patient and family
- Incident reporting and occurrence screening

III. Claims

- The phases in the life cycle of a claim, from investigation to claim closure
- The responsibilities of the risk management office and the health care organization staff in the management of a claim
- The impact of a claim after its resolution, including reporting required by the Health Care Quality Improvement Act of 1986
- Ways to protect the confidentiality of patient information

IV. Risk Management Information Focused on a Specific Clinical Area

- National claims data and in-house claims experience for the clinical area being addressed
- Types of events generating claims in that clinical area
- Suggested interventions to reduce the risk of recognized exposures in that area
- Services the risk manager can offer to specific departments

Focused inservice education should be offered at regular intervals. This type of educational program allows the risk manager to advise the organization of recently identified loss trends, update claim experience, discuss new risk control techniques, or provide an overview of new legislation affecting risk management practices. It is also an opportunity to keep in close contact with and motivate those individuals who must continue to report potentially compensable events. Program format can be varied to include a mock trial, guest speakers from within or outside the organization, and forums with topics determined by the department(s) attending the inservice program.

The orientation or inservice program will provide long-term rewards for the risk manager through the opportunity to deliver first-hand direction to important links in the risk management information network.

Formal and Informal Reporting of Risk Management Activities

The risk manager is a facilitator who must accomplish actions through others in the organization. Information must flow though the risk management office so that knowledge of the need for intervention can be directed to those who can respond and implement changes in the system. To ensure the flow of information, the risk manager must have access to the appropriate channels, both formal and informal.

Formal Reporting System

Formal communications are those established by the organization's policies and procedures and generally follow the chain of command.[1] The risk manager may accumulate incident report data to identify trends that may indicate high-risk areas in the organization. Those data are not limited to the details of incident reports; they should include patient complaints, infection reports, and requests from attorneys for medical records. By allowing an aggressive rather than a reactive approach to loss control, this "near-miss" data information system has substantial value.[2]

Formal reporting may also be accomplished through occurrence screening or generic screening, which is the "early warning system" that alerts the risk manager that a loss-producing event has most likely occurred. This system differs from incident reporting in that the type of event being reported is more than a clinical event with adverse consequences and has probably resulted in a potentially compensable event. The organization's medical staff is given a set of criteria that signify a potentially compensable event. When a member of the medical staff becomes aware of the occurrence of one of these specific events, he or she is required to notify the risk manager as soon as possible. The objective of this information system is to allow the risk manager to begin the investigation immediately. This early signal is also an opportunity to capitalize on any chance of ameliorating the situation before it becomes a claim. Understanding this important benefit may motivate more members of the organization to comply with the requirements of such a system.

Another formal information system, particularly effective in large organizations, is a risk management correspondent network. Correspondents are appointed as representatives of each unit of the organization and are responsible for the flow of information between their departments and risk management. All representatives must be familiar with the overall administration and operation of their unit, as well as with the organization's administrative policies and risk management program.

The risk management correspondent conveys information concerning incidents occurring in the representative's unit to the risk management department. When a potentially compensable event occurs, the correspondent can be called upon to assist in the investigation by obtaining records, arranging for interviews with witnesses, and securing evidence. The correspondents can also act as intermediaries between the unit employees and risk management concerning insurance coverage and risk management policy.

Informal Reporting System

An informal reporting system is equally important to the risk manager. It enables him or her to learn about potentially compensable events through the grapevine or via telephone calls from individuals not involved in the event. The risk manager needs to conduct a careful analysis of the organization to identify all possible sources of informal information. Many areas of the organization, even those not directly providing patient care, can contribute significant information to risk management. For example, the patient accounts department can notify the risk manager about patients protesting the payment of their bills because of dissatisfaction with the care they received. In addition to forwarding record requests to attorneys, medical records personnel can advise the risk manager by phone when a patient's family demands the medical record. Other valuable informants include members of hospital administration, patient representatives, social workers, and the chaplain, all of whom can report patient complaints; pathology personnel, who can report an attorney's request for a patient's slides or blocks; and public relations personnel, who can advise of any media inquiries about patients.

The risk manager must cultivate and maintain the sources of this informally transmitted information by such techniques as paying casual visits to the nursing units, joining a table of anesthesiologists for lunch, or showing interest in a piece of equipment in one of the hospital's labs. The risk manager needs to gain the confidence of personnel so that they will feel comfortable enough to call when a potentially compensable event occurs.

Establishment of the Risk Management Committee

A risk management committee can enhance the effectiveness of the risk manager's activities, as it is another channel for risk management information and it increases the involvement in risk management of key individuals in the organization. Many variables will affect the scope, makeup, and function of a risk management committee in a health care organization. Depending on the size and needs of the organization, activities of this committee can extend to providing input into claims management and selecting a risk financing mechanism. However, the most common element in the charge given to the risk management committee is that of reviewing and evaluating specific incidents and loss trends with the objective of reducing the chance of loss or averting further loss to the organization.

The scope of this committee is broad; therefore, the composition must be multidisciplinary to reach each strategic area. In choosing members, the risk manager's goal should be to select those individuals who are influential in effecting and enforcing change in the organization. Members should also be selected as a result of their linkages to other committees. The following suggests the composition of an ideal risk management committee: risk manager, chief of staff, chief financial officer, in-house legal counsel, director of nursing, hospital director or administrator, member of the governing board, two or three members of the medical staff representing high-risk clinical areas, and the director of quality assurance. It may be difficult to enlist each of these participants. However, it is essential that these individuals be informed of and support the risk management committee's activities, recommendations, and results.

The risk management committee acts to effectuate change in policy and procedure and also can provide guidance and support for the risk management department's efforts. The risk manager can use these committee meetings to educate members about risk management technique and current legislative and regulatory issues that affect risk management activities. The risk manager's participation on this committee also presents him or her with an opportunity to gain greater visibility and credibility in the organization.

The risk manager is the key to the functioning of this committee. In addition to having responsibility for the organization and administration of the committee, many activities of the risk management office will culminate with the report presented to this committee. To effectively prepare for each risk management committee meeting, the risk manager should:

- Review incidents and claims, select those events most appropriate for committee review, and create the agenda using those items
- Develop a capsule summary of each incident to be evaluated and distribute that information to committee members prior to the meeting
- Prepare a report of the status or actions taken following recommendations made at the previous meeting
- Review data accumulated from incident reports and other sources to identify loss trends to be reported at the meeting

- Determine whether other individuals are needed at the meeting to provide additional information concerning an incident or loss trend, and, if so, arrange for them to be present

Of particular importance is the risk manager's transmission of information about the committee's activities, recommendations, and results to the organization's administration and the governing board on a quarterly or annual basis.

☐ Conclusion

The risk manager's role in a health care organization is dynamic and constantly challenged by the diverse components of the risk management program. With the broad scope of activities attendant to that role, the candidate may enter a risk management discipline from a variety of career paths. However, there is one common thread, which is the need for strong managerial skills in this position. Because the practice of risk management encompasses all areas of the organization, the ability to effectively develop systems, coordinate, and plan the risk management effort is critical to this key managerial role.

References

1. Mehr, R. I., and Hedges, B. A. *Risk Management Concepts and Applications*. Homewood, IL: Richard D. Irwin, 1977.
2. Bird, F. E., Jr., and Loftus, R. G. *Loss Control Management*. Loganville, GA: Institute Press, 1976.

☐ Bibliography

American Society for Healthcare Risk Management, Division of Quality Control Management, Office of the General Counsel, American Academy of Hospital Attorneys. *Medical Malpractice Task Force Report on Tort Reform and Compendium of Professional Liability Early Warning Systems for Health Care Providers*. Chicago: American Hospital Association, 1986.

Brown, B. L., Jr. *Risk Management for Hospitals: A Practical Approach*. Germantown, MD: Aspen Publishers, 1979.

Graham, N. O. *Quality Assurance in Hospitals: Strategies for Assessment and Implementation*. Rockville, MD: Aspen Publishers, 1982.

Head, G. *Essentials of Risk Control*. Vol. 2. Malvern, PA: Insurance Institute of America, 1986.

Kraus, G. P. *Health Care Risk Management*. Owings Mills, MD: Rynd Communications, 1986.

Orlikoff, J. E., Fifer, W. R., and Greeley, H. P. *Malpractice Prevention and Liability Control for Hospitals*. Chicago: American Hospital Association, 1981.

Wade, R. D. *Risk Management HPL*. Columbus, OH: Ohio Hospital Insurance Company, 1983.

Chapter 5

The Hospital Governing Board

James E. Orlikoff

The hospital governing board is ultimately responsible and accountable for the operation of the hospital, including, among other things, the quality of care provided, the performance of the medical staff, and the effectiveness of the hospital's risk management and quality assurance programs. The board's accountability for quality and risk management, however, is a relatively recent development. Consequently, few boards understand their accountability and responsibility for risk management, and still fewer effectively oversee and set the direction for their hospitals' risk management programs.

A 1986 survey conducted by the Hospital Research and Educational Trust of the American Hospital Association revealed the top 10 agenda issues that occupied the greatest percentage of a board's time (figure 5-1). The relative importance that boards attached to each issue reflected the amount of time they devoted to the issue. An examination of figure 5-1 reveals that risk management, quality, and insurance, as such, were not among the 10 issues that most frequently occupied a hospital board's time. Further, the three risk management–related issues that tended to be considered by boards—medical staff

Figure 5-1. Agenda Issues That Occupy the Greatest Percentage of a Board's Time

1. Financial viability	29.4%
2. Strategic planning	18.4
3. Diversification/mergers/joint ventures	14.0
4. Capital projects	12.0
5. Competitive position	11.0
6. Medical staff appointments	5.5
7. Other	3.3
8. Patient care standards	2.7
9. Litigation	1.9
10. CEO performance	1.3

Source: Alexander, J. A. *Current Issues in Hospital Governance.* Chicago: Hospital Research and Educational Trust of the American Hospital Association, 1986, p. 5, figure 6.

appointments, patient care standards, and litigation—were given relatively small amounts of board attention. The majority of hospital boards seemed to be unfamiliar with hospital risk management and uncertain as to what their role in risk management should be.

☐ The Board's Role in Risk Management

Risk management preserves and protects the hospital's assets and maintains and improves the quality of care provided by the hospital. Risk management is a critical hospital function and should be an ongoing board priority. The board, however, is not responsible for "doing" risk management; instead, the board's role is to provide direction for the hospital's risk management program and to ensure that the various risk management activities are functioning effectively.

The board's oversight role in risk management includes verifying that the hospital's definition of risk management and the structure and function of the risk management program are consistent with and support the hospital's mission. The board must also integrate risk management into the strategic planning process to ensure that the hospital undertakes new activities in a manner that will minimize liability exposure and maximize high-quality care and asset preservation. Consistent with its oversight role, the board should review and approve the hospital's risk management plan annually and hold the CEO responsible for ensuring that all components of the program are functioning effectively and consistently with the plan.

To help the board to discharge its role effectively, the risk manager must report to the board regularly on the activities of the risk management program and on new developments or major exposures to liability. The risk management reports should be comprehensible, should establish the necessary two-way communication between the board and the risk manager, and should enable the board to understand what is required to provide organizational support and effective resource allocation to the risk management program. This board oversight and support is critical to the ongoing effectiveness of the risk management program.

The importance of effective board oversight of the hospital's risk management program has been recognized by the Joint Commission on Accreditation of Healthcare Organizations. Effective January 1, 1989, the Joint Commission included governing board support for risk management as a required characteristic of the first governing body standard. That required characteristic is stated as follows:

> *GB 1.18* The governing body provides for resources and support systems for the quality assurance functions and risk management functions related to patient care and safety.[1]

In its scoring guidelines for compliance with standards, the Joint Commission is more specific about what a board must do and what reports it must receive to comply with the aforementioned requirement. The elements of satisfactory performance are described below:

1. The governing body requires performance of and has delegated responsibility for the following quality assurance/risk management functions:
   - Identification of general clinical areas that represent actual or potential sources of patient injury
   - Development and use of an indicator-based approach to identifying and evaluating individual cases of undesirable or adverse patient-care occurrences within the general clinical areas
   - Resolution of clinical problems disclosed through data evaluation
   - Provision of education for all staff on approaches to reducing or eliminating potential clinical sources of patient injury

Evidence of the governing body's mandate and delegation of responsibility for these functions may be contained in hospitalwide or (if they exist) departmental quality assurance plans; risk management plans; or administrative, operational, or strategic plans or budgets.

2. The governing body receives reports at least every six months on:
   * The frequency, severity, and causes of undesirable or adverse patient-care occurrences
   * Actions taken and the results of actions taken to reduce the occurrences' frequency and severity or to eliminate their causes

Evidence of compliance may be contained in governing-body-approved minutes of the quality assurance committee, risk management committee, or safety committee; or it may be found in hospitalwide, departmental, or medical staff quality assurance or risk management reports to the governing body.[2]

□ The Board's Knowledge of Risk Management

Notwithstanding the Joint Commission requirements, the board cannot effectively discharge its oversight role in risk management until it knows what its role is and what the purposes, functions, and activities of risk management are.[3] Consequently, the risk manager and the hospital CEO must educate the board about risk management.

One of the basic risk management concepts that the board must be educated about is the difference between custodially related patient injury and iatrogenic (medically related) patient injury. *Custodially related patient injury* is an injury not specifically caused by medical intervention but rather by custodial or administrative action, inaction, or circumstance. Typical examples of custodially related patient injury include slips and falls in wet hallways, falls from bed, falls on the way to the bathroom, and falls within the bathroom. *Iatrogenic patient injury,* on the other hand, refers specifically to those injuries directly related to or caused by medical or professional health care provider action, inaction, or circumstance. Examples of iatrogenic patient injury include a bowel that is perforated during a colonoscopy, an operation performed on the wrong patient, removal of the wrong body part during surgery, an anaphylactic reaction to a prescribed drug or chemical agent, and postoperative infections.

It is important for the board to be familiar with the distinction between custodial and iatrogenic injuries in order to ensure that the resources of the risk management program are appropriately apportioned to focus on preventing each category of injury and on minimizing liability. Although iatrogenic injuries occur much less frequently than custodially related ones, they are generally much more severe and result in much greater liability dollar losses than custodially related injuries do. Consequently, the board may wish to direct that the risk management program devote more of its resources to preventing iatrogenic injury occurrence and liability than to preventing custodially related injury and liability.

In addition, the board must be familiar with the following:

* How risk management is defined and the scope of the hospital's risk management program
* What the role and the job of the risk manager are
* How the insurance and claims functions relate to the risk management program
* How the hospital's quality assurance program and medical staff credentialing function relate to the risk management program
* The data-gathering and risk identification techniques of the risk management program—whether they include incident reporting, occurrence reporting, generic screening, patient complaints, or other methods
* What the highest risk areas of patient injury and malpractice claims within the hospital are and how they compare with national data

- Insurance coverage and costs
- The hospital's claims history
- How the board can help prevent patient injury and malpractice liability and reduce overall liability exposure through effectively discharging its risk management oversight role

These concepts can be communicated to the board through a risk management orientation program conducted by the risk manager, the hospital CEO, the hospital attorney, or the medical staff director or by the regular risk management reports. The risk manager must recognize that failing to educate the board may mean that the board will be unable to oversee the risk management program effectively, may be unreceptive and unresponsive to the risk management reports, and may be unwilling to provide support to the risk manager.

☐ Risk Management Reports to the Board: Content and Format

To be meaningful to the board, the risk management reports should be brief and understandable and should either enhance the board's understanding of an issue or facilitate the board's taking action. The reports should present summary information in a graphic format that compares data over time. For example, a graph of incident report trends by area for the past quarter compared with those trends over the past several years would enable the board to determine whether progress was being made in increasing incident reporting in areas likely to generate medically related patient injury.

To be most effective, the risk management reports should not present too much information and should vary the content presented. For example, one report could present claims information; the next, incident report graphs; the next, insurance information; the next, patient complaint trends. Brief, graphic, and varied reports will best educate the board about the purposes of risk management.

The risk management reports to the board should, at various times, present the following information:

- Analyses of trends identified through incident reports and occurrence screens
- Summary and status of open malpractice claims
- Analyses of trends identified through patient complaints
- An example of the risk management incident investigation and problem resolution process
- Open and closed claims trends and costs of claims
- Actual losses
- Losses by area and physician distribution
- Results of insurance audits, insurance coverages, and costs
- Incident reports compared with claims compared with losses
- Staff turnover trends and patterns of staff complaints

☐ Directors' and Officers' Liability Prevention

Hospital boards increasingly are exposed to directors' and officers' (D & O) liability as D & O insurance becomes more restrictive and expensive. Risk managers can assist their boards in developing a board risk management program to minimize the hospital's and the individual trustee's exposure to liability. In so doing, the board will recognize the importance of risk management and come to regard the risk manager as a valuable resource. This will facilitate effective two-way communication between the board and the risk manager as well as effective board oversight of the hospital risk management program.

A board risk management program starts with the following three-step risk analysis and reduction process:[4]

1. Determination of potential areas of board liability exposure
2. Assessment of the degree of liability exposure in such areas
3. Implementation of corrective action to minimize liability exposure in high-risk areas or activities

Determination of Potential Liability Exposure

To determine potential areas of board liability exposure, the risk manager should first list all D & O insurance policy coverage limitations and exclusions. Next, the risk manager should research the most common types of D & O lawsuits brought against hospitals. Finally, the risk manager should list all current and planned activities that have significant implications for the hospital, its medical staff, its employees, the community, or other area hospitals.

Most insurers have identified the areas of greatest risk of loss and exclude them from coverage or restrict coverage. Common D & O policy coverage limitations and exclusions are as follows:

- Discrimination in employment
- Medical staff appointment and reappointment, including restriction or revocation of staff medical privileges
- Failure to maintain adequate general/professional liability insurance for the hospital
- Hospital pollution, hazardous waste, nuclear perils, and any illegal board activities

Most institutions indemnify their directors and officers through an indemnification provision in the hospital bylaws. An indemnification provision ensures that hospital board members will be compensated by the hospital for losses that trustees are legally obligated to pay and that are related to their being hospital trustees or directors. Indemnification may be used to reimburse a trustee for losses not covered by insurance, or it may be used instead of D & O liability coverage. Governing boards that rely solely on indemnification provisions may be placing their hospitals and themselves at financial risk if the hospital does not have the available funds to cover a large settlement or award. If the hospital cannot pay, the governing board members may be personally liable for the balance. Moreover, most indemnification provisions contain limitations or exclusions of indemnity that may be significant. Those items should also be added to the list of potential areas of board liability exposure.[5]

Another way to determine potential areas of board liability exposure is to list all recent and planned board decisions, noting their implications for any significant groups related to the hospital. As hospitals pursue nontraditional business and marketing strategies, mismanagement allegations against hospital governing boards may increase. Such allegations also are likely to follow from hospital governing board decisions involving closing of facilities, mergers, sales to other organizations, financial failures, elimination of medical staffs, and corporate restructuring.

Assessment of the Degree of Liability Exposure

Once the greatest potential areas of board liability exposure have been identified, the next step is to assess as accurately as possible the degree of the board's liability exposure in each area. This assessment is the most critical step of the risk analysis/reduction process. By honestly assessing each area of potential liability exposure, the board will clarify the most effective means of eliminating or reducing that exposure. This step may be lengthy because it involves a critical review of past and pending board actions for each potential risk area.

For example, a board and a risk manager would review the process the board employs for credentialing and privileging of medical staff applicants and members to confirm that it is based on objective, reasonable, nonarbitrary, and noncapricious criteria and that it is applied equally to all medical staff applicants and members.

Most hospital boards include local businesspeople among their members. Conflicts of interest can arise when the board approves contracts or arrangements with local businesses that are represented on the board. Frequently, local attorneys, insurance agents, or construction contractors who serve as board members may have an interest that conflicts with the hospital's interest. The board should have an approved conflict-of-interest policy that is liberal enough to recognize that such conflicts will exist. At a minimum, board members must be required to disclose potential conflicts of interest and abstain from voting on any issue where there may be a perception that the board member is putting personal interest ahead of the best interests of the hospital. The policy should be reviewed annually, and board members should be given the opportunity to disclose any personal interest that has the potential to conflict with the hospital's best interest. Board members' statements of potential conflicts of interest should be kept on file.

Implementation of Corrective Action

The last step in the risk analysis/reduction process is taking corrective action based on the results of the liability assessment. The board may be advised to revise board policies, procedures, and certain decision-making processes to minimize future liability exposure.

☐ Conclusion

Preventing liability, rather than minimizing it once it occurs, requires an effective governing-board risk management program. Without adequate D & O insurance protection, most board members believe governing-board risk management is a necessity. In today's volatile D & O insurance market, however, governing-board risk management is necessary regardless of a board's insurance coverage. Governing-board risk management will lessen liability exposure, reduce the risk of lawsuit, and diminish the impact of future D & O insurance crises and further narrowing of coverage parameters. Governing board risk management helps to improve the functioning of a board and enables it to protect itself and its hospital. It also heightens the awareness and interest of the board in the hospital risk management program, which facilitates improved communication between the risk manager and the board and improves the board's oversight of the hospital risk management program.

References

1. Joint Commission on Accreditation of Healthcare Organizations. *Accreditation Manual for Hospitals.* Chicago: JCAHO, 1989.

2. Joint Commission on Accreditation of Healthcare Organizations. *Drafting Scoring Guidelines for Hospital Risk Management Activities.* Chicago: JCAHO, Dec. 1988.

3. Veach, M. Minimizing the hospital's risk of liability exposure: the trustee's role. *Trustee* 40(6):16–18, June 1987.

4. Orlikoff, J. E., and Vanagunas, A. M. *Malpractice Prevention and Liability Control for Hospitals.* 2nd ed. Chicago: American Hospital Publishing, 1988.

5. Orlikoff, J. E. Current issues in hospital directors' and officers' liability insurance. Briefing paper for hospital governing boards. American Hospital Association, Dec. 1985.

Chapter 6

The Medical Staff

Jonathan T. Lord

Virtually every facet of health care risk management depends on interaction with medical staff. Although risk management has been an integral element of physician decision making, perhaps one of the most frustrating relationships for the risk manager has been the interface with the medical staff, both individually and organizationally. It is important for the new risk manager to understand the focal role that physicians and other medical staff members play in health care decision making: they make decisions related to the level of care required (hospital admission, intensive care unit therapy, or outpatient management), therapeutic regimen or diagnostic workup, and continued care and discharge of the patient. Every decision requires judgment based on education, training, experience, and current competence. Those decisions must be communicated to others—sometimes in the form of instructions to nursing and support staff, sometimes to other physicians for consultation and continued care of the patient, and sometimes to the patient, family, and others so that they can understand the reasons for treatment and prognosis. Risk management issues are woven into every one of those activities. This chapter explores the role of the medical staff in risk management strategies, ways for the new risk manager to optimize relationships with the medical staff, and techniques for reducing loss in the most common and highest-risk areas of the health care organization.

☐ Role of the Individual Physician

As individuals, physicians are involved in risk management activities on an ongoing basis. The three crucial activities in this area are patient relations, documentation, and staff relations.

Patient Relations

At the heart of the individual physician's role is his or her relationship with the patient. The development of rapport with the patient based on clear discussion of diagnosis, treatment, and potential risks and outcomes is the most effective risk-reducing strategy.

Physicians face several obstacles in this area: time, communication techniques, and, on occasion, their own lack of sensitivity to the importance of the information that they communicate to their patients.

In the rapidly changing environment of modern medicine, the amount of time that physicians are able to spend with patients is decreasing. When this decrease is added to a greater tendency to discontinuity in care, particularly in managed care settings, physicians' potential to develop rapport with patients is diminished. This lack of relationship is frustrating to both parties; patients are already overwhelmed with the complexity and sophistication of modern medicine, and physicians are overly concerned with the potentially litigious posture of their patients. The lack of dialogue tends to reinforce and polarize these positions.

When physicians do discuss issues with their patients, all too often the dialogue is one-sided, hidden in technical jargon, or, at the opposite extreme, condescending. Patients today tend to be enlightened consumers who are aware of many medical issues and have many sophisticated questions that should be answered. Also, physicians' continuous exposure to serious illness has a tendency to make them less sensitive to patients' concerns about less severe disease and routine procedures. However, to patients, everything that affects them is important and significant. The risk manager can work with individual physicians whose patient-communication skills are poor by helping them to understand how patients view their illnesses and the fears and discomforts of treatment.

Documentation

Parallel to good communication is good documentation, in both hospital and office records, of communication with the patient and of the care provided. The documentation in the medical record is primary evidence in litigating or settling claims of a bad outcome. Documentation should include appropriately complete history and physical examinations; frequent progress notes; preprocedure, procedure, and postprocedure notes; discharge notes with outlines for follow-up care; and thorough narrative summaries. Not only are these notes important for good communication among those caring for the patient, but a well-documented chart is easier for risk managers or the defense counsel to use in assessing the strength of their case in the event of a claim.

Noteworthy items for the risk manager to look for in documentation are informed consent and supervision of trainees. Informed consent is more than the witnessed signature on a form; it is the discussion between physician and patient and the patient's voluntary consent based on the information given by the physician. A progress note documenting the discussion of the procedure with the patient should be placed in the record in addition to the signed form. The discussion should include the indications for the procedure, the potential complications and risks, alternate approaches and their associated risks, the risk of not having treatment, and a summary of dialogue with the patient, including the patient's key questions and the physician's responses to them.

Because recent malpractice cases have focused on the supervision of resident physicians, the attending staff physician should document active involvement in the care of patients who are being seen by trainees. The medical staff should establish parameters for the frequency of the attending physician's notes. Many institutions have used the following as guidelines for staff notes:

- Review and justification of admission (within 24 hours)
- Formulation of diagnostic workup or therapeutic plan
- Significant changes in the patient's condition
- Major therapeutic interventions
- Modification of diagnostic workup or therapeutic plan
- Discharge of the patient

Besides communicating those guidelines, the risk manager should discuss with physicians the need for clear, concise, legible, and timely documentation throughout the record. Ideally, all record entries should be dated and timed. Records should not contain pejorative statements about the care provided by nursing or support services, nor should they contain pejorative comments about colleagues who may be providing care to the patient.

Staff Relations

The risk manager also needs to be concerned about the relationships between individual physicians and other members of the health care team. Although many physicians have looked upon themselves as the center of the "universe" of care, in today's complex health care environment, the physician's effectiveness depends on good communication and relations with all care providers. Of incalculable importance is ongoing and open dialogue with nurses involved in the care of the patient. A few minutes' discussion between the nurse and physician at key points during the patient's hospital stay can have the following benefits:

- Assist the nurse in recognizing important changes in the patient's condition (failure to notify the physician of such changes is a frequent malpractice claim against nurses and the hospital)
- Assist the nurse in implementing the physician's plan of care for the patient
- Alert the nurse to timing for diagnostic testing
- Enhance the nurse's ability to establish a dialogue with the patient about care and treatment

Communication between the physician and other "team players," including social workers who ensure timely and appropriate discharges, clinical support staff who provide therapies ordered by the physician, and colleagues who provide support, enhances both the efficiency and the effectiveness of the physician's patient care.

When effectively carried out by individual physicians, these three major activities— patient relations, documentation, and staff relations—are the building blocks of good medical staff risk management. They must be joined with a vigilance and sensitivity to all aspects of the care provided to patients. As Stanley Skillicorn, M.D., said, "The majority of adverse events that occur in hospitals have nothing to do with a lack of knowledge or with a failure to keep abreast of clinical and technological breakthroughs. The bad things that happen in patient care usually result from very ordinary mistakes or oversights, from assumptions that someone else has performed critical duties, from distraction and disruptions, and from a dangerous casualness that tends to accompany repetitive routines."[1]

☐ Role of the Organized Medical Staff

Risk management, quality assurance, credentials review and privileging, and peer review activities, all of which are carried out by the medical staff organization, are key elements in the Joint Commission on Accreditation of Healthcare Organizations' medical staff standards.[2]

The medical staff's bylaws establish the medical staff roles in those functions. The bylaws should describe the following areas pertinent to risk management:

- Credentials review and privileging
- Integrated quality assurance/risk management responsibilities of the medical staff
- Requirements for documentation in medical records (described earlier)
- Policies for the supervision of trainees

Credentialing and Privileging Functions

The credentials review for medical staff membership determines that physicians and other health care practitioners have the necessary qualifications and training and are currently competent. *Credentials* refer to the qualifications that the health care practitioner brings to the hospital; *privileges* refer to the delineated, individually tailored scope of care that an individual may provide based on his or her qualifications, current competence, and the level of support that the facility can provide.

From a risk manager's point of view, the key to effective clinical privileging is current competence. The medical staff bylaws should describe the requirements for application to the medical staff and should explicitly place the burden of providing the required information on the applicant. To ensure that applicants are currently competent, the medical staff should require that letters of recommendation include documentation of performance. All too often, such letters contain only generalities, such as: "Dr. Jones has been a member of our staff for 10 years. He has been a dynamic member of our quality assurance committee, and I'm sure that he will be an asset to your hospital." Rather than relying on useless information, the medical staff should elicit peer and supervisor recommendations that include at least the following:

- Descriptions of scope of practice
- Trends of performance based on results of peer review and quality assurance activities
- Medical staff "citizenship"
- Ethical conduct

As an integral part of this process, all education, training, certifications, and professional licenses from all states should be verified with the granting institution (primary source) or an agency that uses primary sources. ("Certified to be a true copy" stamped on a diploma does not constitute verification.) In accordance with both good practice and the current Joint Commission risk management standards,[3] there should be inquiries into the applicant's involvement in professional liability actions, challenges to and voluntary relinquishment of any licensure or certification, voluntary or involuntary termination of medical staff membership, and voluntary or involuntary limitation, reduction, or loss of clinical privileges at another hospital or health care organization. With the establishment of the National Practitioner Data Bank as a part of the Health Care Quality Improvement Act of 1986, appropriate inquiries should be made at the times of initial appointment and subsequent reappointment.

Once the medical staff and the hospital governing board are convinced that an applicant is qualified, the applicant should be offered a provisional appointment to the medical staff, and clinical privileges should be delineated. Privileges delineation generally is based on preestablished, clinically valid, objective criteria established by the clinical department chairman. Those criteria should be consistently and uniformly applied to all medical staff members, new and existing. The initial phase of appointment to the medical staff should provide for staff surveillance of a new physician appointee; the level of surveillance should be tailored to the type and complexity of the appointee's practice. Such observation ensures that the medical staff has an adequate opportunity to evaluate the appointee's "hands-on" clinical competence. The structure of the period for provisional appointment should be determined in advance, should be objective, and should be uniformly applied to all new members in the same discipline. Many medical staffs have adopted volume-related requirements during the period of provisional appointment. For example, a surgeon may be required to handle 25 major abdominal cases during a probationary period in order for the staff to evaluate current competency and consider a move from provisional to active status.

Surveillance of performance continues throughout the appointment to the medical staff. Reappointment formally takes place every two years at most hospitals; however, evaluation of performance should be an ongoing practice. In order to effectively and consistently monitor performance as well as comply with Joint Commission and other regulatory agency requirements that results of quality assurance activities be considered for reappointment, many hospitals maintain practitioner profiles. These profiles provide a comprehensive and objective look at individual performance. Figure 6-1 is an example of a physician profile that is updated at six-month intervals and is reviewed by both the clinical department chairman and the practitioner.

In addition to examining performance at the time of reappointment, inquiries should be made into the physician's involvement in professional liability actions, challenges to and voluntary relinquishment of any licensure or registration, voluntary or involuntary termination of medical staff membership, and voluntary or involuntary reduction, limitation, or loss of clinical privileges at another hospital. Appropriate inquiries should also be made with the National Practitioner Data Bank.

From the standpoint of reducing risk to the medical staff and the hospital through challenges to the credentials review and privileging process, the keys to success are:

- Defining the process in writing (bylaws)
- Developing objective, clinically valid criteria for privilege delineation
- Uniformly and consistently applying policies and procedures

Evaluation of Allied Health Professionals

Most hospitals use the same credentials review and privileging mechanism to evaluate the qualifications and current competence of nonphysician practitioners who may be allowed to provide independent care (for example, podiatrists and psychologists) as well as allied health professionals such as physician's assistants, nurse practitioners, and nurse midwives. The process for application, review, and approval for all practitioners and allied health professionals is identical to that used for the medical staff. The degree of independence of practitioners in allied health categories will vary based on state laws and hospital policies and procedures. Request forms for special privileges for allied health professionals should list what they may do in the hospital and specify the responsible supervisory staff.

Integrated Quality Assurance and Risk Management Functions

The medical staff organization is created by the governing body and is accountable for the quality of medical care that the hospital provides. This requirement translates into the need for formal quality assurance and peer review programs, inherent in which are risk management activities—risk identification, risk assessment, and risk prevention.

In late 1987, the Joint Commission developed the following 10-step model for monitoring and evaluating the quality and appropriateness of care throughout the institution:[4]

1. Assign responsibility for evaluation
2. Define scope of care/service
3. Identify important aspects of care
4. Establish clinical indicators
5. Establish thresholds for evaluation
6. Collect and analyze data
7. Evaluate care
8. Implement corrective action
9. Evaluate corrective action for improvement in care
10. Integrate results

On the basis of the Joint Commission standards, the medical staff's defined role in evaluating and monitoring activities includes the following:[5]

65

Figure 6-1. Integrated Quality Assessment Practitioner Activity Profile

		Year 1
		Jan-Jun. Jul-Dec.

Volume Data		No. Admissions _____
		_____
Occurrence Screens	Category 1	_____
	Category 2	_____
	Category 3	_____
	Category 4	_____
Specialty-specific	Category 1	_____
Screens	Category 2	_____
	Category 3	_____
	Category 4	_____
Surgical Case Review		No. Deficiencies/No. Cases _____
Blood Usage Review		No. Deficiencies/No. Transfusions _____
Drug Usage Evaluation		No. Deficiencies _____
Prescription Review		No. Deficiencies _____
Medical Records		
	Deliquencies	_____
	Deficiencies	No. Deficiencies/No. Reviewed _____
DRG Violations		_____
PRO Reviews		No. Denials/No. Reviews _____
Focused Review	Category 1	_____
	Category 2	_____
	Category 3	_____
	Category 4	_____
Patient Complaints		No. Validated complaints/Total No. _____
Incident Reports		No. Validated incidents involving practice/Total No. _____
Liability Claims		_____
Safety Issues		_____
Attendance at		
	Required Meetings	_____
	Department Meetings	_____
	Committee Meetings	_____
Continuing Education		No. Hours _____
Morbidity Review		_____
Mortality Review		_____
Utilization Review		_____
Medical Care Evaluation		_____

Source: Reprinted, with permission, from Daniel R. Longo, Kathleen R. Ciccone, and Jonathan T. Lord, *Integrated Quality Assessment: A Model for Concurrent Review* (Chicago: American Hospital Publishing, 1989), p. 188.

- Medical staff monitoring functions
  - Department review
  - Surgical case review
  - Blood usage review
  - Drug usage evaluation
  - Pharmacy and therapeutics
  - Medical record review
- Participation in hospitalwide activities
  - Utilization review
  - Infection control
  - Safety
  - Risk management

All the aforementioned functions have risk management elements that are intimately related to the practices of physicians and other health care practitioners. At the heart of the quality assessment process is the department's review of the quality and appropriateness of care and the peer review necessary to accomplish it. The medical staff must identify important aspects of care, define clinical indicators to measure that care, actively participate in peer review activities, take corrective action within the medical staff organization, and use the results of peer review at the time of reappointment to the medical staff. For clinical departments to carry out those activities effectively, the hospital must provide for staff support in the form of the timely identification of nonroutine events to be reviewed and evaluated by physicians, the collection and display of patient data according to clinical indicators, and communication with the medical staff.

Many hospitals have developed mechanisms for the concurrent review of patient care, allowing for the early identification of high-risk occurrences and permitting the prompt implementation of corrective action to improve patient outcome. In implementing the Joint Commission's 10-step model, hospitals have used risk-sensitive clinical indicators or occurrence screens that are collected concurrently for all hospitalized patients at fixed intervals throughout their stay.

Physicians traditionally have resisted peer review of their cases because of the punitive connotation of having a case "pulled for review." My own experience has shown that in 85 percent of cases identified in a highly structured, mechanical occurrence-screening program, care was found to be both appropriate and of high quality.[6] It is important that the risk manager or quality assurance director emphasize to physicians that peer review results are not always negative and that mechanisms to provide feedback on positive results are developed. In order to add structure and trending mechanisms to the peer review process, some hospitals have developed a formalized process to categorize the results of peer review. Such a process can help eliminate the medical staff's reluctance to engage in peer review while providing an objective and uniform basis for evaluating care.

An example of one such mechanism appears in figure 6-2. Integral to an effective risk management program is the medical staff's participation in the review of nonroutine patient occurrences. Incident reports often are used as an occurrence-screening mechanism. Incident reports related to patient care events may be required by state law or by insurance carriers; however, the same caliber of information can be gathered with enhanced protection from discoverability through the occurrence-screening process. The medical staff should review all medical incidents involving untoward patient outcomes or injuries. Results of significant cases should be presented at medical staff meetings and trended to individuals, departments, or services. Cases involving physicians and having significant potential for becoming a lawsuit should also receive special attention from the medical staff. Often, those cases are reviewed as a part of normal quality assurance mechanisms. Regardless of the means of identification, information that can be used to educate and to preclude recurrence should be disseminated to the appropriate staff members after patient and physician identifiers have been removed.

Figure 6-2. Formal Categorization of Peer Review Findings

- *Not practitioner-related:* These events are causally related to factors intrinsic to the patient (for example, underlying disease, biologic/anatomic variation, hypersensitivity reaction in the absence of allergic history), to institutional support (for example, delay in turnaround time for lab/X-ray studies, unavailability of CT/MRI scans), or to care provided outside the hospital. Trending data from this category would not enhance or identify opportunities to improve practitioner-specific performance but may demonstrate trends useful for departmental or hospitalwide management.
- *Practitioner-related:* The four subcategories listed below should include events that either individually or in aggregate are related to specific health care practitioners. Data derived from these categories will allow department chairpersons and practitioners to identify opportunities to enhance their practice in terms of quality, effectiveness, or efficiency.
  — *Category I. Predictable event within the standard of care:* "Predictable" means that these events are anticipated, well known, widely reported in the literature, and relatively frequent. "Within the standard of care" means that care was provided in accordance with contemporary standards of the specialty and departmental staff.
  — *Category II. Unpredictable event within the standard of care:* "Unpredictable" means that events in this category are infrequent and unanticipated but have been described in the literature (or known by departmental medical staff) to occur in cases where the standard of care is met. *Note:* Category II does not represent an escalation in seriousness over Category I; they are both within accepted standards of care.)
  — *Category III. Marginal deviation from the standard of care:* "Marginal" events in this category reflect care that is minimally outside of the contemporary standards of the specialty or the expected standards of the department staff.
  — *Category IV. Significant deviation from the standard of care:* Events in this category usually speak for themselves. These events represent gross departures from expected standards.

Source: Reprinted, with permission, from Daniel R. Longo, Kathleen R. Ciccone, and Jonathan T. Lord, *Integrated Quality Assessment: A Model for Concurrent Review* (Chicago: American Hospital Publishing, 1989), p. 60.

The Joint Commission standards require that all quality assurance (QA) and risk management activities be discussed at medical staff meetings and documented in minutes of those meetings. The standards provide for flexibility based on the complexity of services rendered, size and composition of the medical staff, and other local considerations. However, they also require the following frequencies for meetings:

- Executive committee of the medical staff (monthly)
- Clinical department meetings (monthly)
- Surgical case review (monthly)
- Blood usage review (quarterly)
- Drug usage evaluation (quarterly)
- Pharmacy and therapeutics review (quarterly)
- Medical record review (quarterly)

The minutes of these meetings should document substantive discussion of QA activities and should include conclusions, recommendations, actions, and follow-up. Risk management activities should be discussed, and attendance by the risk manager is encouraged.

Of particular concern to physicians about quality assurance and peer review are the discoverability of peer review information and, recently, the danger of being sued for violating federal and state antitrust statutes. Most state statutes provide some level of protection for good-faith peer review activities. It is ironic that although many medical staff members use the discoverability of peer review documents as a reason not to do peer review, physicians' casual disclosure of information is the greatest single source of release of information. This is readily apparent in hospital elevators, cafeterias, and hallways. One of the risk manager's major roles in encouraging effective medical staff peer review is to educate physicians on how to protect the confidentiality of information by taking advantage of statutory protection and to caution them about the dangers of gossiping about patients and peers.

Supervision of Trainees

Supervision of trainees is an important issue because it is a frequent theme in lawsuits involving teaching hospitals. Recently, the New York State Department of Health established far-reaching regulations for limiting the working hours of trainees and establishing a process that parallels clinical privileging.[7] Effective July 1989, trainees in most specialties are not allowed to work more than 24 scheduled, continuous hours in regular duty nor more than 12 hours in an emergency room that sees more than 15,000 patients annually. New York teaching hospitals are also required to define the scope of activities and the level of supervision required for each trainee, factors dependent on individual competencies.

No matter what state the hospital is located in, the medical staff, working with the administration and the governing body, should establish policies and procedures for the adequate supervision of trainees. Included in those policies should be the following:

- Procedures for admission and discharge, including the level of staff involvement
- Procedures and requirements for documentation in the medical record
- Minimal required levels of supervision for major procedures
- Policies on work schedules
- Mechanisms for selecting, reviewing and evaluating, and terminating trainees
- Mechanisms to ensure that patient care is always accountable to a staff physician and that the patient is aware of who that physician is

When reviewing the quality and appropriateness of care, as well as when reviewing medical records for clinical pertinence, medical staffs at teaching hospitals should focus on supervision of trainees to reduce the predictable exposure related to the lack of adequate supervision.

☐ Strategies for the Risk Manager

To win the confidence of the medical staff, the risk manager must demonstrate knowledge and competence. The risk manager should focus on developing goal congruence—that is, the goals of the hospital's risk management function should be aligned with the medical staff's risk management needs. Besides becoming familiar with the concerns of the medical staff, the risk manager must educate the medical staff about the risk management requirements of both the medical staff and the hospital. It is essential that dialogue begin through both formal and informal mechanisms shortly after the new risk manager assumes his or her position. For example, the risk manager could do the following:

- Develop a five-minute introduction for presentation at a medical staff meeting. The introduction should focus on the role of the risk manager, how the risk manager can assist the medical staff, and how effective risk management can benefit the medical staff.
- Arrange for time on the agendas of meetings of the medical staff executive committee, major clinical departments, key committees, joint conference committees, or boards.
- Schedule one-on-one meetings with the president or chief of the medical staff and with the chairman of each major high-risk department.

- Walk through the hospital frequently and at different times of the day, engaging physicians, nurses, medical assistants, clerical staff, and administrators in informal conversation.
- Be available by keeping flexible or unusual hours to accommodate the complex, highly structured schedules of the medical staff.
- Speak with confidence. Medical staff members are professionals who will respond and listen to others who present themselves as professionals.
- Listen carefully in order to elicit the primary concerns of *all* members of the medical staff.
- Be responsive and keep commitments by establishing realistic time frames.
- Develop a strategic plan for risk management with involvement of the medical staff, the nursing staff, the hospital administration, and the governing board. The plan should be based on a common vision of the goals of the program, with short-term, mid-term, and long-term objectives clearly identified. Issues that should be addressed include program structure, communication, responsibilities, education, and ongoing assessment of the program's effectiveness.
- Educate. The medical staff's educational needs will encompass a wide range of topics, including the requirements of health care regulators, feedback from the hospital's liability carrier, lessons learned from occurrences and claims, summaries of medicolegal court decisions, and changes in hospital policies.
- Remain flexible. The risk manager should be able to develop innovative ideas for fitting the hospital's risk management goals into a series of different organizational and personal agendas.
- Remain patient. How quickly the risk manager accomplishes his or her goals depends on the "horsepower" of that position within the organization, the level of support from the CEO, the board, and the medical staff, the relative "external pressure" on the risk management program, and the traits that the risk manager brings to the position.

Risk Management and Quality Assurance in the Emergency Room

The emergency room is the primary route of entry for hospital admission, and an emergency admission often is the first time a patient has ever encountered a hospital. It is imperative that the emergency room reception area and reception/triage staff convey an image of caring because that will be the image that the patient retains throughout his or her hospital stay. Because most patients seen in the emergency room usually have to wait their turn for treatment, the risk manager should work with emergency room staff to ensure that patients who are waiting are checked frequently, that their vital signs are monitored, and that they are reassured. When working with the emergency room medical staff, the risk manager should take time to discuss the importance of good patient relations and precise, comprehensive, and timely documentation. Good risk management is particularly important in the emergency room setting because the patient and the practitioner do not have an ongoing relationship.

To monitor and improve quality and lessen the likelihood of claims, the medical and nursing staffs of the emergency room need to develop a series of indicators that would alert them, as well as the risk manager, to any important occurrence. Such indicators may include the following:

- Any unexpected, unplanned return of a patient who was seen in the emergency room in the past 48 hours
- Any discordance in the interpretation of diagnostic tests or X rays between the emergency room staff and the pathologist or radiologist
- Any failure to follow up promptly on an abnormal test result
- Any resuscitative effort in the emergency room

- Any death in the emergency room
- Any patient leaving against medical advice
- Any patient complaint

As noted earlier, the specialty societies have developed a number of additional screens that may be useful. The relationship between the hospital and the emergency room staff has become a concern, particularly in hospitals with contracted emergency room services. Continuity of practitioners and nursing staff is important for the appropriate flow of patients and utilization of support services and hospital consultants.

Risk Management and Quality Assurance in Anesthesia

Risks associated with the practice of anesthesia are unique because patients generally have no choice or even knowledge of their anesthesiologist. In addition, anesthesia is an inherently high-risk area, and although untoward outcomes are rare, they result in severe impairment or death. Other concerns for the risk manager are that one anesthesiologist may supervise a number of anesthetized patients simultaneously and that an increasing number of procedures are being performed on an ambulatory basis. The Joint Commission has focused special attention on anesthesia because of this variety of factors. As a part of the Joint Commission Agenda for Change, a task force was established that developed the following risk-sensitive clinical indicators:

- Mortality within a specified time following anesthesia care
- Failure to emerge from general anesthesia within a specified time
- Development of injury to the brain or spinal cord within a specified time following anesthesia care
- Development of a peripheral neurologic deficit within a specified time following anesthesia care
- Cardiac arrest within a specified time following anesthesia care
- Clinically apparent acute myocardial infarction within a specified time following anesthesia care
- Fulminant pulmonary edema within a specified time following anesthesia care
- Respiratory arrest within a specified time following anesthesia care
- Aspiration of gastric contents with development of typical X-ray findings of aspiration pneumonitis within a specified time of anesthesia care
- Development of postdural puncture headache within a specified time following anesthesia care
- Dental injury during anesthesia care
- Ocular injury during anesthesia care
- Unplanned hospital admission within a specified time following an outpatient procedure involving anesthesia
- Unplanned admission to an intensive care unit within a specified time following administration of anesthetic

Analysis of data derived from the use of these risk-sensitive indicators would require stratification by covariants such as age, sex, weight, and type of procedure (including emergency status), as well as type and duration of procedure. The risk manager will note that anesthetic records are considerably different from other hospital records. They normally include graphs, large volumes of data, and very limited areas for narrative documentation.

It is not uncommon for anesthetic records to be marginally legible or incomprehensible. The risk manager should work with the medical records staff and the chairman of the anesthesiology department to develop policies, procedures, and forms that provide for clear documentation of anesthesia care. In addition to records of care, other important documentation related to anesthesia includes records of preanesthesia and post-anesthesia evaluation.

Since the mid-1980s, a considerable volume of surgical work load has shifted to the ambulatory care setting. This shift has affected anesthesiology practice, particularly as it relates to the physician's "control" of the patient. Patients no longer are readily available the night before surgery for preanesthesia evaluation and counseling and, instead of staying "in-house" for postanesthesia monitoring, patients are discharged from the recovery room to home. The risk manager should work with the staff of the ambulatory surgical facility, the anesthesia staff, and the nursing staff to ensure comparable levels of preand postanesthesia evaluation, policies and procedures for release of patients, and methodologies to document postanesthesia instructions to patients.

Another issue in the ambulatory setting is the administration of anesthetic by physicians who are not anesthesiologists, particularly for procedures such as endoscopy, bronchoscopy, and other invasive diagnostic procedures. If nonanesthesiologists are administering anesthetic in these areas, the risk manager should work with the professional staffs of the involved departments and the anesthesia staff to develop policies and procedures for pre- and postanesthesia evaluation, monitoring of patients during anesthesia, and clinical indicators to monitor and evaluate the quality and appropriateness of anesthesia.

Risk Management and Quality Assurance in Obstetrics

The risk management focus in the labor and delivery room should be on building a team approach among all care givers in the labor and delivery area and on building the patient's knowledge of and confidence in the team members. The risk manager can work with the obstetricians in the community to suggest techniques to strengthen their relationships with patients, such as the full disclosure of who will actually perform the delivery of the baby, introductions to group practice members who may cover for the patient's physician at delivery, coordination of patient education activities between the group and the hospital during prenatal care (such as Lamaze classes, tours of the labor area, films about vaginal deliveries and cesarean sections, and anesthetic choices), and integrated postdelivery education (surgical wound care, parenting, and choices for feeding babies). Ideally, there should be a close working relationship between the medical staff and the nursing staff in the labor and delivery area. The risk manager can help foster this strong relationship by encouraging frequent interdisciplinary meetings and educational sessions.

Medical record documentation in obstetrics also should be a risk management concern. "Routine" obstetrics patients may be admitted to the hospital on an abbreviated medical record form; frequently the level of documentation and the legibility of these "short forms" is of poorer quality than those of other records. Other records unique to obstetrics that require special mention are fetal monitoring recordings and records of deliveries. All fetal monitoring strips should be maintained along with "real time" entries (casual notes placed on strips) made by medical and nursing staff monitoring the patient. As in the case of anesthetic records, records of delivery have a jargon of their own and in general have a tendency to be short on space and marginally legible. The risk manager should work with the obstetrics staff, the labor and delivery nursing staff, and the medical records department to establish guidelines and forms to ensure the best possible documentation.

Obstetrics is a place where quality assurance and risk management functions can be brought together. The Joint Commission has convened a task force to develop clinical indicators in obstetrics, and the American College of Obstetricians and Gynecologists has been very active in it. On the basis of initial work by the Joint Commission task force, the following risk-sensitive clinical indicators (occurrence screens) may be used to support both quality assurance and risk management:

- Induction of labor for indications other than diabetes, premature rupture of membranes, pregnancy-induced hypertension, intrauterine growth retardation, cardiac disease, isoimmunization, fetal demise, or chorioamniotis
- Primary cesarean section for failure to progress
- Successful or failed vaginal birth after cesarean section
- Delivery of an infant weighing less than 2,500 grams, or with hyaline membrane disease, by planned repeat cesarean section
- Delivery of an infant weighing less than 2,500 grams, or with hyaline membrane disease, following induced labor
- Eclampsia
- In-hospital initiation of antibiotics 24 hours or more after term vaginal delivery
- Excessive maternal blood loss except with abruptio placenta or placenta previa as evidenced by a red cell transfusion, a hematocrit less than 22 or a hemoglobin less than 7, or a decrease in hematocrit of more than 11 or of hemoglobin more than 3.5
- Maternal length of stay of more than five days after vaginal delivery or seven days after cesarean section
- Maternal readmission within 14 days of delivery
- Maternal death up to 42 days postpartum
- In-hospital intrapartum death of a fetus weighing more than 500 grams
- Perinatal death of an infant weighing more than 500 grams
- Neonatal death of an infant with a birth weight of between 750 and 999 grams who was born in a hospital with a neonatal intensive care unit

A key issue in applying those indicators is the consistent evaluation of care regardless of the category or discipline of the practitioner. In order to meet the concept of "one level of care," the outcomes measured through this process need to be used by obstetricians, family practitioners, and nurse midwives performing deliveries at the hospital.

References

1. Skillicorn, H. *Risk Management*. Minneapolis: St. Paul's Insurance Company, 1984.

2. Joint Commission on Accreditation of Healthcare Organizations. *Accreditation Manual for Hospitals*. Chicago: JCAHO, 1989.

3. *Accreditation Manual for Hospitals*.

4. Joint Commission on Accreditation of Healthcare Organizations. *Perspectives*. Chicago: JCAHO, Jan. 1988.

5. *Accreditation Manual for Hospitals*.

6. Lord, J. T. Personal experience.

7. *New York State Code of Rules and Regulations*, Part 405.

Chapter 7

Nursing and Patient Care Staff

Paul A. Greve, Jr.

Nursing staff members are quite literally the eyes and ears of the risk management program. Because nurses are always present in patient care areas, they can be excellent sources of information on risk management problems. Their timely reporting of problems and injuries of patients will help the risk manager take action to minimize liability.

Nurses can also cause risk management problems, however. Deviation from appropriate nursing practice may result in liability for both nurses and employers. As the scope of nursing practice has expanded, nurses have become more visible and accountable for their actions. The risk manager must know the risks associated with the nursing function. The nursing staff, especially nursing administrators, must actively participate in the risk management program.

☐ Determination of Nursing Malpractice Liability

The American justice system is divided into *criminal law,* which exists for the protection of society, and *civil law,* which allows citizens to redress actual or perceived wrongful acts by others. A malpractice case is a matter of civil law. *Malpractice* means the negligence or carelessness of a member of a recognized profession. Nursing is a profession recognized by the courts and legislatures in most jurisdictions.

In order to recover damages from the nurse and/or the nurse's employer, the patient must prove that there was a deviation from accepted nursing practice that caused injury to the patient. The burden of proof in almost all malpractice actions lies with the patient. In a criminal case, the state must prove its case against the accused beyond a reasonable doubt. In civil cases, plaintiffs have a lesser burden. They must prove their case by only a preponderance of the evidence, which means that the judge or jury must conclude that the plaintiff's proof is at least slightly better than the defendant's.

The one rare exception to the requirement in malpractice lawsuits that the patient must bear the burden of proof is the legal doctrine of *res ipsa loquitur* (a Latin phrase meaning "the thing speaks for itself"). In malpractice lawsuits, the plaintiff may use that doctrine in situations in which there is no direct evidence as to how an injury occurred but the nature of the injury implies that it would not have occurred absent a negligent act. When courts permit use of the doctrine of *res ipsa loquitur*, the burden of proof shifts to the defendant. Courts have been reluctant to apply the doctrine except in cases where negligence is obvious. The retention of foreign objects such as sponges, instruments, and needles after surgical procedures is a common fact pattern in which the doctrine has been applied.

In a malpractice case against a nurse, the plaintiff must prove each of the following elements:

- A legal *duty* owed to the patient
- A *breach* of that duty (deviation from the nursing standard of care)
- *Damages* (injury)
- *Causation* (the injury was directly caused by the defendant nurse's breach)

Duty

Whether the nurse owes a legal duty to the patient depends on the existence of the nurse–patient relationship. This issue will be examined in each malpractice case to determine whether the nurse had sufficient control over the patient to owe the patient a duty of care. If such a relationship exists, the nurse's duty to the patient can be stated as follows: The nurse may not carelessly cause harm to the patient in carrying out patient care responsibilities. In most cases where patients have been admitted to an institutional setting, it is quite clear that the nurse is obligated to the patient to use care in performing assigned duties.

Breach of Duty

Whether the nurse breached the duty of care is the most frequently disputed element in malpractice cases. The test of whether the nurse adhered to the appropriate nursing standard of care is what a reasonable and prudent nurse would have done in the same or similar circumstances. Both plaintiff and defendant must determine what the applicable nursing standard of care is and whether the nurse in question adhered to that standard.

For example, a key issue in a case involving an IV infiltrate injury to surrounding tissue is what the nursing standard of care is for monitoring the appearance of the IV site. If a drug or fluid known to be caustic is being administered to the patient, the nursing standard of care will usually require the nurse to observe the appearance of the IV site more frequently than when a noncaustic drug or fluid is used.

Courts almost always require the use of expert witnesses to testify on behalf of the patient to establish what the standard of care is and that a breach of duty occurred. The defendant is also permitted to use expert witnesses to demonstrate to the jury that the nurse adhered to the nursing standard of care. The expert witness will be a nurse if the nursing standard of care is at issue.

Ultimately, the jury must weigh the evidence. In doing so, it may consider the credentials of the expert witnesses and the experts' credibility.

Damages

Patients may seek financial compensation, called "damages," for injuries sustained. In order for the patient to recover damages, there must be discernible injury of at least a temporary nature caused by the defendant's breach of duty. Historically, courts required proof of a physical injury before patients could recover damages. Today, patients in many jurisdictions can recover damages for nonphysical injuries, such as anxiety and emotional stress, caused by negligent or intentional conduct of the defendant nurse or physician. For example, if a nurse in a newborn nursery inadvertently discharges an infant to the wrong mother, even though the infant is safely returned to its natural mother, either or both mothers can recover money damages for the anxiety and emotional distress they suffered because of the nurse's carelessness.

Patients receive damages for emotional, physical, or financial injuries. In rare cases where a nurse's actions are reckless or grossly negligent, patients also can recover punitive damages, which are intended to punish the defendant for outrageous conduct. Such damages are awarded in addition to other compensable damages.

Causation

In order for the patient to recover damages, the patient must show that the injury was a direct result of the nurse's carelessness. The element of causation will almost always require a physician's expert testimony. Yet even with expert testimony, this element can be difficult for patients to prove because there may be many reasons for the injury besides the nurse's negligence. For example, the parents of an infant who dies only hours after birth may allege that the obstetrical nurse failed to respond to signs of fetal distress. If the autopsy shows that the infant had a chromosomal defect that is incompatible with survival, the cause of the child's death is the chromosomal defect, not the nurse's negligence. Therefore, because the element of causation is lacking, the parents of the child cannot recover damages.

☐ Employer's Liability for the Nurse

Under the law of agency, an employer is "vicariously liable" for the negligent acts of an employee. Vicarious liability, or *respondeat superior,* permits injured patients to sue the employer for damages based on the employer's actual control or right to control the activities of its employees. *Respondeat superior* means "let the master respond" for the negligent acts of the servant. The legal theory of the vicarious liability of the employer does not absolve the nurse of negligent conduct. Technically, the plaintiff has a right to seek damages from any defendant or from all defendants and thus can name the nurse as a party defendant in addition to the employer. In today's litigious climate, the plaintiff's attorney will attempt to sue as many parties as possible, and nurses are named more frequently now than ever before. The employer's responsibility is limited, however, to those acts performed within the scope of employment.

Employers generally are not liable for intentional acts committed by employees. If a nurse, for example, learns that a patient admitted to the unit is being treated for a sexually transmitted disease and subsequently divulges that information to neighbors of the patient at a party, the employer is not liable for breach of confidential patient information. The nurse is personally liable for that intentional act.

The risk manager must learn what the employer's policy on defense strategy is when employees are named as codefendants. Adding employees to lawsuits as codefendants or even seeking contributions to settlements from their personal insurance may cause employee-relations problems. The risk manager will want to be able to assure nursing staff and other employees involved in lawsuits as named defendants that the employer will support them if a lawsuit is filed. It will be the risk manager's job to coordinate defense of lawsuits with affected employees and to make sure that they are informed of all developments in the litigation.

☐ Nursing Standard of Care

In a malpractice lawsuit, the nursing standard of care usually will be the issue that receives more focus than any other because the plaintiff must prove that the nursing standard of care was not met. The legal system looks to the nursing profession to set its standard of care. The nursing standard of care is a yardstick by which the nurse's legal duty to the patient is measured. The standard of care is not static; as nursing practice evolves, the standard of care reflects the changes in practice. A nurse is held legally accountable for conforming to the standard of care that was in effect at the time of the alleged patient injury. For example, a lawsuit that is filed in 1990 alleging nursing malpractice arising out of an incident occurring in 1988 must focus on the standard of care that was in effect in 1988.

There are many ways to determine what the nursing standard of care is for a particular fact pattern. The risk manager must be familiar with all of them so that he or she can determine whether there is liability for actions of the nursing staff, whether he or she is involved in managing a claim or in assessing nursing practices to prevent incidents. The risk manager and nursing administrators need to work closely in reviewing the safety standards for new nursing functions. This assessment will involve determining what the nursing standard of care is and how to ensure conformity to it.

The nursing standard of care that is applicable is specific to the type of nursing unit. For example, nurses in an intensive care unit will be required to observe patients more frequently and take their vital signs more often than nurses on a general nursing floor. Therefore, if the nurse is functioning in a specialty setting, such as the operating room, emergency department, or labor and delivery room, the question of the applicable standard of care becomes what the reasonable and prudent nurse in the specialty area will be required to do in the same circumstances. If there are professional organizations that establish standards for specialty areas, such as Nurse's Association of the American College of Obstetrics and Gynecology (NAACOG) does for labor and delivery nurses, the risk manager must become familiar with those organizations and their standards. They will be cited by plaintiff's attorneys as establishing the nursing standard of care.

Policies and Procedures

The institution's administrative policies, and particularly its nursing policies and procedures, can be determinative of the standard of care. In many malpractice cases, these policies and procedures are crucial in analyzing liability because they are evidence of the nursing standard of care that has been set by the hospital and/or the specialty nursing unit where the patient's injury occurred. In managing a claim involving nursing malpractice, the risk manager must be able to find any nursing policies and procedures in effect at the time of the incident that describe the nursing standard of care. The risk manager can assist the nursing staff to write policies and procedures that reflect the minimum current nursing standard of practice. Policies that state goals for "high-quality" patient care may result in unattainable standards that create potential legal defense problems. Policies should set a standard similar to the standard in like settings, but nurses should be able to perform according to the standard set by the policy in every instance.

Journal Articles and Textbooks

Nursing journal articles and textbooks can be factors in determining the standard of care. Nursing staff should be encouraged to read journals. Along with attendance at continuing education programs, nurses can demonstrate an awareness of current practice through faithful reading of at least one nursing journal.

Custom and Practice

Custom and practice in a similar setting can also determine the standard of care. Courts in most jurisdictions have moved away from the "locality rule." In effect, this rule means that across the country there is a certain minimum standard of care. However, it can be helpful to survey other area hospitals informally whenever issues of custom and practice are being examined.

☐ Regulatory and Accrediting Bodies

State and federal agencies can directly or indirectly affect nursing practice. Legislatures have granted those agencies the authority to make rules and regulations that have the force of law. The state legislature controls the practice of nursing by enacting nurse practice acts and by granting authority to the state nursing board (a state agency) to make rules and regulations that will carry out and interpret the nurse practice act. One key function of the nursing board is the licensure of nurses; another is disciplinary action against nurses for substance abuse or unsafe practice. Other state agencies may affect nursing practice by regulating public health, maternity units, and hospitalization of the mentally ill and mentally retarded. Certain federal agencies, such as the Food and Drug Administration and the Department of Health and Human Services, also affect the practice of nursing, at least indirectly.

Accrediting bodies (such as the Joint Commission on Accreditation of Healthcare Organizations and the American Osteopathic Association), which set compliance standards, can also directly or indirectly affect nursing practice. Knowledge of nurse practice acts, rules and regulations of the state nursing licensure agency (nursing board), and accreditation standards can assist the risk manager in analyzing or determining liability.

☐ Recurring Causes of Nursing Liability

Nursing liability has always been a significant area of focus for health care risk managers. An article published in 1989 in *Forum*, the publication of the Risk Management Foundation of the Harvard Medical Institutions, stated that there has been an increase in the number of lawsuits in which nurses are named as defendants.[1] Open and closed claims and suits over a 12-year period from April 1, 1976, to December 31, 1987, were reviewed. During that period, nurses or nursing services were named in 178 cases, representing 7.8 percent of the total number of cases at the Risk Management Foundation. In the 178 cases, nurses were the primary or only named defendants in 59 cases; the institution was the sole defendant in 108 cases. In 11 cases, multiple parties were named. Figure 7-1 lists the most common claims involving nurses at Harvard-affiliated institutions participating in the Risk Management Foundation. This listing reflects nursing errors that would be found in almost any institutional setting. The remainder of this section discusses recurring types of nursing errors and patient injuries.

Falls

In many institutions, patient falls are the most frequently recurring patient incident. They occur most often with elderly patients, patients under sedation or other medication that causes disorientation or dizziness, and patients whose disease process causes disorientation or dizziness. Nursing staff must be alert to conditions that can cause falls. For patients with those conditions, there must be nursing policies or protocols on the use of bed or cart rails, restraints, intermittent or continuous patient observation, and assistance with ambulation, especially between bed and bathroom. Such measures may significantly reduce the number of falls.

Many institutions have established fall-prevention programs that assist nursing staff in identifying and monitoring those patients at particular risk for falls. Fall-prevention programs attempt to heighten the nursing staff's awareness of fall safety by identifying such patients on admission to the floor or unit and by distinguishing the chart, the

Figure 7-1.   Top Ten Primary Allegations for Nursing Cases

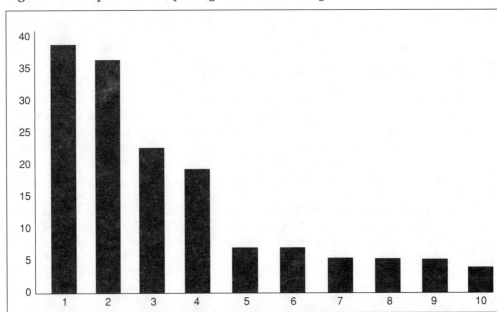

Source: Reprinted, with permission, from W. J. McDonough and M. Rioux, *Forum* 10(1):5, Jan.–Feb. 1989.
Note: This chart represents data from the Risk Management Foundation of the Harvard Medical Institutions, April 1,
1976–December 31, 1987. It does not include 33 cases with less frequent allegations.
Allegation Category Codes: 1, fall/hospital negligence; 2, failure to monitor; 3, failure to ensure patient safety; 4, improper
treatment/performance; 5, failure to respond to patient; 6, medication error; 7, wrong dosage administered; 8, failure to
follow hospital procedure; 9, improper technique; 10, failure to supervise treatment.

patient's wristband, the patient's room, or some combination thereof. A nursing care
plan is then developed to minimize the chance of falls.

In reviewing incident reports or investigating claims involving patient falls, the risk
manager should be alert to the following trends and patterns:

- Type of unit
- Time of day (shift)
- Nurse staffing of the unit
- Presence or absence of physician orders on patient activity such as ambulation
- Use or position of bed rails
- Use of restraints
- Type of medications and/or patient conditions that could have resulted in the
  patient's dizziness or loss of orientation
- Whether or not the patient requested nursing assistance by use of a properly func-
  tioning call-light system
- Applicability of any nursing policies and procedures
- Condition of floors at the time of the incident

In developing a fall-prevention program, the risk manager should also consider
environmental factors, such as the call light's accessibility to the patient in bed or in the
bathroom, lighting in the patient's room and bathroom, and accessibility of grab bars
in the toilet and shower.

Medication Errors

Medication errors by nursing staff can occur in many ways and are another frequently
recurring patient incident. Errors in medication administration often result from failure

to follow basic medication safety. For example, nurses should always read labels on medication containers before administering the medication. However, nurses can become hurried, distracted, or careless, and may thereby administer wrong medications. Nurses have a legal duty to administer medications accurately and in a timely manner. Nurses also have a legal duty to defer executing all physicians orders that they know to be clearly contraindicated. Nurses who administer medication that they know or should have known is clearly contraindicated have the same liability as physicians who improperly prescribe medication. Medication errors can be categorized in the following ways:

- Mistaken patient identity
- Administration of a wrong medication
- Administration of a wrong dosage
- Administration of a wrong concentration of a medication
- Incorrect route of administration
- Failure to read labels on vials, syringes, IV fluid bags, and so on
- Improper injection technique
- Transcription mistakes
- Misreading written orders
- Misunderstanding written or verbal orders
- Omission of medication administration
- Untimely administration of medication

In reviewing incident reports and investigating claims involving medication errors, the risk manager, with the assistance of the nursing staff, should attempt to categorize the type of medication error that was made. The risk manager may also seek assistance from the appropriate managers and the staff nurse responsible for the medication error. In addition to categorizing the error, the risk manager should also consider the following factors:

- Type of unit
- Time of day (shift)
- Nurse staffing of the unit
- Correctness, completeness, or ambiguity of physician orders
- Legibility of physician orders
- Any failure to follow basic medication safety procedures

Many medication errors result from a series of failures in the chain of communication that links the physician, the nurse, and the pharmacist. Therefore, the risk manager may need the assistance of nurse managers and hospital pharmacists to analyze and correct possible medication administration system failures. Patterns of medication errors should also be reported to the pharmacy and therapeutics committee for discussion and suggestions of remedial measures.

Equipment Injuries

Patient injuries caused by the nursing staff's use of equipment usually fall into two categories: (1) improper use of equipment, and (2) use of equipment that is obviously defective. As to the first category of equipment injury, the hospital has a legal obligation to provide adequate training and education in the use of patient equipment. This training and education should be provided at nursing orientation for all staff nurses, on the specific unit of assignment, and whenever the hospital purchases new equipment. The nursing staff and other care givers should not be required to use equipment for which they have not been provided proper instruction. For example, physicians and other care providers should not be allowed to use new equipment on trial without following a hospital protocol designed to ensure patient safety. The hospital must have a system in place to screen new equipment and perform safety tests, usually by biomedical engineering personnel.

As to the second category of equipment injury, use of defective equipment, the nursing staff is not liable for hidden defects that cause patient injury. In the case of an equipment shortage, nurses may be tempted to continue to use defective equipment; however, unsafe or broken equipment should be clearly marked as such and removed from the patient unit. The nursing staff should be taught to save all pieces of equipment that break while in use. Without all pieces, it may be impossible to ascertain that the equipment was defective rather than used improperly by the nurse.

Burns

Through carelessness, nurses can cause patients to be burned in many different ways. Cautery devices, hot-water bottles, heating pads, ultraviolet and warming lights, vaporizers, warming mattresses, caustic solutions, and hot water all can cause patients to be burned.

Nursing staff must be properly trained in the use of any electrical devices that have the potential to cause burns. This is especially true in operating rooms and intensive care units. Such devices may also require periodic visual inspection by nursing staff and scheduled preventive maintenance checks by biomedical engineering personnel. Nursing staff in the operating room must be aware of the dangers that prep solutions can present if allowed to pool under a patient's body or when inadvertently heated by electrical devices such as cauteries or warming mattresses.

Many burn injuries are caused by nurses who fail to exercise due care in treating patients who are unconscious, under anesthesia, paraplegic or quadriplegic, elderly, or debilitated—patients who may not react in pain to a burn injury but who sustain significant tissue damage from the burn. Many burn injuries can be treated successfully, and the immediate and ongoing application of therapy by experienced physicians and nurses can help minimize physical injury, especially scarring. In the case of a patient burn injury, the risk manager should ascertain that burn therapy has commenced.

Lack of Adequate Patient Supervision or Monitoring

Nursing staff are responsible for monitoring the patient's mental as well as physical condition. Nursing intervention may require the nurse to take reasonable steps to promote patient safety through various methods, such as using restraints or bed rails, assisting with ambulation, observing the patient constantly or periodically, accompanying the patient to ancillary departments, and using suicide precautions.

In addition to fall-prevention measures mentioned previously, all institutions should have written protocols on the use of restraints. Such protocols should be flexible enough to allow nursing staff to exercise clinical judgment in their use. For example, nursing staff must have the ability to intervene immediately to restrain patients before a physician signs such orders. It is justifiable for nurses to restrain patients who are a danger to themselves or others. The justification should be written in the nursing notes section of the patient's medical record. Nursing staff need not fear liability for using restraints except in the following instances:

- When clearly excessive force is used (such as sitting on a patient's chest)
- When patients are not checked as frequently as their condition warrants (especially patients who have also been medicated)
- When the condition of the patient's skin and circulation is not assessed

The risk manager should know the protocol for use of restraints and also should periodically review protocols, policies, and procedures on the use of bed rails, accompanying patients to ancillary departments, and suicide precautions.

Another recurring cause of nursing liability that falls under the category of failure to monitor is tissue injury that results from IV infiltrations. Nurses are responsible for checking the appearance of IV sites as frequently as indicated by protocol. The more caustic the solution, the more frequently the site must be observed. Nursing staff must document the frequency of checks and the appearance of the IV site. Bandages and tape can prevent observation, so checking under bandages is required; the use of clear tape will assist in preventing IV infiltrates.

Failure to Follow Institutional Policies and Procedures

As discussed previously, nursing department policies and procedures indicate a standard of care for the institution. Whenever the possibility exists that a member of the nursing staff has caused a patient injury, the risk manager must inquire as to the existence of any written policies, procedures, guidelines, or protocols. A key issue may be whether the nurse's actions complied with institutional standards.

In writing or updating policies and procedures, the nursing department must use care that the standards set are not so high or unrealistic that the nursing staff cannot meet them, nor so low that the institutional practice is below that in other similar settings. The risk manager or hospital legal counsel can perform an important risk control function by reviewing institutional standards for language that sets unrealistic and unattainable patient care goals. For example, a policy requiring that all patients who are sent to the radiology department must be accompanied by a member of the nursing staff may be unrealistic, given staffing levels and the stable condition of certain patients. Nursing staff must have the flexibility to exercise clinical judgment in any given situation. Therefore, policies and procedures must be clear and realistic, reflect current nursing practice, and not be too restrictive. Outdated policies and procedures should be preserved for a period that is equivalent to the malpractice statute of limitations for the jurisdiction because they may be needed as evidence of the applicable nursing standard of care during that period.

Improper Technique

Another frequently recurring incident is the improper administration of an injection, causing tissue and/or nerve damage. For example, an injection that should properly be given in the upper outer quadrant of the buttocks may instead be given improperly and the needle may enter the sciatic nerve, causing permanent injury. There are many ways in which a risk manager can determine whether or not improper technique was used. Nursing administrators, nursing educators, clinical specialists, and other staff nurses assigned to a similar unit could be asked for their opinion. Nursing textbooks and journal articles can be consulted. Also, the risk manager should know of any institutional policies and procedures that may help determine whether or not the nurse used improper technique.

☐ Documentation

The medical record provides a means of communication to all health care team members that helps ensure continuity of patient care. The patient's chart becomes a permanent record of the treatment provided and the role of each provider. Because it is a record of the patient's care and treatment, it becomes important to third-party payers, in personal injury suits, in criminal prosecutions, in workers' compensation cases, and in will contests, among many uses. It is always admissible in court under the rules of evidence in malpractice lawsuits. Because the way in which nurses document patient care is critical in defending claims, the risk manager must provide education programs on proper nursing documentation.

Documentation is the nurse's best way to demonstrate that the nursing standard of care was met. The absence of nursing documentation, especially at critical points during the course of care and treatment, makes defending malpractice suits much more difficult and may have been the reason that a lawsuit was first filed. Even though nurses are permitted to give oral testimony, the time lag between the event and the nurse's testimony makes such testimony far less reliable than good descriptive charting.

Part of the nurse's legal duty to the patient is to chart the care given to the patient accurately and in a timely manner. Because the chart's primary use is to communicate among care givers, patients can be harmed when charting is not accurate or timely.

Gaps and Omissions

The major problem that risk managers face in managing malpractice claims is gaps or omissions in the patient's record. Such omissions make it difficult to reconstruct what happened when a patient was injured. The following are three key nursing functions that should be documented but often are not:

- *Nursing assessment:* For example, electronic fetal monitoring strips that display tracings that the nurse should interpret as evidence of fetal distress
- *Nursing intervention (and patient response):* For example, an injection of a drug that may relieve the patient's pain
- *Patient education:* For example, giving instructions for a parent whose child has suffered head trauma to watch for signs of potential complications after discharge from the emergency department

There are patient care situations where gaps or omissions in the chart are likely to occur. These include failure to note:

- Nursing response during cardiorespiratory arrest and resuscitation
- Abnormal patient vital signs
- Nursing response during labor and delivery to fetal monitoring strips that revealed fetal distress
- Nursing care as patients are being transferred to the recovery room from surgery
- Nursing assessment on patient admission
- Nurse's observation of an IV site when a vesicant (agent that can cause blistering) is being infused

Other Deficiencies

Other nursing documentation deficiencies can create difficulty in the defense of litigation, including the following:

- Obliterations or erasures. Obliterations or erasures may appear to be an attempt to alter the record. A plaintiff's attorney can argue that the nurses made obliterations or erasures in an attempt to avoid liability. Nurses should be taught to draw a line through information written in error so that it can still be read, and then initial the change.
- Illegibility
- Ambiguous abbreviations. For example,"PE" may mean "physical examination" or "pulmonary embolus." Nursing staff should use only institution-approved abbreviations. A copy of those abbreviations should be available in every patient care area.
- Absence of date, time, and signature. Each page should be dated, each entry timed to the minute whenever possible, and each signature should include the initial of the first name, full last name, and professional designations of the writer.

- Missing pages.
- Lack of chronology in recording patient information.
- Placing blame on other professionals. Jousting in the medical record may make litigation more likely. For example, if a physician does not respond to a call, it is not appropriate for the nurse to chart "Dr. Jones did not respond to the call." It is appropriate for the nurse to list in chronological order each time the physician was called. If the record does not show a physician response, it will speak for itself.

Improvement of Charting

The elimination of charting deficiencies should be one important goal of risk management educational programs. The other important goal is to improve charting by making appropriate recommendations to the nursing staff. Suggestions include the following:

- *As nurses chart, they should remember that they are telling a story—the patient's story.* By reading the medical chart, the risk manager must be able to recreate the course of the patient's medical care. More important, so must all other care providers.
- *Charting should be clinical, objective, and descriptive.* Although nurses are pressed for time and must deliver patient care before they write on the chart, they must develop a charting style that is concise yet provides a clear, factual description of the course of patient care.
- *Documentation of nursing assessments should reflect a blending of sensory and clinical skills.* Nurses should chart what they *observe*. When they observe bleeding or discharge from a wound, charting should include a clinical description of that observation. Nurses should chart what they *hear*. Patient complaints should be recorded, in the patient's own words when possible. Nurses also should chart what they hear while assessing a patient with breathing irregularities. Nurses should chart what they *feel*, as when palpating an area of the patient's abdomen. Nurses should chart what they *smell*, as when the nurse smells alcohol on the patient's breath, for example.
- *Documentation of nursing interventions should note what has been done to or for the patient and the patient's response.* When the nurse observes a patient's abnormal vital signs, the chart should show that the nurse called a resident or paged anesthesia in response. When the patient appears likely to fall, patient safety measures such as the use of restraints or side rails or assistance with ambulation should be charted. Psychosocial assistance, such as calling a social worker or chaplain, should be charted. If a patient appears likely to develop a pressure sore, the use of special equipment, such as a decubitus mattress, should be in the chart. Examples of patient response to nursing intervention that should be charted include relief of pain when traction is applied, refusal to cooperate with nursing instruction, or reactions to drugs.
- *Documentation of patient education should show what information has been provided to the patient or to the family member or other person responsible for an outpatient, and that the person instructed understood the information.* Examples of patient education include admission instructions; information for orienting patients to the room; activity orders, particularly restrictions on activity; booklets or printed instruction sheets for home care; follow-up instructions upon discharge, including signs that may signal complications and thus necessitate a return to the emergency department or physician.
- *Charting should be contemporaneous to the nursing action.* Each nursing action should be recorded as soon as possible after it is completed. Nursing assessments and interventions should be in chronological order. When nurses wait until the end of the shift to complete all patient charts, charting tends to be incomplete, out of sequence, and less meaningful.

- *Verbal (unwritten) orders should be kept to a minimum.* The nursing department's policies and the medical staff bylaws should have statements on the use of verbal orders. Some hospitals prohibit nurses from accepting the verbal order of a physician who is physically present, except in an emergency. Telephone orders should be repeated verbatim to the physician for the sake of clarity before being accepted, carried out by the nurse, and then charted. Verbal and telephone orders entered on the chart require the physician's signature, usually within 24 hours.

□ Nurse Staffing Issues

There are significant risk management issues related to adequate nurse staffing, floating of nursing personnel from one unit to another, and use of agency nurses. The health care employer has a corporate legal duty to provide adequate staff. If it fails to do so, it can be held legally accountable on a theory of corporate negligence.

In a malpractice case, the plaintiff's attorney may seek to prove that the institution failed to meet the standard of care if a patient is injured as a result of understaffing. The attorney may use staffing measurement methods that take into account such factors as the type of nursing unit, patient activity, and shift. The Joint Commission on Accreditation of Healthcare Organizations has nursing service standards that apply to hospitals that seek accreditation.

Nursing administration is delegated management control over nursing resources. Essentially, staffing is a function of balancing patient needs and available nursing resources. Nursing administration carries out this function by considering such things as the following:

- Available staff (number and quality, including allied medical professionals)
- Patient acuity levels
- Type of unit
- Nursing care plans
- Hospital policy on staffing
- National practice on staffing of a similar unit
- Closing beds in units that cannot be adequately staffed
- Applicable state regulatory standards
- Joint Commission standards
- Nurse staffing measurement programs
- Assignment of priorities in order to defer certain patient care procedures that can be safely postponed

What are the risk management issues related to staffing? Patient safety must be of paramount concern to nursing administration. There are few reported cases in which a hospital was found negligent because nurse staffing was deficient. One case from New York involved circumstances in which the priority assigned to nursing tasks was deemed negligent. In *Horton v. Niagara Falls Municipal Medical Center,*[2] the patient was admitted with high fever and delirium. On the day in question, a charge nurse, a licensed practical nurse (L.P.N.), and one aide were assigned to 19 patients. The patient became disoriented and went out onto a balcony outside his room. After the patient was initially returned safely to his room, the attending physician wrote orders that the patient needed to be observed. The charge nurse phoned the patient's wife, telling her to come to the hospital because no staff was available to observe the patient. The charge nurse, citing insufficient staff, refused the wife's request to have a staff member remain with the patient until a family member could arrive. Before the wife arrived, the patient fell from the balcony and was injured. The court reviewed the staffing issue and held that the nursing staff was engaged in routine duties that could have waited. At trial there was testimony that the L.P.N. had left the floor to eat supper at the time the patient fell.

The practice of floating nurses to units other than their regular assignment is a necessity in many institutions. The potential for conflict exists here because the institution has a legal duty to staff its units using available nursing personnel, yet the nurses have a legal duty to avoid assuming tasks for which they are unqualified. Supervisors should check the qualifications and experience of those asked to float to a particular nursing unit. Once the decision is made to float a nurse, the supervisor or unit staff should provide a brief unit orientation and make the patient assignment fit the float nurse's training and experience, whenever possible.

The employer has the ultimate control of and accountability for the activities of its employees. There are cases that support the employer's right to discharge nursing personnel who refuse an assignment. Nurses who leave a patient care area in anger or frustration could also be liable for abandonment. The best advice a risk manager can give staff nurses is to accept float assignments. Staff nurses who are asked to float should state any limitations of their qualifications and experience to supervisory personnel, clarify responsibilities of the patient assignment, request a unit orientation if needed, and identify a resource person who is regularly assigned to the unit. All those measures will demonstrate that the float nurses acted reasonably under the circumstances. Staff nurses are never excused from exercising care, skill, and diligence, but if patients are injured because of inadequate staffing and there has been no failure of basic nursing skills, the employer is ultimately liable, not the individual staff nurses.

Contracting with an agency for nursing staff is another method that hospitals use to maintain adequate staffing. If the hospital uses agency nurses, the risk manager should review all the contracts with the agency to make sure that the hospital is protected from liability for the negligence of an agency nurse. The contract should require that the nursing agency provide adequate insurance coverage. The risk manager may wish to consider such risk transfer methods as indemnity and hold harmless clauses or having the institution made a named insured to the agency's professional liability policy. The contract should specify the minimum qualifications of staff provided by the agency, proof of current valid licensure, and the right of the institution to refuse agency personnel who have demonstrated practice problems. The institution should check the credentials of agency nurses assigned to it. The institution must provide agency nurses with an orientation to its policies and procedures and to the patient unit.

☐ Nurse Insurance Issues

The risk manager should be prepared to respond to questions from nursing staff on whether or not nurses should carry their own personal liability insurance policy. The best response to this question is that the decision to carry personal liability insurance is an individual one. The risk manager should then present reasons to carry personal liability coverage, as well as reasons not to carry it.

Reasons to Carry Insurance

Nurses who carry personal liability insurance have their legal expenses covered should they be held liable for their own acts of negligence at work or outside the employment setting. Other advantages of having such coverage include the certainty of coverage associated with a personal policy, the assurance of personal legal representation, and the protection of personal assets.

Personal Liability of Nurses for Negligence
Nurses may be held personally liable for their own acts of negligence. The hospital or another codefendant has a legal right to seek a contribution to a settlement from the

nurse's carrier or to sue the nurse for reimbursement after a settlement with the plaintiff. In either case, the nurse's policy provides payment of legal expenses and settlement or judgment amounts for which the nurse is personally liable.

Potential Liability Outside the Employment Setting

Nurses who serve as volunteers at church or at school athletic functions, for example, should maintain their own coverage. Although there are no known cases against nurses for negligence in rendering professional services to friends or neighbors, physicians have been sued in similar circumstances.

Certainty of Coverage

If the nurse has any doubt that the employer will provide coverage through its insurance program, the purchase of a personal liability policy may provide relatively inexpensive peace of mind.

Personal Legal Representation

The nurse's insurance carrier will be obligated to provide the nurse with an attorney whose sole interest is in representing the nurse in the event of a lawsuit. The nurse then has assurance that his or her personal interests are paramount in the defense of a lawsuit.

Protection of Personal Assets

Although it is extremely unlikely, a plaintiff could satisfy a judgment through forcing the sale of a nurse's personal property or attaching bank accounts. Realistically, physicians and institutional employers such as hospitals are the targeted defendants of plaintiffs' attorneys.

Reasons Not to Carry Insurance

Nurses may elect not to carry insurance for fear of being sued more frequently or because insurance is costly. Coverage may be unnecessary if nurses are protected by the insurance policies of their employers.

Frequency of Lawsuits

Nurses may be sued more frequently in today's litigious environment. Although a plaintiff's attorney is not likely to know that any particular nurse involved in a patient incident is carrying insurance, the fact that nurses may be more likely to carry insurance now than in the past may make them more inviting targets as defendants.

Coverage by Employer's Policy

Generally, institutions provide insurance coverage for their employees. Coverage includes all costs of settlements and judgments, costs of investigating the allegations, all court costs, attorneys' fees, and all costs of defense. The institution's employees will have no out-of-pocket expenses if named personally in a lawsuit. Employers are aware that it would be extremely short-sighted to refuse to provide coverage, even in those circumstances where the nurse does not follow hospital policies and procedures.

Many nurses do, however, carry their own insurance. The risk manager may be required to rein in hospital defense counsel who seek contributions from a nurse's personal insurance carrier. If the institution seeks contributions from employees who are involved in lawsuits, it will not only have employee morale problems, but the nursing staff may no longer trust the risk manager, who must depend on the nursing staff's cooperation to maintain a successful risk management program.

Pricing of Personal Liability Premiums

In recent years, some insurance carriers have significantly raised premiums for nurses. The rates vary, depending on the specialty unit of the nurse. Nurses in such high-risk areas as obstetrics, emergency services, and surgery may be paying much more than they have in the past. In 1989, many specialty nurses paid an annual premium of $800, depending on the carrier. Curiously, some carriers have raised their rates just slightly, if at all. It may be excessively costly for nurses to purchase personal liability policies when coverage already is provided through the employer's insurance program.

☐ The Risk Manager and Nursing Administration

The risk manager must interact closely and often with nursing administrators, the director of nursing, head nurses and assistant head nurses, and charge nurses. The interaction should occur in formal and informal ways. Formal interaction occurs through committee meetings, inservice programs, and through the incident-reporting system. Informal interaction can occur while making rounds on patient care units. Rounding gives the risk manager visibility and accessibility to nursing leadership. The information that the risk manager gathers on rounds will assist in the concurrent review and management of adverse occurrences and will encourage nurses to notify the risk manager of such occurrences before they become claims. The risk managers should go on rounds at least weekly, if not daily. In addition, the risk manager should consider using a pager in order to be accessible at all times to nursing administrators, medical staff, and administrative staff.

Incident reports are initiated primarily by nursing personnel, and nursing administrators must be educated in their proper use. Incident reports call attention to situations that may require corrective action. They help identify trends and patterns of unsafe practices. They may aid nursing staff in recalling an incident years after it occurred. Most important, they alert the risk manager to individual adverse occurrences that may become claims. Because the risk manager needs this information, nursing staff must be encouraged to report adverse patient occurrences. The use of incident reports by physicians and nursing administrators as a means of punishing nurses should be discouraged.

The risk manager should be involved with the nursing quality assurance function. If the risk manager compiles incident report data from nursing units, these should be reviewed by the nursing quality assurance coordinator or committee, as should trends in nursing malpractice claims, so that corrections can be made to minimize incidents. The nursing quality assurance coordinator can also provide the risk manager with nursing systems analyses such as staffing patterns or error trends in medication administration. With this information, the risk manager and nursing administration can do a better job of risk prevention. Other nursing risk-prevention activities that can be undertaken with the assistance of nursing administration include fall-prevention programs and high-risk surveys on such specialty units as labor and delivery, surgery, emergency service, and intensive care.

The risk manager must provide the nursing staff with inservice education programs. All new nursing staff should be provided an orientation to the risk management program. Other educational programs can focus on such topics as nursing documentation, consent issues, malpractice prevention, and withdrawal and withholding of life-sustaining technology.

The risk manager can assist nursing administration with writing and review of nursing policies and procedures, especially those concerned with patient safety. The risk manager also must recommend a policy on retention of outdated policies and procedures and other nursing documents, such as patient assignment sheets, that may be essential in the defense of claims and suits.

The cooperation of nursing administration is essential to the success of the risk management program. Nursing administration must view the risk manager as an ally in the delivery of safe patient care. The risk manager must view nursing administration and the entire nursing staff as the eyes and ears of the risk management program. Perhaps more than any other department, nursing can provide the risk manager with timely information on adverse patient occurrences.

References

1. McDonough, W. J., and Rioux, M. Increasing number of nurses named as sole defendants in malpractice suits. *Forum* 10(1):4–5, 12, Jan.–Feb. 1989.

2. *Horton v. Niagara Falls Memorial Medical Center,* 380 N.Y.S.2d 116 (N.Y. App. Dir. 1976).

□ Bibliography

Calloway, S. D. *Nursing and the Law.* 2nd ed. Eau Claire, WI: Professional Education Systems, 1987.

Creighton, H. *Law Every Nurse Should Know.* 5th ed. Philadelphia: W. B. Saunders Co., 1986.

Chapter 8
External Relationships

Frances Kurdwanowski

Because risk management is a discipline that cannot be mastered in isolation, it is necessary to forge good communication lines with attorneys, insurance brokers and carriers, police, prosecutors, and regulatory agencies. Also, colleagues in risk management will serve as advisors and share valuable information. How does the new risk manager establish solid working relationships outside the hospital? This chapter will touch briefly on each of these communication links and offer some guidelines.

☐ Health Care Attorneys

The risk manager will need to interact with the corporate attorney, the defense attorney for a particular case, and sometimes the plaintiff's attorney.

Hospital (Corporate) Attorney

The hospital attorney serves as corporate counsel to the hospital, its board, and its management. If the corporate attorney is not an employee of the hospital, that role may be fulfilled by one multidisciplinary firm or by a number of firms, each with a different specialty. Most health care institutions will have relationships with more than one outside attorney. The hospital's outside attorney will assist with business relationships, contracts, legal issues involved in patient care, labor issues, hospital finance, Medicare reimbursement, physician bylaws, disciplinary issues, and credentialing matters. Hospital counsel may attend meetings of the board of trustees and board committees and, sometimes, meetings of the medical staff or medical executive committee. The hospital's attorney will handle legal matters involving the medical staff, except in rare instances when a particular issue necessitates hiring separate legal counsel for the medical staff.

Some examples of hospital attorney–risk manager interaction include the following:

- Reviewing informed consent process and necessary forms
- Reviewing certain policies and/or procedures that have potential for liability
- Advising on legal problems involved with the care of patients

- Providing legal guidance to various committees
- Sharing information about upcoming or current legislation that will affect risk management decisions
- Reviewing hospital contracts
- Advising on confidentiality issues
- Advising on peer review, credentialing, and privileging issues
- Establishing physician disciplinary procedures
- Responding to subpoenas for records and witnesses

The risk manager will meet with the hospital counsel regularly to decide what areas will be important for each to best serve the other. If the attorney acts as coordinating legal counsel for the hospital, he or she may request monthly reports on the status of open malpractice case files.

There are areas of exposure where damages awarded in a successful lawsuit may not be covered by insurance. Among those are antitrust, environmental impairment, physician credentialing, discrimination, and wrongful termination. Punitive damages are not covered by insurance. In these instances, the hospital counsel will defend against such action but may bring in cocounsel who specializes in the area being litigated.

A cost-effective approach to communication with the hospital attorney is to set up a protocol that hospital staff call the risk manager when legal advice is required. The risk manager then consults with the attorney and assists hospital staff in resolving the problem. The risk manager must have a written policy for handling these matters and educate hospital staff accordingly.

Defense Attorney

If a hospital is self-insured, the risk manager will have considerable input into the selection of defense attorneys for the hospital. It may also be part of the risk manager's role to monitor defense's handling of each case and evaluate the fees in relation to the amount and quality of the work. That particular aspect will assist in keeping legal expenses within reasonable limits. This monitoring by the risk manager is particularly important for self-insured hospitals because no one else may be overseeing the handling of the case.

For those institutions that are fully insured, the insurance company will select the defense attorney(s). However, insurers generally are willing to listen if the risk manager requests that certain attorneys do the hospital's defense work. It is very helpful to establish a collegial relationship, because risk manager and defense counsel will be working very closely on each case. In defending claims, the risk manager coordinates the gathering of information, investigates the claim internally, and interacts with hospital personnel.

The risk manager is a liaison between the defense counsel and the hospital. After the risk manager has interviewed the staff involved in a reported incident, there should be full discussion of the case with the defense counsel. In fact, any sensitive information should be communicated to the defense attorney. In planning defense strategies, the defense counsel will rely heavily on the risk manager. As both learn more about the case, they will be able to advise the insurer about whether there is liability, the value of the case, and possibilities of settlement. This evaluation of liability is an essential part of the risk manager's role.

When plaintiff's counsel issues interrogatories, the risk manager must answer them in a timely fashion. By completing them promptly, the risk manager helps not only the institution but also the defense attorney, who will have time to modify the responses, assert privileges of nondiscoverability, and address the legal issues raised by the interrogatories. Defense counsel will then return them for certification by either the risk manager or the designated hospital authority. The risk manager should feel comfortable calling the defense attorney to ask questions or share new information.

Another way in which the risk manager assists the defense attorney is by scheduling depositions. To minimize disruptions in scheduling hospital employees and to make hospital witnesses more comfortable, it is more orderly and less time-consuming if depositions are scheduled at the hospital rather than at the attorney's office. At the deposition, the risk manager's presence provides moral support to witnesses and helps the defense attorney gain insight into their responses.

When it comes time for trial, it is part of the risk manager's function to arrange for the witnesses to be on call and to obtain the original medical record and any other documents that might be needed for the case.

What should the risk manager expect of the defense attorney? Besides the two-way communication already discussed, the defense attorney should seek the risk manager's advice on proposed interrogatories or before deposing plaintiff's witnesses. As the case progresses, counsel should provide reports of expert witnesses, status reports on the progress of the case, and summaries of depositions of plaintiff's witnesses.

The defense attorney is best qualified to discuss damages, legal proofs, and possible defenses.

Plaintiff's Attorney

Unless it is approved by the defense attorney, the plaintiff's attorney should not be communicating with the risk manager or with anyone else in the hospital. Any request for documents, information, or addresses of possible witnesses should be directed to the defense attorney, who will in turn convey that information to the risk manager. In rare instances, the defense attorney might allow direct communication.

☐ Insurance Broker or Agent

It is the risk manager's responsibility to report claims to the broker or agent. The insurance broker is a real partner to the risk manager and can be of invaluable assistance throughout the risk manager's tenure. The new risk manager should meet with the insurance broker and ask what services are available to support the program. For instance, the insurance broker should be able to provide:

- A loss run of all prior professional and general liability lawsuits that the hospital has been involved in that were covered by the present insurance carrier.
- A history of prior insurance carriers and the coverages.
- Information on who is covered by the hospital's policies and what the property coverages are. The risk manager can provide the agent or broker and defense counsel with information on insurance coverage of codefendants, physicians, and nurses who carry their own insurance.
- Advice on insurance issues as they arise.
- Assistance with claims-handling matters.
- Interpretation of the insurance contracts.
- Loss-prevention educational material.
- A loss-prevention survey of the hospital with recommendations for loss-prevention activities.
- Participation in the hospital's safety committee meetings.
- Participation in safety inspections.
- Review of insurance clauses in contracts or agreements.

Questions often arise about insurance matters, and no one is better able to answer those than the informed insurance broker. Therefore it is helpful to have a broker who is well versed in medical liability insurance. Needless to say, the broker should also have a proven record in property, fire, and other types of insurance.

The broker sends applications for insurance renewal to the risk manager, who completes them. Later the risk manager will meet with the broker to discuss changes in the hospital's bed complement or services that require changes in insurance coverage. The insurance broker, insurance company risk service representative, risk manager, and hospital administration should meet quarterly to discuss reserves, the status of open cases, the disposition of closed cases, and any other matters that might optimize the broker's representation of the hospital.

☐ Insurance Carriers

Generally, the insurance company representing the hospital or other health care institution will have a person, called a risk service, or claims, representative, who is designated as the contact for the risk manager. The new risk manager should arrange an initial meeting with that person to discuss open cases and determine from the risk service representative exactly what the carrier expects from the risk manager and what services and information the risk manager needs from the risk service representative. After this initial meeting, it will be necessary, generally, to meet at least once a month—perhaps even weekly if the caseload is very heavy. The risk service or claims representative has many other health care institutions as clients and will depend heavily upon the risk manager to do the preliminary setting up of a case. The risk manager will conduct initial interviews of people involved in incidents and make arrangements with hospital personnel for the claims representative's investigation.

The risk service representative is critical to the communication between risk manager and broker because he or she provides information regarding the status of open suits and claims, any negotiations that might be taking place with regard to settling a suit, and reserves for open claims when the quarterly review of cases and claims is done. The risk service representative is the person to whom the risk manager reports a potential claim as soon as the risk manager has completed an initial investigation to determine what happened. After reviewing the medical record and speaking with any witnesses, the risk manager will be in a very good position to discuss the situation with the risk service representative.

The risk service representative usually is the link between risk management and the underwriting department of the insurance company, which determines the hospital's premium. The risk service representative's help is vital in planning educational programs for hospital staff because he or she knows the types of claims that the insurance company is seeing from other hospitals. The representative is also the liaison to the insurance company's loss-prevention section. Loss-prevention consultants can serve as resources for educational programs for hospital staff or will advise the risk manager as to where to obtain speakers and/or educational materials.

It is also helpful to risk managers to develop a rapport with other major carriers that insure the medical staff members. Usually the doctor-owned insurance companies have excellent resources for assisting with medical staff education, and they should be used. The physicians will be even more likely to appreciate the advice of a representative of their own insurance carrier. Other contacts at the insurance company might include an underwriter, if information is needed about premium cost or if the risk manager wishes to find out whether a certain resident or physician had been covered in prior years on the hospital insurance policy. An insurance carrier that specializes in medical malpractice work will generally have educational seminars about loss prevention and other risk management activities.

If the institution does not have excess insurance coverage with its primary carrier, the risk manager should establish contact with the insurance company that provides this coverage, even though the excess carrier is involved in cases less frequently than the primary carrier. Usually the primary carrier will take care of this type of communication, or the hospital insurance broker should be of assistance, but the risk manager needs to know that someone has notified the excess carrier if there is a possibility that a judgment or settlement will exceed the limits of the hospital's primary coverage.

Because the risk manager coordinates the defense of claims against the hospital, he or she will interact with other insurance companies, such as insurance carriers of codefendants, workers' compensation carriers, and insurance carriers that cover companies with which the hospital does business. The rule in all such communications is to be polite, knowledgeable, businesslike, and helpful.

In addition to coordinating medical malpractice matters, the risk manager also will be handling general liability, auto, fire, boiler and machinery, and other types of claims. There may be different insurance representatives handling those matters, or the insurance broker might act as intermediary. The risk manager needs to establish clear communication lines for all types of claims.

☐ Police

Emergency room personnel usually deal with police when crime victims or prisoners are brought into the emergency room. However, they may call on the risk manager when they need assistance.

Many states have legislation regarding the collection of specimens that are to be provided to the police, and it is essential that the risk manager be aware of what those laws require. Generally, they involve blood alcohol and drug testing. The risk manager should be aware that although the function of the police is to protect the public against those who commit crimes, the hospital's charge is to provide care and treatment to patients and protect the confidentiality of patient information. Because these interests sometimes cause conflict between care givers and police, it is important to develop policies and procedures outlining the responsibilities of each. The risk manager should review the hospital's policies regarding blood for alcohol testing and recommend changes if needed.

When crime victims are brought to the emergency room for treatment, emergency room personnel must preserve any evidence, which could include victims' clothing, hair under the victims' fingernails, possessions found on the victims or brought in by them, weapons, and so on. Proper procedure might be as simple as not cutting the clothes of a person who has a gunshot or knife wound so that the fabric around the wound can be preserved properly. The best course of action in such situations is to make sure that the emergency room staff is aware of the importance of preserving evidence and documenting the chain of custody in giving this material to the police officer who either comes in with the patient or will be called by emergency room personnel. The police officer should sign for everything that is being given to him or her. State law governs the responsibility of the hospital in treating criminals and crime victims. The risk manager can assist the hospital in balancing those responsibilities with its responsibilities to these patients as well as its need to minimize disruption of service. To assist in police investigations, the risk manager will facilitate interviews and help obtain specimens or reports regarding them from the laboratory. The method of obtaining and preserving evidence in rape cases should be detailed in a hospital policy according to guidelines acceptable to the police and the hospital. In all such matters, the risk manager must respect the confidentiality of patient information and know under what circumstances it can be released, even to the police.

In conjunction with the risk manager, the security and nursing staff will call upon the police for assistance with patients who have eloped, visitors who have weapons or exhibit disruptive behavior, or simply to identify or locate patients' families.

Some matters must be reported to either the police or other social service agencies. For example, hospital personnel are required to report suspected child abuse or elder abuse, gunshot wounds, and suspected felony. The best guideline for the risk manager in these matters is to follow hospital policy and state law.

☐ Prosecutor and Other Court Officers

When a hospital patient has been involved in a crime, the hospital should have a clear policy on how to deal with requests from the prosecutor's office. If those contacts fall within the risk manager's role, an easy way to handle any communications with that office is to set up protocols for handling certain situations.

In these situations, as well as others, hospital staff will be served with subpoenas. Allowing staff to accept subpoenas disrupts patient care and poses a security problem when the persons attempting to serve them seek out staff members who are working. Therefore, one person, with an alternate, should be delegated to accept all subpoenas. The risk manager or other person delegated to receive a subpoena will find out whether the person being served is still employed at the hospital, or whether it is an attending physician whose office is not in the hospital.

The risk manager should set up a procedure with the prosecutor's office so that subpoenas may be served without disruptions. There is very little need for "emergency" subpoenas to be issued; court cases are scheduled and the investigator at the prosecutor's office is well aware of when that case is set for trial. The hospital should have ample notice of any witnesses who might be needed for testimony at trial. It should be agreed that witnesses be scheduled "on call" so that they need not waste time in the courthouse waiting to testify.

The procedure for accepting civil action summonses is basically the same as in prosecutor cases: one person plus an alternate should be designated to receive summonses and complaints (see figure 8-1 for a sample policy).

☐ Regulatory Agencies

Risk managers may have contact with regulatory agencies such as the state or local department of health, the board of medical examiners, the board of nursing, or the office of the ombudsman. The risk manager may wish to find out from the board of medical examiners the latest information regarding certain regulations that apply to physicians. Similarly, the risk manager may wish to ask the board of nursing a question regarding nursing practice.

In most cases, simply knowing that those agencies can be of assistance is enough. The office of the ombudsman may be conducting an investigation into some reported incident or perception of an incident by either a hospital patient or a nursing home resident, and the risk manager should cooperate fully with agency investigators. The risk manager should also stay abreast of the findings of investigations or routine surveys as well as the hospital's filed responses, because those are public records that may be admissible in a later lawsuit.

Other regulatory agencies include the Occupational Safety and Health Administration, the Food and Drug Administration, and the Joint Commission, to name a few. The extent to which the risk manager interrelates with them will be determined by the administrative directives of the hospital.

☐ Other Risk Managers

By becoming involved in local, state, and national risk management societies, the risk manager has access to ready knowledge and expertise. The new risk manager should develop a network of other risk managers with whom he or she can discuss common problems or who can offer help in difficult situations. Other colleagues may be able to share policies or procedures that have worked well for them.

Figure 8-1. Civil Action Summonses Policy

SUBJECT: Civil Action Summonses

PURPOSES: To establish the policy and procedure for accepting Summonses and Complaints in civil actions against the hospital, its employees, residents, attending physicians, and patients.

SCOPE: This policy is applicable to all Civil Action Summonses and Complaints and to all employees, residents, members of the attending staff, and patients.

Policy

No Civil Action Summons or Complaint against _____ Hospital is to be accepted by any employee, resident, attending physician, or patient. All court officers attempting to serve such papers should be directed to the *delegated authority,* who is the only individual authorized to accept same on behalf of the Hospital.

 With respect to Civil Action Summonses and Complaints against parties other than the Hospital, service of these papers is not permitted on the Hospital's premises. Court officers will be directed to the *delegated authority,* who will assist them by confirming the current addresses of such individuals.

 Any employee or resident who is served at home with a Civil Action Summons and Complaint should review these papers immediately. If he or she appears to be named in the lawsuit because of his or her status as an employee of _____ Hospital, the papers should be brought immediately to the *delegated authority.* Expeditious processing of such papers is of utmost importance because failure to file an answer within the time allowed by law can result in the entry of a judgment by default.

Source: Reprinted, with permission, from *Administrative Policy Manual* of St. Joseph's Hospital and Medical Center, Paterson, NJ.

☐ Bibliography

Boone, R., and others. Tips on holding down spiralling hospital defense costs. *Hospital Risk Management* 6(3):29–32, Mar. 1984.

Cooke, P. I'll never forget that face. *Hippocrates,* Nov.–Dec. 1988, pp. 106–108.

Fetzer, B. Early investigation of incidents important in malpractice defense. *Perspectives* 8(3):5–9, Summer 1988.

Irwin, J. Wanted: top-notch medical counsel to survive malpractice era. *Hospital Risk Management* 10(10):128–30, Oct. 1988.

Jeddeloh, N. P. Attorney recommends cooperation, mutual respect for effective risk management-JD relationship. *Hospital Risk Management* 9(7):94–95, July 1987.

Troyer, G. T., and Salman, S. L. *Handbook of Health Care Risk Management.* Rockville, MD: Aspen Publishers, 1986.

Willmarth, R. R. Retain hospital attorney carefully to save time, money. *Hospital Risk Management* 7(10):133–36, Oct. 1985.

Part Three

Related Functions

In order to accomplish risk management goals, the risk manager must coordinate with other key managers and important committees within the institution, such as the quality assurance and safety committees. In some institutions, the risk manager either performs or supervises one or more of these related functions or chairs these committees. In others, the risk manager establishes operational links with key functions and serves on the committees. The chapters in this section explain why each function is critical to the success of risk management and how the risk manager interacts with each to accomplish risk management goals.

Chapter 9
Quality Assurance

Peggy Berry Martin

Quality assurance is a formal, systematic program by which care rendered to patients is measured against established criteria. The program performs the following functions:

- Identifies problems in patient care
- Designs activities to overcome those problems
- Performs follow-up monitoring to ensure that no new problems have been introduced and that corrective steps have been effective[1]

The primary goal of any quality assurance activity is to improve the quality of patient care. Many hospital activities have the purpose of monitoring and improving the quality of care, such as medical staff or hospitalwide committees involved with surgical case review or tissue review, infection control, medical records, utilization review, credentialing, drug utilization review, and morbidity and mortality review. Information gathered in any of those activities can be useful in the problem-identification phase of the quality assurance process.

In its 1990 quality assurance standard, the Joint Commission on Accreditation of Healthcare Organizations states that there should be "an ongoing quality assurance program designed to objectively and systematically monitor and evaluate the quality and appropriateness of patient care, pursue opportunities to improve patient care, and resolve identified problems."[2]

To comply with those standards, a quality assurance program must have the following components:

- A mandate for a program from the governing board, as well as active participation and review of the program
- Monitoring of the quality and appropriateness of patient care and clinical performance by clinical and administrative staff
- A written plan that describes the program's objectives, organization, scope, and mechanisms for overseeing the effectiveness of monitoring, evaluation, and problem-solving activities

- Documented improvement in patient care as a result of the monitoring activities
- Annual evaluation and periodic revision of the program as a result of evaluation[3]

☐ Structure of the Quality Assurance Program

It is a myth that one department, one individual, or one group of individuals "does" quality assurance. The monitoring and improvement of the quality of patient care is the responsibility of all hospital employees and all members of the medical staff. However, for purposes of efficiency, accountability, and effectiveness, there must be some structure to support the function and someone who is responsible for making sure that all the steps in the process are accomplished.

The responsibility for developing and maintaining the quality assurance function may rest within a designated department of quality assurance or may be combined, especially in smaller hospitals, with other "monitoring responsibilities" such as infection control, utilization review, or medical records. Quality assurance programs can be structured in a variety of ways, depending on the needs, resources, and philosophy of the institution and the personnel qualified and available to perform the tasks. The proposed structure shown in figure 9-1 can be adapted to all sizes and types of health care organizations.[4] The basis of this structure is a central data-collection function from which data can be directed to the appropriate department head, chief of service, peer review chairman, or review committee. This kind of structure could eliminate some duplication of effort, especially in the area of risk identification.

Criteria concerning what data to collect must be chosen by individual hospital departments and clinical services. The director of quality assurance and the risk manager can assist in selecting criteria, based on their knowledge of institutional claims experience, institutional and national quality assurance data on high-risk areas of practice, clinical standards set nationally or locally, and legislative and/or accreditation requirements set by external organizations. Physician-specific results of monitoring should be used in the reappointment process. Criteria can also be revised according to the results of monitors (that is, results may suggest other potential problem areas that should be monitored).

☐ The Quality Assurance Plan

Although the institution must make some decision about the structure of the quality assurance program, the program's structure is not as important as its function. How problems are identified, addressed, and resolved and how the program is evaluated must be outlined in a written plan. The sample quality assurance plan in figure 9-2 (pp. 104–6) is an example of a plan that describes the necessary elements of a formal program, its objectives, the authority for it, and how it is to be evaluated.[5]

With this type of detailed plan as a blueprint, some specific job descriptions and policies and procedures can be developed to address the daily activities of the program. For example, a procedure should be developed to define how and by whom data are collected, who reviews the data, and how that is documented. It would be useful also to describe the quality assurance responsibilities of various hospital departments and clinical services and how they relate to the hospitalwide quality assurance program. Formats for reporting to various medical staff committees and the governing body can be developed and appended to the plan.

After such a plan is developed with the input of a variety of medical staff and administrative personnel and committees, the plan should be shared with all departments, services, and committees so that they are aware of their role in the program. Individual hospital departments and clinical services should write their own quality assurance plans to complement the hospitalwide procedures.

Figure 9-1.   Proposed Structure of Quality Assurance

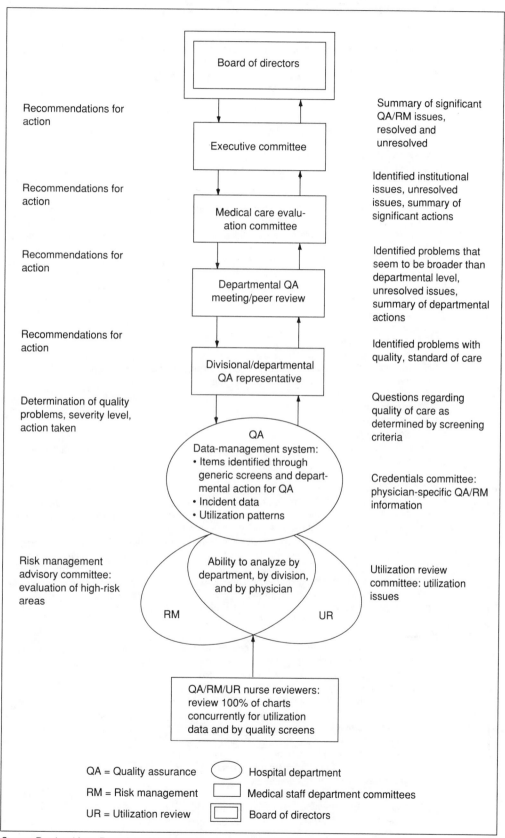

Source: Reprinted from *Essentials of Hospital Risk Management* by B. J. Youngberg (ed.), p. 47, with permission of Aspen Publishers, Inc., © 1989.

Figure 9-2. Sample Quality Assurance Program Plan

(Name) Hospital Medical Center, through the board of trustees, medical staff, and administration, is dedicated to the provision of quality care to all its patients. In order to ensure that quality care is provided, an ongoing quality assurance program has been established. The program includes an effective mechanism for monitoring patient care and responding to problem areas in an appropriate and timely manner.

I. Objective of the Quality Assurance Program
    A. To ensure the provision of high-quality patient care through objective care evaluation and other quality assurance activities.
    B. To ensure coordination and integration of all quality assurance activities by establishing a quality assurance committee as the focal point through which all quality assurance information will be exchanged and monitored.
    C. To identify and correct patient care problems by assessing their cause and scope and implementing actions to resolve them.
    D. To prioritize identified problems so that those directly affecting patient care can be resolved in a timely manner.
    E. To ensure communication and reporting among quality assurance personnel, administration, department heads, medical staff, and board of trustees.
    F. To ensure that all JCAH quality assurance requirements are met, the following departments will participate in evaluations as recommended:
        1. Activities services
        2. Dental services
        3. Dietetic services
        4. Housekeeping and laundry services
        5. Medical services (medical staff services/departments will conduct ongoing evaluation and monitoring of patient care by means of clinically valid criteria)
        6. Nursing services
        7. Pharmaceutical services
        8. Rehabilitation services
        9. Social services
    G. To ensure that all PRO quality assurance requirements are met, *(Name)* Hospital Medical Center will participate in all areawide audits generated by area PRO.

II. Authority for Quality Assurance Program
    A. The final authority to ensure that quality patient care is provided rests with the board of trustees. By approval of this program plan, the board of trustees authorizes the administration and the medical staff to establish a quality assurance program.
    B. The hospital administrator, by approval of this program plan, authorizes all hospital departments, their directors, and their members to participate in the quality assurance program.
    C. The executive medical board, by approval of this program plan, delegates authority to the medical staff departments, their chairpersons, and their members to participate in the quality assurance program. The authority of the executive medical board to direct participation in a quality assurance committee is defined in the medical staff bylaws.

III. Organization
    A. The focal point of the quality assurance program is the quality assurance committee, whose primary responsibility is to monitor the quality of care provided within the hospital. This committee is authorized as a standing committee of the executive medical board with direct reporting responsibility to that body. The executive medical board, in turn, reports to the executive director of the hospital and the board of trustees.
    B. The quality assurance committee is composed of the following members:
        1. Representative from the surgery department
        2. Representative from the medicine department
        3. Representative from the family practice department
        4. Representative from the obstetrics/gynecology department
        5. Representative from the pediatrics department
        6. Director of medical education
        7. Chairperson of the medical care evaluation committee
        8. Chairperson of the utilization review committee
        9. Chairperson of the risk management committee
        10. One representative from the board of trustees

Figure 9-2. (Continued)

> 11. One representative from the administration
> 12. Director of nursing or representative
> 13. Coordinator of quality assurance
> C. The chairperson of the quality assurance committee is appointed by the chief of staff for a term of one year.

IV. Hospital Organization
   A. The development and implementation of this plan necessitates the establishment of a quality assurance department that includes a director of quality assurance and a data retrieval specialist/typist.
   B. The department will provide support services for all quality assurance activities:
      1. Preparation and analysis of monthly statistics
      2. Research in development of review criteria
      3. Development of review methods
      4. Staff support to medical staff committees, hospital departments, and administrative committees involved in quality assurance activities
      5. Maintenance of quality assurance records

V. Program Description
   A. The quality assurance committee will identify problems based on analysis of monthly trends, statistics collected from hospital incident reports, generic screens, critical events monitoring criteria (see Attachment 1), quarterly reviews of responses to patient questionnaires, and input from other medical staff and hospital committees. These committees include, but are not limited to:
      1. Utilization review committee
      2. Infection control committee
      3. Pharmacy and therapeutics committee
      4. Tissue committee
      5. Transfusion committee
      6. Surgical chart review committee
      7. Risk management committee
      8. Medical records committee
      9. Medical education committee
      10. Tumor board
      11. Clinical department committees
      12. Safety committee
   B. The quality assurance committee will prioritize problems that most directly affect patient care.
   C. The quality assurance committee will refer identified problems to the appropriate medical staff committee, hospital department, or administrative committee for action. One individual representing a department or committee will be selected as a liaison to the quality assurance committee. The medical staff committee, hospital department, or administrative committee will:
      1. Identify the method to be used to assess the problem
      2. Set criteria
      3. Evaluate findings
      4. Make recommendations for action to correct the problem
      5. Implement the action
      6. Report findings and problem resolution to the quality assurance committee through the liaison
   D. The quality assurance committee will monitor the progress of the various committees to which problems have been referred toward solution of the problems.
   E. The quality assurance committee will recommend additional corrective action when needed.
   F. The quality assurance committee will report monthly to the executive medical board for transmittal to the executive director and/or board of trustees.
   G. The quality assurance committee will obtain documentation that substantiates the effectiveness of the overall program.

VI. Evaluation of the Quality Assurance Program
   A. The medical executive committee or outside consultants will evaluate the program to determine its effectiveness on an annual basis.
   B. Measures to be used to determine the program's effectiveness will be:
      1. Reduced incident reporting

(continued on next page)

Figure 9-2.   (Continued)

2.   Downward trends in critical events statistics
3.   Reduction of patient complaints
4.   Review of major problem resolution

_____   _____
Executive Director   Chairperson, Board of Trustees

_____
Chief of Staff

_____
Date

Attachment 1
Critical Events Monitoring

Objective

The intent of this monitoring system is to identify potential problem areas and trends. As trends develop, specific critical events will be assessed to identify specific problems and determine solutions.

Definition

A critical event is defined as:

1.   All second admissions on the same audit to a critical care unit
2.   All admissions to the critical care unit from the floor
3.   All second surgeries during the same hospitalization
4.   All readmissions with same diagnosis within one month (excluding cancer)
5.   All hospital-acquired infections
6.   All discharges against medical advice
7.   All drug reactions
8.   Patient accidents

Process

1.   The medical records coders will code these critical events.
2.   Each month a trend report will be presented to the quality assurance committee for review and follow-up.
3.   Formal assessments may be developed from this information.
4.   All information regarding critical events will be kept in the office of the director of quality assurance, and only those who have the authorization of the director will have access to the information.

Source: Reprinted from *Risk Management: A Guide for Health Care Professionals* by J. F. Monagle, pp. 76–79, with permission of Aspen Publishers, Inc. © 1985.

☐ Relationship between Quality Assurance and Risk Management

Quality assurance and risk management are not the same set of activities, but they do have similarities. The risk management process of identification, analysis, treatment, and evaluation looks very much like the quality assurance process described in the previous section. To be effective, both must address the greatest risk that exists in a health care facility—the risk of patient injury. Both quality assurance and risk management serve risk-prevention functions; if care can be improved, some injuries that give rise to claims can be prevented. It seems logical then to have quality assurance and risk management functions work closely to identify and resolve problems that could lead to financial loss for the institution and individual providers.

In some institutions, quality assurance and risk management do not routinely work together and, as a result, monitoring functions may be duplicated and important information overlooked. The different origins of the two programs may account for some of this lack of integration. In the mid-1970s, the Joint Commission began to encourage health care facilities, primarily hospitals, to formalize the process of reviewing and improving the care rendered by a variety of health care providers. Hospital employees (usually those with clinical experience, such as nurses) were designated to develop and maintain review systems that included considerable documentation of the process. It is only recently that the Joint Commission has developed risk management standards as an extension of the original quality assurance standards and narrowly defined the aspects of the risk management process that they survey during the accreditation process—that is, the risk of patient injury.

Risk management, on the other hand, was transplanted from industry by way of commercial insurers who, in addition to selling insurance, provided some risk-prevention services to client hospitals to help them prevent occurrences, hence reducing the insurance company's payout. If institutions had their own risk managers in the mid-1970s, they usually were safety engineers rather than personnel involved directly with patient care. When programs "grew up" separately, there was little sharing of information.

Quality assurance and risk management functions do not overlap in all areas. Figure 9-3 illustrates the relationship.[6] The area of circle unique to risk management with some, but minimal, effect on quality assurance contains such functions as risk financing, employee benefits, and general liability issues. The greatest area of overlap involves the sharing of data between quality assurance and risk management—the problem identification functions.

Current wisdom in the field, reflected in the Joint Commission's risk management standards, acknowledges that although quality assurance and risk management are not the same function, both can benefit from cooperative efforts. However, there has been some confusion and discomfort on the part of both quality assurance and risk management with the term *integration*. For some professionals on both sides, integration means that one function envelops and subsumes the other—a circumstance that would not be in the best interest of either function. In an effort to avoid such territorial struggles, the Joint Commission uses the term *operational linkages* to describe the working arrangement between quality assurance and risk management.

Operational linkages is a term that is vague enough to allow for a variety of organizational models, reporting relationships, and data flow. For example, one model used by a number of hospitals has both the risk manager and the quality assurance director

Figure 9-3.   Risk Management and Quality Assurance Overlap

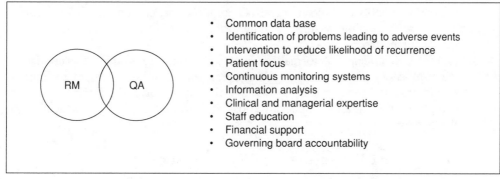

- Common data base
- Identification of problems leading to adverse events
- Intervention to reduce likelihood of recurrence
- Patient focus
- Continuous monitoring systems
- Information analysis
- Clinical and managerial expertise
- Staff education
- Financial support
- Governing board accountability

Source: Reprinted, with permission, from Kibbee, P. *Quality Assurance, Utilization, and Risk Management, 1989.* Deerfield, IL: National Association of Quality Assurance Professionals, 1989, p. 58.

reporting to the CEO or to another administrative person. In another model, the quality assurance director reports to the medical director and the risk manager reports to the CEO. Data flow between the two functions is shown on an organizational chart and described in the quality assurance/risk management plan. Yet another model has the functions of quality assurance and risk management directed by one individual who reports to the CEO. Clearly, the model should be based on what will best enable the available personnel to perform the functions in the most effective manner.

Quality Assurance Enhancing Risk Management

The following list summarizes the ways in which quality assurance activities can most benefit the risk management function in health care institutions:

1. *Data sharing.* Data generated on patient care issues and provider performance are important to the risk management process. The problem-identification function of a quality assurance program may be the most important component for loss-prevention and loss-control efforts. The biggest losses in health care involve patient injuries and provider performance. Data sharing between quality assurance and risk management, mandated by the Joint Commission, can be accomplished in several ways. If the structure of the quality assurance program provides for a central collection of data, whether it be for quality assurance, utilization review, or risk management purposes, it is easy to direct the potential liability issues directly to the risk manager. Data can be conveyed by physician-specific reports, departmental reports, minutes of peer review bodies containing quality/potential liability issues, or summary reports that include results of all monitoring done within a particular time period. It is important that quality assurance personnel and risk managers be cognizant of applicable state statutes involving discoverability of peer review data and design procedures that will afford the data the necessary protection from discovery.
2. *Framework.* Quality assurance programs in hospitals were established before risk management programs. Until the mid-1970s, many hospitals were commercially insured for professional liability, and risk management services were often provided by consultants from the insurance company. The emphasis was usually on the environmental safety losses. It was only when health care institutions were forced to enter into other insurance arrangements, such as self-insurance, that internal risk management programs were strengthened and become more clinically focused to address the risks that provider performance could bring to bear on the financial resources of the institution. Because quality assurance programs are concerned with the identification and resolution of problems in patient care, they can provide a framework, at least, for the clinical aspects of a health care risk management program.
3. *Physician support.* Quality assurance by necessity and design has had at least some physician support. An effective risk management program must have physician support to identify and resolve areas of high risk of patient injury. Working cooperatively with quality assurance may bring more physician support to risk management.
4. *Requirement fulfillment.* A formalized quality assurance program fulfills an increasing number of regulatory and accrediting requirements. There is risk to the financial and intangible (public relations) assets of the institution if the institution fails to comply with standards (especially those affecting quality of care issues) set by the regulators.

Risk Management Enhancing Quality Assurance

The hospital's risk management program can enhance the quality assurance program in the following ways:

1. *Physician motivation.* The risk management function may give the physicians more motivation to address the difficult problems identified through the quality assurance process. Although physicians are sensitive to quality issues, they may be more motivated to change particular behaviors and may respond more quickly when dollar loss and loss of reputation are real possibilities.

2. *Data sharing.* The risk manager will be able to give the quality assurance function some specific data about what needs to be monitored. For example, the risk manager may provide excellent data showing that claims have been brought in the past year regarding informed consent for a particular surgical procedure. A quality assurance monitor of the informed-consent process (perhaps performed by quality assurance personnel during record review for another monitor) may reveal a more extensive problem or may pinpoint one physician as having difficulty in that area. Every problem addressed jointly and resolved lends credibility to both the quality assurance and risk management processes.

3. *Policy assessment.* The risk management programs can be a check on whether policies and procedures are realistic. Claims data or incident-reporting data may reveal that some policies and procedures are rarely followed and, as a result, that the institution is putting itself at risk by having policies that cannot or will not be followed. For example, if hospital policy specifies that only physicians can change ventilation settings, but in reality nurses routinely change them, a potential liability situation is created. If it is appropriate for nurses to perform that task under specific circumstances, the policy should reflect that information. Quality assurance and risk management can work together with the care givers involved to create more reasonable policies that can be followed without compromising the quality of patient care.

4. *Bridge with safety programs.* The risk management program can be a bridge between the quality assurance functions and the safety functions. The Joint Commission's new Plant Technology and Safety Management standard has been rewritten for the 1989 edition of the *Accreditation Manual for Hospitals.*[7] The purpose of the revision seems to be to bring safety back into the quality assurance and risk management systems within health care institutions. The risk management function in many facilities originally was under the supervision of or actually performed by safety personnel. Now safety has once again been recognized as fulfilling an important role in quality assurance and risk management programs—that of providing a safe environment for patients, visitors, and staff.

5. *Team responsibility.* The risk management program can help the quality assurance program to emphasize the team responsibility for quality of care (and therefore, risk reduction) shared by every member of the hospital and medical staff. Quality assurance programs have long been preaching, for very good reason, that achieving and maintaining high-quality care is the responsibility of everyone in an institution. By coordinating efforts with the risk manager, the team effort will be visible and credible.

Putting the Two Programs Together

The benefits to each program of working together have been discussed. The process of creating the "operational linkages," as the Joint Commission recommends, needs to be engineered carefully.

The first step in designing an effective cooperative program should be the somewhat arduous and often-overlooked task of assessing any existing structure or functions or data-collection efforts to see if they can be used to design and maintain a workable, coordinated program. There is no doubt that such a survey will be time-consuming and fairly labor-intensive, but done as a joint quality assurance–risk management effort, the rewards may be worth the effort.

There are several references to help plan and execute a survey of existing quality assurance and risk management activities. Stern and Fox published an article that describes how to determine what data sources are being used, who is collecting and reviewing the data, to whom it is reported, and where it is stored.[8] The results may reveal overlapping responsibilities and services; lack of clear lines of reporting, authority, and accountability; and potential confidentiality problems. They may also reveal some gaps in the information flow and data collection that the risk manager may be able to fill.

The survey process may also send the message to hospital administration, medical staff leadership, hospital employees, and the governing body that the motivation for coordination of all risk identification and resolution activities has never been greater. The Joint Commission's risk management standards recommend such coordination of effort, some state licensing boards require it, and some insurance companies look for it at premium-setting time. Coordination of effort in the quality assurance/risk management area can also demonstrate a willingness to avoid duplication of effort and additional expenditure for personnel—a message that will certainly please administration in this time of cost containment. Coordination of effort, especially the functions associated directly with producing and reviewing sensitive data, can reassure hospitals' legal counsel that the paper flow can be protected as much as possible under existing regulation and legislation.

One welcome byproduct of effective coordination of the quality assurance and risk management functions directly involves the medical staff: a well-coordinated program can save providers' time. If data are collected efficiently, reviewed properly, and presented coherently, practitioners' time can be devoted to the tasks most suited to their expertise—making appropriate clinical judgments that enhance the quality of patient care.

By far, the greatest benefits of a coordinated quality assurance/risk management program to a health care facility are the enhancement and increased efficiency of all functions involved. Duplication can be eliminated, the medical staff–administration gap can be bridged, the governing board can get better data on actual problem resolution, and compliance with accrediting and regulatory bodies can be demonstrated.

References

1. Kibbee, P. *Quality Assurance, Utilization, and Risk Management, 1989.* Deerfield, IL: National Association of Quality Assurance Professionals, 1989, p. 1.

2. Joint Commission on Accreditation of Healthcare Organizations. *Accreditation Manual for Hospitals.* Chicago: JCAHO, 1990, p. 211.

3. Kibbee, p. 1.

4. Lee, E. A. Risk identification strategies in hospitals. In: B. J. Youngberg, editor. *Essentials of Hospital Risk Management.* Rockville, MD: Aspen Publishers, 1989, p. 47.

5. Monagle, J. F. *Risk Management: A Guide for Health Care Professionals.* Rockville, MD: Aspen Publishers, 1985, pp. 76–79.

6. Kibbee, p. 58.

7. Joint Commission on Accreditation of Healthcare Organizations.

8. Sterns, G., and Fox, L. A. Assessing quality assurance and risk management activities: a profile analysis. *Quality Review Bulletin* 5(10):26–29, Oct. 1979.

☐ Bibliography

Longo, D. R., Ciccone, K. R., and Lord, J. T. *Integrated Quality Assessment: A Model for Concurrent Review.* Chicago: American Hospital Publishing, 1989.

Meisenheimer, C. G., editor. *Quality Assurance: A Complete Guide to Effective Programs.* Rockville, MD: Aspen Publishers, 1985.

Rowland, H. S., and Rowland, B. L., editors. *Hospital Quality Assurance Manual.* Rockville, MD: Aspen Publishers. Looseleaf manual updated annually.

Troyer, G. T., and Salman, S. L., editors. *Handbook of Healthcare Risk Management.* Rockville, MD: Aspen Publishers, 1986.

Chapter 10
Related Committees and Programs

Ann Helm

Health care risk management is intricately related to the processes, goals, and activities of many committees and programs in health care settings, in addition to the quality assurance function described in the preceding chapter. Those various committees and programs are essential to an effective and integrated risk management program; an apt analogy would be with a wheel, with risk management as the hub and the various committees and programs as spokes.

This chapter describes some of those related committees and programs; they can vary greatly, depending on the type of health care facility. The core group would most likely consist of pharmacy and therapeutics review, infection control, tissue committee, blood usage review, medical records review, morbidity and mortality review, credentials and privileges review, utilization review, and discharge planning.

☐ Pharmacy and Therapeutics Review

The review of pharmacy and therapeutics can be done either by an individual or by a committee. It usually is done by an interdisciplinary committee whose membership includes physicians, nurses, and pharmacists. The committee has three major responsibilities: (1) drug utilization review, including developing physician profiles and assessing the efficacy of drug therapy for particular patients; (2) formulary or cost reviews; and (3) review of all adverse drug reactions of patients, including allergic reactions and drug contraindication. The drug-utilization–review process assesses the efficiency, cost, and efficacy of particular drugs. Usually a high-use and/or high-cost drug is reviewed. Potentially risky drugs, such as warfarin, are also reviewed because of the potential for complications.

The committee serves in an advisory capacity to the pharmacy, medical staff, and nursing departments, monitoring prescribing, dispensing, and administering practices. This function, particularly the adverse-drug-reaction review, is a risk management activity that can identify, trend, and respond to drug-related patient occurrences.

The committee may also review medication errors that occurred during the month, again identifying trends by the nurse or individual who administered the drug, the order, the reactions, the time of day, the ward, and so forth, for appropriate follow-up. This information may then be given to the hospital's risk management or quality assurance committee.

The risk manager's role with this committee, as with many others, is to ensure that this information is given to and coordinated among the appropriate staff members in the facility.

Even in health care settings with a small patient population, there may be a large number of prescriptions because patients may have many prescriptions from more than one physician. Computerized drug profiles can help the pharmacy and therapeutics function by identifying synergistic and contraindicated agents, including potentially dangerous over-the-counter remedies.

☐ Infection Control

This function includes the surveillance, prevention, and control of infections of patients, employees, and volunteers in the health care setting. Infection control also monitors employee infections and provides educational programs for staff and patients. A large facility may have one or more full-time nurses to monitor infections, or it may have a physician epidemiologist. In small facilities, the infection control nurse may also be the employee health nurse. Effective infection control can prevent the spread of minor to life-threatening infections in patients and staff. The process involves the entire health care setting, from the emergency department, operating room, and patient rooms to the kitchen and biological-waste area. Activities that minimize infection involve the clinical staff, dietetics, pharmacy, laundry, housekeeping, supply and distribution, engineering, and administration.

The risk manager must see that strict infection control policies are in place and enforced in order to prevent employee infections. Not only do employee infections endanger patients and hospital personnel, but employees who acquire a disease on the job qualify for workers' compensation if they can show that they abided by the established policies.

The reporting of infectious disease must adhere to confidentiality laws and policies to minimize additional risks to patients, staff, and the facility. The staff is entitled to confidentiality, just as the patients are.

☐ Tissue Committee

This activity determines whether tissue or an organ was unnecessarily removed; the physician may have believed it to be cancerous when in fact it was not. The tissue committee (typically consisting of several surgeons, one or more pathologists, and the risk manager) reviews the pathologist's reports of tissue taken during surgeries and autopsies. When the pathologist's report does not agree with the surgeon's presurgery diagnosis, the risk manager should ensure that there is appropriate follow-up in the surgery department and with the medical staff.

The tissue committee's review includes inpatients and outpatients and cases with both tissue and nontissue specimens submitted for review, and it feeds into medical staff peer review. The review can assess whether procedures are being performed by practitioners with appropriate privileges for those procedures.

Trends or patterns of inappropriate surgery may be identified. If they are, the risk manager or quality assurance director should initiate a focused evaluation of either a particular procedure or of a physician's practice patterns.

Autopsies can identify unsuspected conditions, assess the effectiveness of therapeutic measures and the thoroughness of patient care, and confirm or identify the cause of death. They can also ascertain whether certain procedures or hospital or physician practices contributed to death. That information can reduce risks to other patients and can provide information about genetic or contagious disease to staff and families.

☐ Blood Usage or Transfusion Review

This function monitors all blood or blood component usage for appropriateness of clinical indications, accuracy of cross-match and appropriate administration, untoward reactions, contraindications, errors, safe storage and transfer, and ratios of ordered to used blood. Variations from predetermined criteria are reviewed for justification by clinical circumstances. All departments that order blood components are included in the review, including ambulatory surgery and the emergency department. Members of the blood usage committee include a pathologist, a surgeon, one or more nurses, a blood bank staff/supervisor, and other physicians. The Joint Commission mandates specific blood reviews, as do other accrediting bodies, such as the College of American Pathologists.

The committee's risk management function is to prevent inappropriate administration of blood or blood components, untoward reactions, and inappropriate utilization of this scarce resource. Physician-profile information on blood-ordering practices is given to the quality assurance department. The committee will thoroughly review any blood transfusion error, from labeling to administration, and assess the patient's reactions. Corrective efforts should be made immediately to prevent repeat errors. This committee may be involved with the national "look-back" program, which attempts to identify recipients of blood donated by someone who later tested positive for AIDS or AIDS-related complex.

☐ Medical Records Review

The members of this committee include physicians, nurses, medical records technicians, and other record users. This committee reviews medical records to determine whether they are being completed within the time frame established by the medical staff bylaws. The review also monitors the access, security, and confidentiality of records. Clinical information is extrapolated to assist with peer review functions, including documentation of house staff supervision, appropriate workup, treatment, and outcomes of patient care. Thoroughness of the record is reviewed, as well as appropriate filing in the chart for quick retrieval. Key components, such as patient consent forms, autopsy reports, operative reports, and medication sheets, are assessed for completeness of the record. The Joint Commission requirements for medical records review, follow-up, and reporting to the medical staff are very specific. Objective review of the record can help identify iatrogenic events, unreported incidents, unnecessary procedures, or excessive or inappropriate lengths of stay.

One source has stated, "Medical liability experts estimate that 35 to 40 percent of all medical malpractice suits are rendered indefensible by problems with the medical record".[1] For that reason, ensuring that there is an ongoing review of the facility's medical records is a key element of a successful risk management program.

☐ Morbidity and Mortality Review

Morbidity is defined as an undesired and/or unexpected complication; *mortality* is death (usually unexpected). Morbidity and mortality conferences are held in the various medical departments, including medicine, surgery, neurology, and psychiatry. Departmental morbidity and mortality conferences can identify facilitywide opportunities to improve patient care, including such issues as timeliness of treatment; appropriate choice of treatment; accuracy of diagnosis; adequacy of skill, judgment, or performance;

functioning of equipment; and responses to medications. Physician-specific information can then be put into physician profiles for reprivileging. Departmental trends can be developed using morbidity and mortality information. Morbidity and mortality conferences are the essence of peer review if agreed-upon criteria and standards are developed at the outset. The risk manager should ensure appropriate follow-up with physicians, such as counseling, education, restriction of privileges, and changes in procedures.

☐ Credentials and Privileges Review

Quality assurance activities and the many reviews discussed in this chapter provide information for the credentialing and privileging process. Initial confirmation of professional credentials protects the facility against the risks involved in allowing imposters to gain medical staff privileges. This review includes obtaining documents from the physician; communicating directly with educational institutions, certifying boards, previous employers, and hospitals where medical staff appointment previously was held; contacting references; and gathering information about current and prior malpractice insurance carriers. Not infrequently, this review will identify physicians who have privileges for procedures that they have not performed for years. As part of the privilege-renewal process, there is a comprehensive review of the physician's blood usage patterns, infection rates, prescriptive patterns, lengths of stay, complications, tissue and diagnostic agreement, medical record documentation, closed malpractice claims, patient and family complaints, and departmental quality assurance monitors.

☐ Utilization Review

This function assesses how efficiently resources are used in the facility. Because both over- and underutilization can expose patients to many unnecessary risks, the utilization review process is an integral component of the risk management program.

The utilization review process reviews lengths of stay against preestablished criteria for severity of illness or intensity of service. It also reviews unnecessary or delayed procedures, duplicative efforts, and unnecessary inpatient admissions. Premature discharge can result in accidents at home, burdens to care givers in the home, and other complications. On the other hand, unnecessary days in the hospital dramatically increase the incidence of falls, hospital-acquired infections, unnecessary and inherently risky tests, pneumonia, and loss of mobility. Utilization review develops physician profiles of utilization practices; those profiles are assessed when renewal of privileges occurs.

☐ Discharge Planning

This function is closely related to utilization review in that it strives to ensure timely discharge, prevent unscheduled readmissions and postdischarge complications, and provide appropriate patient education through the coordinated efforts of many providers, including medical staff, nursing, pharmacy, rehabilitation, dietetics, and home-based care. Discharge planners not only must have a thorough knowledge of the hospital, but also a realistic knowledge of the patient's home environment and resources. A particularly challenging aspect of this activity is locating appropriate placement in a timely fashion.

☐ Other Committees, Programs, and Functions

The following additional programs may exist, depending on the scope of services provided by the facility.

Product Standards Review: Biomedical and Other Equipment

This program reviews requests to purchase new equipment and the performance of equipment already owned. The hospital can minimize its exposure to product liability claims through the effective monitoring of biomedical equipment. In most institutions, the biomedical division of the maintenance department evaluates biomedical equipment. Timely acquisition of state-of-the-art equipment and adequate maintenance are key elements of a safe environment. Some facilities have computerized systems that keep detailed maintenance records for selected, if not all, pieces of biomedical equipment. Repair trends can pinpoint vulnerable pieces of equipment.

The product standards function reviews more than just biomedical equipment; it also reviews other kinds of equipment and supplies used in the hospital. The function strives to standardize those items so that the hospital can get the most efficient use of resources in the most cost-effective way and so that personnel do not have to become familiar with a variety of vendors and the uniqueness of each different brand. An additional component of a product standards program is a reliable staff education effort to ensure that equipment is used correctly.

Radiation Safety Committee

This committee reviews the diagnostic, therapeutic, and research application of radioactive substances and, as indicated, establishes a radiation safety program for patients and staff in accordance with guidelines set by the Nuclear Regulatory Commission. Evaluation of radiation exposure against preestablished criteria can reduce the likelihood that patient and staff will be overexposed. The functions of this committee include reviewing the calibration of equipment and the disposition of waste and evaluating new equipment or proposed purchases and employee exposure to radiation. Members of this committee typically include the safety manager, the risk manager, nurses, a radiation physicist or radiation safety officer, and physicians.

Laser Committee

This committee reviews the use of laser equipment, including privileging of physicians for using such equipment. Its activities include monitoring for clinically indicated use and complications and providing educational programs to ensure patient and staff safety. Because laser usage is extremely sophisticated, physicians typically are privileged to use a specific type of laser and must seek expanded privileges for other types of lasers.

Emergency Preparedness Committee

This committee assesses the medical readiness of the facility to respond to emergency situations in the community, including internal disasters and loss of services. Through this process, treatment for victims of such disasters as hurricanes, floods, and civil disasters can be done efficiently by planning, coordination, and trial exercises.

The facility should have several practice exercises to familiarize the staff with the speedy and safe evacuation of the premises in the event of fire, earthquake, flood, civil disaster, tornado, hurricane, or even volcano eruption. This requires a community effort for the citywide coordination of available beds and staff.

AIDS Programs

Some facilities have established AIDS committees or programs to review care and risks associated with AIDS. This can clearly serve a risk management function, given the risks associated with detection, appropriate treatment, confidentiality, and reporting of AIDS. The AIDS programs are closely related to infection control, patient education, and employee wellness functions.

Bioethics Committee

Not all hospitals have a bioethics committee, although the number is growing quickly. This committee typically serves three areas: staff education, policy development, and case consults. *Bioethics* includes the ethical and clinical dimensions of complex and uncertain arenas, such as informed consent and refusal, organ transplantation, surrogate decision making, do-not-resuscitate orders, withdrawal or withholding of life support, living wills, scarce resources, confidentiality, and the duty to warn third parties.

Goals usually include enhancing an effective physician–patient relationship, ascertaining the patient's wishes, and, if necessary, reconciling those desires with futile treatment while respecting patient self-determination. Issues brought to a bioethics committee may range from withholding scarce resources to reports of provider incompetency; recent issues have included arguments for and against active euthanasia. The role of the bioethics committee is intimately related to risk management. Before difficult decisions are made regarding termination of treatment, the perceptions of people in a variety of disciplines are shared. Such a process also is recommended by many court decisions, as well as by a presidential commission.[2]

Public Relations Department

This function is closely associated with marketing and should be monitored by risk management for exposures generated through information released by the public relations department. Close and frequent communication between the risk management and public relations departments can minimize risks to the facility associated with the rushed release of inaccurate, incomplete, or confidential material. Risk managers should also review advertisements for elements that could be construed as guarantees.

Patient Representative

This function promotes physician–patient communication, resolves patient complaints (thereby preventing or reducing the likelihood of litigation), and markets the facility. The patient representative identifies many imminent and potential risks through contact with patients, families, and staff.

This position can provide much data that the risk manager can use to identify or confirm areas of concern. Tabulating the information gathered by the patient representative can provide a baseline against which the facility's ability to resolve patient concerns can be measured. Some studies have indicated that using a patient representative to facilitate provider–patient communication can help prevent malpractice claims. The patient representative may be the first to identify risk to the patient and/or institution; for instance, the patient may report to the representative that he or she is having difficulty in getting the physician to answer questions. The risk manager or patient representative can follow up with the physician to resolve the problem before the patient becomes angry enough to find reason to bring a claim.

Employee Wellness Program

An effective employee wellness program can enhance the delivery of patient care. For example, if staffing is reduced because of a high incidence of employee injuries or illnesses, patient care will suffer. If morale is low for any variety of reasons, patient care may also suffer. If employees have low resistance to disease and/or lack knowledge regarding general job safety, communicable disease, or safe use of equipment, they are at risk for illnesses, some of which could be transmitted to patients. An effective employee wellness program can help to avert these situations. It can also help prevent provider burnout and occupational stress. The initiation of an employee wellness or fitness program is an indication of management's concern for its employees.

Some facilities have introduced special "value added" programs that strive to promote not only a healthy and energetic work force, but also positive attitudes, sensitivity toward patients and staff, and true caring. The axiom that employees treat patients as supervisors treat employees gives special significance to "value added" and employee wellness programs.

Research and Development/Human Studies Review

Typically referred to as the institutional review board, this function reviews human research proposals for compliance with specific regulations of the Food and Drug Administration and the U.S. Department of Health and Human Services to ensure safe research in the institutional setting. These regulations mandate close scrutiny of experimental drugs and therapies; they may be complemented by local and state regulations. The federal regulations contain preestablished standards to ensure appropriate protocol, informed consent, timely review of the research, release of validated findings, and approval from other areas, such as the radiation safety committee, the laser committee, or animal studies groups. This provides a crucial check-and-balance system to prevent an overzealous researcher from losing sight of the patient's best interests.

Education Committee

This committee serves, among other functions, as a resource to the risk manager when other committees have identified the need for staff or patient education. The education committee is in a unique position to develop training in areas identified by other committees, ranging from safe lifting techniques and stress management to dealing with ethical dilemmas. The risk manager may propose topics to the committee. The presentations may be for clinical staff or may be facilitywide.

Behavioral Committees

Some facilities have other functions or committees unique to their setting or patient population.

Behavioral Emergency Committee
The Portland Veterans Administration Medical Center has a behavioral emergency committee,[3] which identifies patients who are known to be potentially violent to themselves or other patients or staff. The hospital computer flags those patients as a precautionary warning to admissions clerks and health care providers. The committee has developed a training program to assist staff members in identifying safe approaches to dealing with this population. All staff members can report episodes of significant violent behavior on a special form to the quality assurance office. The committee reviews, trends, analyzes, and monitors this population to recommend appropriate preventive measures.

Drug-Seeking Behavior Committee
A similar process is in place with the drug-seeking behavior committee, which identifies patients who seek or obtain habituating drugs from physicians in the facility, outpatient clinic, nursing home, other Veterans Administration medical centers, or the private sector. This activity also flags the patient population to alert providers and the pharmacy department. The process has become an actual component of therapy and is a risk

management activity that prevents accidental and intentional overdoses and potential illicit drug traffic to third parties. It also serves as a monitor of prescribing practices.

References

1. Rasinski, D. G. *Risk Management in Practice.* Publication No. 353 RSM 4/84. Washington, DC: American Society of Internal Medicine, 1982.

2. *Deciding to Forego Life-Sustaining Treatment.* President's Commission for the Study of Ethical Problems in Medicine and Biomedical and Behavioral Research. Washington, DC: U.S. Government Printing Office, Mar. 1983, pp. 153-70.

3. Sparr, L. F., Drummond, D. J., and Hamilton, N. G. Managing violent patient incidents: the role of a behavioral emergency committee. *Quality Review Bulletin* 14(5):147-53, May 1988.

Chapter 11

Hospital Safety and Security

Leilani Kicklighter

If hospitals are to survive the demands of government and business for lower-cost health care, they must reduce costs while delivering high-quality patient care. One way to do that is with a well-structured, well-administered safety program. Such a program can prevent the loss of physical assets and reduce loss resulting from work-related injury or illness.

An added benefit of good safety performance is the positive effect that control of employee incidents can have on staffing. When employees are not able to work because of occupational injuries or illnesses, they must be replaced in order to maintain adequate staffing levels, which places an added burden on supervisors and employees. Safe working conditions and procedures contribute significantly to a reduction in employee absences resulting from workplace injuries and illnesses.

From a business standpoint, a safety program contributes toward conservation of financial resources. The frequency and severity of accidents, injuries, and occupational disease affect workers' compensation insurance premiums. By controlling the number of employee incidents and illnesses, a health care facility reduces its cost of insurance through improved experience modification rates, which lowers premiums. As an employer, every health care facility is mandated by federal and state law and private accrediting agencies to develop and implement an employee safety program, the goal of which is to provide safe working conditions and procedures for all employees. Although all the states had passed worker's compensation laws by 1948, it was not until 1970 that Congress passed Public Law 91-596, known as the Occupational Safety and Health Act. The agency charged with implementing the legislation is the Occupational Safety and Health Administration (OSHA).

Every employer whose business "affects commerce" is subject to OSHA regulations. A business "affects commerce" if any of the tools, equipment, materials, or devices used in it were manufactured in another state. Employers are subject to either civil or criminal sanctions for OSHA violations.

In addition, the Joint Commission on Accreditation of Healthcare Organizations requires hospitals to have "a safety management program that is designed to provide a physical environment free of hazards and to manage staff activities to reduce the risk of human injury."[1] That program is to include "a system for reporting and investigating all incidents that involve patient, personnel, or visitor injury, occupational illness, or property damage."[2] In addition, the hospital's governing body is to strive to ensure "a safe environment for patients, personnel, and visitors by requiring and supporting the establishment and maintenance of an effective safety management program,"[3] and there shall be "the provision of employee health services. . . ."[4]

☐ Function of an Employee Health Program

An employee health program is a strategic component of an effective safety program. The hospital may be able to realize substantial savings and generate employee goodwill by having programs that enhance employee health.

Health education, wellness promotion, preplacement medical examinations, and initial treatment and follow-up of occupational injuries and illnesses are the basics of an employee health program. Health care facilities increasingly are staffing their employee health offices (EHOs) with advanced registered nurse practitioners (ARNPs), a practice that can result in cost savings. By diagnosing and treating certain injuries and illnesses, ARNPs can reduce the need for the more costly services of physicians.

An EHO staffed with an ARNP can provide routine immunizations; perform scheduled preplacement and other medical examinations; screen and refer non–job-related injuries and illnesses; evaluate, treat, or refer job-related injuries and illnesses; and monitor the care and rehabilitation of employees who have suffered job-related injuries or illnesses that resulted in time lost from work.

Through such a program, the institution can stay in contact with the employee and, when appropriate, bring the employee back to work in a capacity that is physically compatible with his or her job-related functions. Maintaining contact with the employee and the appropriate physician to monitor the employee's recuperation assists in planning the need for additional or substitute personnel or reassignment of duties.

The employee health records kept in the EHO are valuable sources of information on the frequency and severity of injuries suffered by individual employees. Administration may address the problem of repetitive "accidents" through counseling or retraining.

☐ Safety Programs and Insurance and Workers' Compensation

The premium for the institution's workers' compensation insurance policy is calculated by a formula set by each state. An individual business's "modification factor" is used in the calculations. The modification factor is based on experience—the frequency and severity of employee injuries and illnesses that occurred during the previous policy period. Therefore, the insurance premium is directly affected by an effective safety program coupled with an aggressive employee health program to prevent and control employee occupational accidents and illnesses.

☐ One Hospital's Safety and Security Program

Guidelines for developing and maintaining a hospital safety program are set forth in the following model. Such factors as size, range of services, number of employees, and management structure, among others, affect how a safety program is set up; this program is one example. The commitment and involvement of management, supervisors, and employees provide the necessary ingredients for the success of the program.

Policy

A highly visible program shall be established throughout the hospital to emphasize and maintain safety and security practices as they relate to patients, medical staff, employees, visitors, equipment, and property on an ongoing basis. Additionally, this program will be concerned with loss control and the prevention of incidents that relate to safety and security. This program will be coordinated with, and an integral component of, the overall risk management program.

Methods of Implementation

The Safety and Security Committee membership shall be constituted according to the guidelines outlined in the Joint Commission Standards for Functional Safety and Sanitation. This committee will meet at least monthly—more often when the agenda shows that problems need to be addressed in a more timely fashion. The institution's board will review and approve annually a resolution granting the safety committee the authority to act in the event of an emergency. The committee operates as follows:

- The chair of the Safety and Security Committee will be appointed by the executive director of the hospital. The chair will be responsible for setting the agenda of the meetings and for monitoring to ensure implementation of the actions taken by the committee.
- The Safety and Security Committee will determine the safety and security in-service program. That is, if a problem is recognized as relating to particular departments or groups of employees, programs addressing that problem will be developed and presented for those employees.
- As necessary, the chair may assign individuals or ad hoc committees to investigate or more thoroughly analyze identified problems and charge them with reporting back to the committee.
- On an ongoing basis, the committee shall be kept abreast of all new and modified standards, statutes, and regulations that affect the safety and security programs.
- As necessary, the committee will use the expertise in the community, state, and nation to supply references, ideas, or in-service programs when available and pertinent.
- The risk manager or safety officer will serve as administrative staff to the committee and work closely with the chair, with input from the safety and security officer(s).
- The minutes of the committee meetings will be forwarded to the executive director, administrative management group, and executive medical staff committee for information and/or action on pertinent points, as necessary.

Safety Officer Functions

The functions of the safety officer are:

- To monitor employee injuries in a timely fashion by implementing and maintaining a log of all employee injuries by individual, pay classification, unit or department, summary of incident, contributory negligence or determination of cause of incident, and time lost to date.
- To analyze employee injuries and provide information to the divisions, units, and departments involved so that they can implement programs to resolve identified problems.
- To investigate all employee injuries, including viewing the site of the accident and interviewing the employee and witnesses involved and devise prevention strategies or educational programs.
- To develop a method to track and trend an individual employee's accident record and to provide any necessary counseling and retraining through the appropriate department head.

- To maintain a working relationship with the state workers' compensation offices.
- To be knowledgeable in the field of safety as it relates to medical institutions and as required by the Joint Commission, the applicable state hospital licensing agencies, OSHA, and other applicable federal, state, and local regulations.
- To make routine monthly rounds of all nursing units and other hospital departments to view each area for potential safety-related problems. Recommendations resulting from those surveillance rounds will be documented and referred to the appropriate director of the area for implementation within 10 days (or for feedback to the safety officer as to why implementation is not feasible at the time).
- To ensure that fire drills are held on a timely basis in each nursing unit and hospital department and that appropriate documentation is provided.
- To maintain adequate documentation of safety education programs to comply with Joint Commission standards, applicable state hospital licensing standards, and OSHA, as well as other federal, state, and local regulations, as required.
- To maintain a close working relationship with the workers' compensation claims-handling agency.
- To keep administration advised of the status of reserves for employee injuries and of payouts for medical expenses and salary reimbursement.
- To facilitate and coordinate identification of all substances governed by the right-to-know regulations, ensure reporting to proper authorities, and maintain all material safety data sheets, in-service programs, and other records.
- To identify hazardous waste in the facility, monitor and evaluate its disposal, and take corrective action, as necessary.

☐ The Hospital Security Program

The goal of the hospital's security program is to provide a safe environment for patients, employees, and visitors, including business invitees. Security officers protect the patients', employees', and visitors' valuables and other property. The presence of narcotics, other controlled substances, and syringes poses an additional burden of surveillance and protection on the security personnel of a health care facility.

☐ Security Program Staffing

The structure of the security program depends on the location of the facility, its management philosophy, and the organization's particular needs. The effectiveness of the security program depends on many variables, one of the most important of which is personnel.

Some organizations choose to contract with an independent agency to provide security personnel. Should the organization choose to contract for security services, the risk manager must review the contract carefully for risk exposure, hold harmless and indemnification clauses, and adequate insurance requirements to make sure that the risks are appropriately transferred. The contract should also require that the security personnel provided by the contractor meet any state statutory guidelines for security personnel and that the security personnel be required to participate in appropriate inservice programs at periodic intervals.

Some organizations augment their security personnel with off-duty law enforcement officers. Even though off-duty law enforcement personnel are governed by their sworn duty to uphold the law, the health care organization employer might have risk exposure if those officers handle their duties differently than the organization wishes. The risk manager must be able to recognize and manage these exposures.

Small or rural health care organizations may not have a security department, either because they are unable to afford such programs or because they do not perceive the need. In such instances, the risk manager can develop relations with the local law enforcement agency so as to enhance the visibility of its officers and vehicles on the hospital's grounds. For emergencies, a "hot line" or "panic button" system connected directly to the law enforcement agency can be installed. Free coffee and pastries, particularly on the late-evening and night shifts, made available in the emergency room and other strategic areas, will encourage visits by law enforcement officers. Their visibility both deters trouble and provides a sense of security for evening- and night-shift personnel.

In instances where there is no separate security department, the staff of the entire organization will need to assume responsibility for being observant and protective of patients, visitors, and property.

☐ Functions and Activities of the Hospital Security Program

Whether the security program is in-house or is provided by a contract service, certain functions are to be performed by the person who is accountable for the institution's security. These are as follows:

- To establish a system for surveillance throughout the facility on all shifts and on all days of the week so that areas will be monitored to prevent bodily harm and loss or damage of property
- To devise and implement a system for prompt reporting of all losses of or damage to property and to implement corrective or preventive action
- To monitor unauthorized ingress to and egress from the facility
- To provide support personnel to subdue patients who may cause harm to themselves, others, or property
- To develop and implement a monitoring system to prevent loss of hospital supplies and equipment
- To develop and implement inservice programs to enhance employee sensitivity to security problems and teach employees how to act in specific situations
- To maintain appropriate documentation to ensure compliance with Joint Commission standards, applicable state hospital licensing regulations, and OSHA and other federal, state, and local regulations, as required
- To develop and maintain a working relationship with all applicable law enforcement agencies
- To maintain current knowledge, theoretical and practical, so as to conduct a program and manage a staff with the ability to respond and interact appropriately in any situation that threatens people or property
- To provide to the safety and security committee monthly reports of incidents and recommend appropriate correction or prevention

Use of Weapons

If security personnel use guns, nightsticks, KEL/MAG lights, stun guns, or handcuffs, they need additional training in the use of those weapons. The security director and the risk manager should establish guidelines for who may carry weapons, circumstances for the use of weapons, and training for each type of weapon. Training guidelines should be the same as for local law enforcement personnel. When use of weapons is permitted, background and character investigation of security personnel is imperative. Other issues to be decided are policies on weapon inspection, whether the employee owns the weapon, and whether weapons may be carried off the premises when personnel go off duty. Each officer authorized to carry a weapon should be responsible for the care and upkeep of that weapon.

The risk manager should discuss the organization's policy on weapons with the insurance agent/broker or carrier to verify that there is coverage available should a claim arise as a result of the use of such weapons. Endorsements or additional coverage may be needed to provide coverage for such exposures. Some carriers consider use of a weapon to be an intentional tort and exclude such incidents from coverage. The risk manager should evaluate the risk benefit to the organization of the use of weapons and provide that analysis to senior management.

Handling of Arrests or Detention

Some jurisdictions provide that security personnel can be deputized and are able to make arrests. The risk manager who is knowledgeable of those laws can develop policies and procedures regarding the circumstances under which officers should make arrests. The risk manager should be notified, verbally or on an incident report, of any arrests in the facility so that claims of injury from an arrest or allegations of false arrest can be investigated before suit is brought.

Handling of Combative or Disturbed Persons

Security personnel often are called on to assist in handling combative patients and visitors. Staff members have a responsibility, when subduing a patient or visitor, to use care and reasonable force to prevent injury to other patients, staff members, and visitors who may be in the immediate area. All efforts should be made to protect property.

Security personnel and strategic nursing personnel should be trained how to subdue a combative individual using proper technique and without being injured. Evidence of the successful completion of such training should be maintained in the individual's personnel file. Should a claim be asserted against the institution and its personnel for injuries suffered as a result of such handling, evidence thus will be available that the employee was trained to use techniques in keeping with the established policies and procedures to protect the individual and others from harm.

Use of Restraints

Security personnel are often called on to assist in restraining patients and should be trained in the application of both soft and leather restraints. Documentation of attendance at inservice programs on the proper use of restraints should be maintained in the personnel files for reference. Policies regarding restraints should emphasize that restraints are applied only at the direction of nursing or medical personnel.

When security personnel are called on to subdue a patient or visitor, risk management should be made aware either verbally or through an incident report. Whether the risk manager is notified when restraints are applied depends on whether a claim may be brought because of the incident.

Use of Shift Reports

Some security supervisors require security officers to keep a log or shift report that notes all activities, observations, and circumstances that were out of the ordinary during a shift. In addition to the time and date, each entry includes a brief description of the situation, the location, the persons involved, and how the situation was handled. No reference should be made in the log as to whether an incident report was completed.

Patients Who Are Prisoners

Patients who are prisoners pose special problems for security and risk management, especially if the patients are shackled or under police guard. The institution's policies regarding the care of prisoners must be developed in cooperation with area law enforcement agencies. Policies should include the requirement that a key to the prisoner's shackles be accessible to nursing personnel in case of fire or other emergency. The key may be maintained in the narcotic cabinet and accounted for on each shift. When the patient is discharged, the shackle key should be returned to the appropriate law enforcement agency and a receipt should be obtained.

For patients who are not shackled but who are subject to police holds under state or local law, other policies should address how or whether these patients may be discharged.

Patients Who Are in Protective Custody

Patients who are in protective custody pose yet another challenge to security and risk management. These patients should be assigned to rooms that are easy to secure; for example, they should *not* be located near an exit stairwell or an elevator, or on an outside wall by a window if there is a building next door. These patients should not have roommates. Security or police guards, if used, should be posted inside the patient's room, not in the corridor. Consideration might be given to registering the patient under an alias, but all the medical records should reflect the patient's real name after he or she has been discharged.

Loss or Theft of Property

Patients who lose property may bring a claim against the hospital for the lost property and may be more likely to bring a claim for malpractice if an incident occurs. Therefore, developing ways to manage claims for lost property, especially dentures, is an important function of risk management and security departments. The responsibility for investigating lost patient, employee, hospital, and visitor property belongs to the security department. The risk manager is notified when trends are identified, when items of significant value are lost, or if there is criminal activity or negligence on the part of the hospital. Working together, security and risk management can develop and implement appropriate loss control measures.

To assist the security department, the risk manager can provide educational programs to teach the principles of investigation and interviewing. Improper methods of investigation or delay in reporting a loss may result in denial of coverage for a claim.

To manage claims appropriately, the risk manager should develop policies whereby loss of property above a designated amount is reported to the risk manager. The risk manager then determines how to handle the claim. In any case, if reimbursement is appropriate, the risk manager should authorize it. The patient should submit proof of value before any reimbursement is made. The risk manager may decide to replace the item, reimburse the patient for the cost of replacement, or reimburse for its depreciated value. In those instances where the loss or theft is a result of negligence by the facility or staff, the payment should be applied against the budget of the unit that is responsible for the loss or theft. It might be advisable to obtain a release in such situations, too. In some instances, the patient can be advised to file a claim against a homeowner's policy.

Thefts of patient property may be more likely during visiting hours, especially in the obstetrics unit, where patients and visitors frequently leave patient rooms to go to the nursery windows to look at the babies. During those hours, increased rounds by staff and security personnel may serve as a deterrent to theft.

The institution should have policies and procedures for staff to follow for handling patients' valuables and belongings and the property of deceased patients. The hospital's attorney and the risk manager should assist in drafting or reviewing those policies. See figures 11-1 through 11-7 on the following pages for sample policies and procedures and forms for handling lost and found articles, investigating reported losses, and securing patients' valuables.

Figure 11-1.   Policy and Procedure for Investigation of Reports of Loss, Theft, or Damage of Patient's Property or Belongings

Policy

Although Hospital X does not assume responsibility for patients' property or belongings, the security department of Hospital X will investigate any appropriate report of loss, theft, or damage of patient's property or belongings.

Procedure

1. Upon notification by a patient or visitor of loss, theft, or damage of personal property or belongings, the nursing staff shall immediately place a phone call to the security office to notify them of the report.
2. Security personnel will respond in a timely manner to interview the patient, visitors, roommate, and nursing personnel, as appropriate.
3. If security personnel are unable to respond before the end of the shift of notification, the head nurse or nurse completing the report will pass the information to the next shift at the time of shift report.
4. The person investigating will complete a Report of Loss, Theft, or Damage of Personal Property form. The original will be given to the patient, and the copy sent to the security department. (The original report will be needed if the patient makes a claim under his or her homeowner's insurance policy.)
5. A copy of the completed report will be forwarded to the risk management office by the security department.
6. Should the patient request it, the city police department will be called by the security department to complete a police report of loss.
7. An incident report will be completed by nursing personnel and sent directly to the risk management office.

Visitor Control

Visitor control can be another challenge to both risk management and security personnel. Many health care facilities have liberalized their policies on visiting hours. In obstetrical units, the practice of rooming-in by family members means that policies on visiting hours and who may visit may be even more liberal than on other units.

The facility may choose not to monitor visitors during the day and early evening shifts. Some facilities use badges with the date and unit to be visited as a means of identifying visitors.

Access to the facility by outsiders after visiting hours is another challenge and poses a significant exposure to employee and patient safety. One suggestion to control visitors after hours is as follows: After the end of visiting hours is announced, security personnel will make rounds on each patient care unit. Visitors and family members who remain must have doctor's orders allowing them to do so. Those visitors who may not remain will be escorted out by security. Those who are allowed to stay must abide by these rules:

- After-hours visitors will be logged in by security. This log will contain the date; patient's name, unit, and room number; and name of visitor.
- Visitors will be issued a dated stick-on badge with the name of the unit and the room number prominently displayed. Each visitor will be given a list of after-hours visiting rules.
- Visitors must remain on the patient's unit, or in the closest vending machine area or cafeteria. If such visitors are found in any other area, they may be challenged or ejected from the facility.

Because all employees should be required to wear their name badges and all after-hours visitors should be required to wear stick-on badges, unidentified individuals will be readily recognized. Security can then intercede to determine whether the individual is on the property appropriately and handle the situation accordingly. This after-hours visiting procedure can be of great assistance to the late-evening and night nursing staff and can convey a sense of security to night-shift personnel.

Many health care organizations require that vendors have an appointment and a permit issued for that appointment only before they can enter the facility. Stick-on badges that clearly identify the department with which the vendor has an appointment can be used. All vendors should be advised of the appointments-only policy and that violation of that policy will result in termination of visiting privileges.

Preservation of Evidence

When a crime suspect is treated in a hospital, security personnel may need to assist local law enforcement agencies with preserving evidence for the prosecution of that crime. Auto accident victims may have their blood tested for levels of alcohol or controlled substances. Patients may be brought to the facility's emergency department for the removal of bullets and other projectiles or for the removal from body cavities of condoms filled with cocaine or other controlled substances. Law enforcement officers may require that they be allowed to observe the removal and take immediate possession of the removed object. Having policies in place to deal with such issues is advisable. The policies should be developed in cooperation with local law enforcement agencies.

Preserving the chain of custody of the evidence should be part of those policies and procedures. The procedures to maintain the chain of custody should be developed with the assistance and input of the local law enforcement agencies and risk management personnel. In prosecuting crime, law enforcement officers must be able to identify evidence and demonstrate that it has been in continual custody since the crime. Hospital personnel often are an essential link in the chain of custody, particularly when law enforcement officers are not in attendance or when evidence is introduced in places other than the operating room setting.

When the procedures are established, all patient care personnel, including physicians—especially in the emergency department, the operating room, and pathology—should receive inservice education.

Figure 11-2. Report of Loss, Theft, or Damage of Personal Property

Patient's name: _____ Room #: _____
Date of report: _____ Alleged date of loss: _____
Security notified by: _____
Date: _____ Time: _____
Item(s) allegedly lost:

Do not write below this line
_____

(For Security to complete)

Report completed by: _____ Date: _____ Time: _____

(Original to Patient—Copy to Security)

Figure 11-3.   Policy and Procedure for Handling Patients' Valuables or Belongings

---

Policy

Hospital X will not be responsible for any personal property or other belongings of patients admitted unless surrendered to be secured in the hospital safe.

Procedure

A.   Admission

During the admitting procedure, the patient must be given the Patient Valuables Declaration Form (figure 11-6) to sign. The admitting clerk will explain the form to the patient.

If the patient has no valuables/belongings to declare for safekeeping in the hospital safe, the patient will so indicate on the form and sign, with the admitting clerk signing as witness. The patient will be given the carbon copy; the original will be placed in the patient's chart.

Should the patient have valuables/belongings to declare, he or she is encouraged to give such to family members, only if present, for safekeeping. If the patient declines to surrender valuables to accompanying family members, or if none are present, the valuables will be listed item by item (figure 11-4) and placed in a valuables envelope. The patient will be given a carbon copy of the itemized list after signing both copies to validate the listing. The original listing will remain attached to the sealed envelope, which will be placed in the security file in the safe.

The admitting clerk will indicate on the Patient Valuables Declaration Form that the itemized valuables/belongings have been secured in the safe. The patient will also sign the form. The original will be placed in the patient's chart; the carbon will be stapled to the copy of the listing and given to the patient.

If the patient should give the valuables/belongings to an accompanying family member, the name of that individual should be entered on the Patient Valuables Declaration Form, along with a notation that such was done, accompanied by the patient's signature and denial of valuables. The patient will be given the carbon copy and the original will be put in the patient's chart.

All luggage will be identified/tagged in the admitting office. Luggage identification strips should be used.

B.   Nursing Units

When a patient arrives on the nursing unit, nursing personnel must emphasize to the patient and accompanying family members that Hospital X will not be responsible for personal belongings that are not locked in the safe for safekeeping.

Should the patient have eyeglasses, contact lenses, dentures, or a hearing aid that must be kept at the bedside, this must be noted on the nursing admission assessment record. The patient should be provided with the appropriate receptacle (for example, denture cup), if necessary.

C.   Preoperative—To Return to the Same Room

When it is known that a patient is scheduled for surgery, the nursing staff is to provide a plastic valuables bag, in which the patient should pack his or her belongings. This bag should be labeled with the patient's ID label. This packed valuables bag should be sent home with a family member the night before surgery, to be returned when the patient has returned to his or her room.

The nurse's notes should reflect that the patient packed his or her own belongings and to whom they were given.

If the patient is unable to pack his or her own belongings (because of mental or physical impairments), the family member should do the packing. If there are no family members available, but the patient is capable of packing his or her own belongings, the packed bag will be labeled and stapled closed in front of the patient and taken to the personal property room and logged in. The nurse's notes and the personal belongings list (figure 11-5) should reflect this.

Figure 11-3. (Continued)

If the patient is mentally or physically unable to pack his or her belongings and there are no family members available to give the patient's belongings to, two members of the nursing unit staff will pack the valuables bag, listing each item. Both staff members will sign, date, and time the list; the original will go with the chart, and the copy will be given to the patient. The nurse's notes will reflect the names of the individuals who signed the form and the disposition of the bag to either the valuables safe or the personal property room. The packed valuables bag will be stapled shut in the presence of both staff members and the patient.

D.   Preoperative—To Be Transferred from Operating Room

When it is known prior to surgery that the patient is to be transferred from the operating room to another unit (for example, the intensive care unit), the night prior to surgery the patient will pack his or her belongings in a valuables bag. This bag will be given to a family member to take home until the patient is alert and able to have his or her belongings.

In the event that there are no family members with whom to send home the patient's belongings, the bag should be packed by the patient, if he or she is able, and handled as described in C.

If the patient is mentally or physically unable to pack his or her belongings and no family members are available to do so, two members of the nursing staff will do so as described in C.

E.   Transfers—Internal or to Another Facility

As in C and D above. However, if it is known where the patient is being transferred internally, the staff members shall take the sealed bag to the new nursing unit and give it to the receiving staff members, who shall sign on the nurse's notes and the itemized listing receipt of sealed bag, which shall be countersigned by the deliverer.

F.   Storage of Belongings Not Sent Home

If there are no family members available to take home the patient's belongings after they have been packed and secured as described above, a member of the nursing staff shall call the security office to request that he or she be met at the personal property room.

The sealed bag will be logged in by both deliverer and security receiver at the personal property room as to time, date, receiver, and deliverer. The bag will then be placed on the appropriate shelf in the secured area.

G.   Return of Patient Belongings

1. From hospital valuables safe: This may be accomplished Monday through Sunday between 8:00 a.m. and 5:00 p.m. only. The staff member will take the chart copy of the secured items to the admitting office. The patient will indicate on the form that he or she wishes to have his or her belongings retrieved. The staff member will sign the log book with date and time of retrieval of the secured envelope.

Upon return to the nursing unit, the patient and staff member will open the secured envelope and identify and check off all items contained in the envelope against the listing. When all items are accounted for, the patient and staff member will sign the original, which will be placed back in the patient's record. The nurse's notes will reflect his return of valuables to the patient.

Should a patient request return of a specified amount of money or items secured in the valuables safe, the patient request for release of valuables (shown below) must be signed by the patient and the name of the individual to whom the items are to be given. The cashier will retain the request for release of valuables form. The valuables envelope will reflect the amount or items released, the date of the release, and the name of releasing cashier.

(continued on next page)

Figure 11-3. (Continued)

Request for Release of Valuables

I, _____ , request you release to _____ the following items or money from the envelope you have secured in your safe in my name.

_____
Patient name

_____
Date

_____
Witness

    2.   From the personal property room: The staff member will follow the steps outlined previously, with the exception that if the patient or family members packed the patient's belongings, the staff member need not verify the items contained therein with the listing. However, the nurse's notes will contain such information regarding the retrieval of property.

H.   Discharged Patients

On discharge, the patient will be asked to pack his or her belongings: if the patient is physically or mentally impaired, a family member should pack the patient's belongings. If no family member is available and the patient is unable to pack his or her belongings, two staff members will list the items found in the patient's bedside stand, closet, and general area, pack the items in the belongings bag provided, and both sign the list. The original of the list will go in the patient's chart; the carbon will go inside the patient belongings bag. The nurse's notes will reflect which activities were undertaken regarding the patient's belongings.

Before the patient is discharged, a nursing staff member will check the patient's medical record to ascertain whether any belongings are in the valuables safe or in the personal property room; if so, they will be retrieved, and the retrieval will be documented in the nurse's notes.

Note:

1.   At no time will Hospital X staff members lock up valuables or other belongings in such areas as the nurse-server or narcotic cabinet. Valuables will be sent either to the hospital safe or home with the patient's family members.
2.   Paper bags of any sort will *not* be used at any time.
3.   Family members and patients are encouraged not to bring in personal or valuable belongings. Whenever possible, such items should be sent home with family members.
4.   The nurse's notes should clearly reflect all interactions with patients and/or families regarding the handling of valuables and other belongings.

Searches

Searching private belongings of the hospital's patients and employees is generally an acceptable practice if done as advised by hospital legal counsel. Procedures for searches of employees for stolen hospital property may differ from procedures for searches of patients for weapons or drugs. Therefore, policies specifying who is authorized to conduct searches, circumstances under which searches may be conducted, involvement of the security force, and other issues related to searches that involve patients, visitors, and employees should be developed with the guidance of legal counsel and risk management personnel.

Security Surveillance

Routine surveillance of the hospital grounds, including the parking lots and the facility's doors, is important for the security of property and the safety of personnel. When doors that should be locked are found unlocked, these incidents should be logged. A short-form notice regarding unlocked doors should be sent to the department head. If the same door is found unlocked more than once, increased surveillance may be justi-fied. If security personnel notice as they make rounds that personal property of patients, employees, or visitors is unattended or left in an unsecured place, they may leave a warning on a brightly colored two- by three-inch card or sticker that says, for example, "If I were a thief, this would be gone! Your friendly security personnel of Hospi-tal X."

Figure 11-4. Form for Securing Patient Valuables

Valuables Envelope
Sealed Securely in Presence of
Person Depositing Valuables

No. 0000
To be signed when valuables
  are deposited
Name of Patient _____
Signature of
Depositor _____
Received by _____
Date _____ 19 _____

Contents to be surrendered to owner
only after signature on depositor's
receipt has been witnessed and
compared by custodian.

Contents

_____
_____
_____
_____
_____
_____
_____
_____
_____
_____
_____
_____
_____
_____
_____
_____
_____
_____

Personal Property Room
Sealed Securely in Presence of
Person Depositing Valuables

No. 0000
To be signed when valuables
  are deposited
Name of Patient _____
Signature of
Depositor_____
Received by _____
Date_____ 19_____

Contents to be surrendered to owner
only after signature on depositor's
receipt has been witnessed and
compared by custodian.

Contents

_____
_____
_____
_____

It is understood and agreed that Hospital X
maintains a safe for the safekeeping of
wallets and their contents, jewelry, money,
and religious medals only. The hospital also
maintains a personal property room for all
other property requiring safeguarding. The
hospital shall not be liable for loss or
damage to any valuable or personal property
unless deposited with the hospital for
safekeeping.
_____ No declared valuables
_____ Valuables given to
  family member

_____
Name

_____
Relationship

_____
Patient or Authorized Representative

Figure 11-5. Valuables Form for Transferred Patients*

Name of Patient _____
Signature of
Depositor _____
Received by _____
Time _____ Date _____ 19 ___

Contents to be surrendered to owner only after signature on depositor's receipt has been witnessed and compared by custodian.

Contents:

_____
_____
_____
_____   Name
_____
_____   Relationship
_____
_____   Verification
_____
_____   Position
_____
_____
_____
_____
_____

Disposition of valuables:
_____ Remained in room
_____ Transferred to floor
_____ Transferred to personal
          property room
_____ Packed at discharge
_____ Given to family member

Patient Label Here

*To be used only in cases where the patient cannot pack his or her belongings.

Figure 11-6. Patient Valuables Declaration Form

Name of Patient (affix patient identification label here)

Personal valuables: It is understood and agreed that Hospital X maintains a safe for the safekeeping of money and valuables, and that Hospital X shall not be liable for loss of or damage to any money, jewelry, glasses, dentures, documents, furs, fur coats, fur garments, or other articles of unusual value and small compass unless placed therein, and shall not be liable for loss of or damage to any other personal property unless deposited with the hospital for safekeeping.

_____ I have read the above statement and have no valuables to declare.
_____ I have read the above statement and wish to have my valuables locked
          in the hospital safe.

Patient Signature _____
Witness (optional) _____
Date _____

Figure 11-7. Policy for Lost Items

Policy

Items found on hospital premises will be sent to the Lost and Found area via the security department to be kept for claiming.

Procedure

1. Items left by patients or otherwise found on hospital premises will be sent to the Hospital X security department to be stored in the Lost and Found area.
   A. The item will be logged into a Lost and Found log. The information entered in the log will include a brief description of the item, date and location where the item was found, name of owner, if known (sometimes items are left by patients upon discharge and ownership can therefore be determined), and disposition and date thereof.
2. When ownership of an item is known, the address of the owner will be obtained from the medical records department or the business office. A form letter notifying the owner of our possession will be sent. The letter will designate a time limit after which Hospital X will donate the article to Goodwill (or other charity).
3. Alternatively, the article can be mailed, if not too large, to the owner in lieu of the aforementioned letter.
4. All items sent to Lost and Found will be kept a minimum of six months from date sent to Lost and Found.
5. Periodically security and risk management will review the Lost and Found log to determine whether a pattern of locations or items can be identified for loss control actions.

Escort Services and Parking Surveillance

Many security departments offer staff and visitors an escort service to parking areas. If such a service is offered, notice of its availability should be posted and circulated. Forty-five minutes to one-half hour prior to and after each shift change, security should increase surveillance of all parking areas. This surveillance increases the safety—both actual and perceived—of employees who are going off duty, especially at night.

Key Control

Responsibility for key control should be delegated to the security department. Dispensing of keys, especially masters and submasters, should be *strictly* controlled. A policy that keys are turned in upon separation from employment should be enforced.

Human Resources Issues

If the institution plans a layoff of a large number of people, the security department should be notified to be alert to potentially violent situations. In instances of individual terminations, security personnel may be called on to give assistance should the individual become hostile.

Another service that security may perform for the human resources department is to do background checks on applicants for employment, especially for those positions where cash handling or access to the storeroom is included in job responsibilities.

Protection of Money

Security personnel protect those areas of the facility where money is handled, such as the cashier's office, the cafeteria, the gift shop, and so on. Consideration should be given to the installation at each cashier's location of silent alarms that connect either to the local police department or the hospital security department. When hospital personnel take money to the bank, risk management principles dictate that the trips be made at staggered times, by different personnel, using different vehicles over different routes. The ideal way to transport money to and from the bank is by armored car; however, when a contract service is unavailable or undesirable, *not* establishing a routine is one of the best loss-prevention methods.

Fires, Disasters, and Traffic Control

Security personnel play a major role in traffic control in the event of fires, other disasters, and even when a Code Blue occurs. Security personnel should participate in disaster planning, and all security officers should receive inservice training as to their responsibilities during a disaster.

☐ Use of Local Agencies

Local law enforcement and fire departments can help health care facilities to enhance their safety and security programs. For example, police officers can conduct inservice education programs for hospital staff on self-defense, and firefighters can instruct on home fire prevention. Development of positive relationships with these public service agencies and their respective personnel also can enhance the health care facility's public and community image.

☐ Conclusion

The assistance provided to the risk management and safety activities by security personnel is invaluable. Security officers patrol all parts of the facility's building and grounds and interact with the hospital's staff, patients, and visitors. The extra eyes and ears can only enhance the overall effectiveness of the goals of the risk management program.

References

1. Joint Commission on Accreditation of Healthcare Organizations. *Accreditation Manual for Hospitals, 1990 edition.* Chicago: JCAHO, 1989, p. 195.

2. Joint Commission on Accreditation of Healthcare Organizations, p. 196.

3. Joint Commission on Accreditation of Healthcare Organizations, p. 195.

4. Joint Commission on Accreditation of Healthcare Organizations, p. 75.

☐ Bibliography

Ashley, J., and others. *Study of Hospital Injury Prevention Program.* Silver Spring, MD: U.S. Department of Commerce, Applied Management Services [no further information available].

Bailey, M. J. *Reducing Risks to Life, Measurement of the Benefits.* Washington, DC: American Enterprise Institute for Public Policy Research, 1980.

Buchan, R. M. Evaluating health, safety services' cost-effectiveness to small business. *Occupational Health and Safety* May 1984.

Capell, M. The stress-loss connection. *Professional Safety* 30(3), Mar. 1985.

Chaffin, D. B., Herrin, G. D., and Keyserling, W. M. Preemployment strength testing–an updated position. *Journal of Occupational Medicine* 20, 1978.

Cheio, E. F., and Gordon, M. S. *Occupational Disability and Public Policy.* New York City: John Wiley & Sons, 1963.

Cowles, S. How to manage occupational health programs. *National Safety and Health News* May 1985.

Emergency Care Research Institute (ECRI). Risk analysis: hospital relations with police. *Hospital Risk Control* (Plymouth Meeting, PA), Sept. 1988, pp. 1–7.

Emergency Care Research Institute (ECRI). Violent crime in hospitals: a security issue. *Hospital Risk Control* (Plymouth Meeting, PA), July 1987, pp. 1–5.

Fielding, J. Effectiveness of employee health improvement programs. *Journal of Occupational Medicine* 24(11), Nov. 1982.

Gelb, B. Preventive medicine and employee productivity. *Harvard Business Review* Mar.–Apr. 1985.

Gilmore, C. L. *Accident Prevention and Loss Control.* Saranac Lake, NY: American Management Association, 1970.

Guthier, W. E. Accident causation data: putting the pieces together. *Risk Management* Dec. 1983.

Handbook of Occupational Safety and Health. 2nd ed. Chicago: National Safety Council, 1976.

Heinrich, H. W. *Industrial Accident Prevention—A Scientific Approach.* 4th ed. New York City: McGraw-Hill, 1959.

Jones, D. Back injury prevention—are our programs adequate? *Professional Safety* 39(2), Feb. 1985.

Levin, L., Ober, J., and Whiteside, J. Injury incidence rates in a paint company on rotating production shifts. *Accident Analysis and Prevention* 17(1), 1985.

Markham, S., and Scott, D. Absenteeism, linked to job satisfaction. *Personnel Administration* Feb. 1985.

Public Law 91-596, 91st Congress, S. 2193, *Occupational Safety and Health Act of 1970,* Dec. 29, 1970.

Robinson, J. C. Racial inequality and occupational health in the United States. *International Journal of Health Sciences* 15(1), Jan. 1985.

Ruchlin, H., Finkll, M., and McCarthy, E. Containment programs can brake steamrolling health care costs. *Intracorp Report* (Wayne, PA): Spring 1983.

Schenkelback, L. *The Safety Management Primer.* Homewood, IL: Dow Jones-Irwin, 1975.

Security update, 1983. *Hospitals,* Nov. 16, 1983, pp. 76–79.

Smith, R. S. *The Occupational Safety and Health Act—Its Goals and Its Achievements.* Washington, DC: American Enterprise Institute for Public Policy Research, 1976.

Starr, S., Shute, S., and Thompson, C. Relating posture to discomfort in VDT use. *Journal of Occupational Medicine* 27(4), Apr. 1985.

Chapter 12

Occupational Risk Exposures

Guy Fragala

Accidents involving patients can result in general liability, professional liability, or products liability claims, whereas accidents to an employee can result in workers' compensation claims or employer liability claims. Also, under the dual capacity doctrine, a health care institution may be liable in the area of professional liability if the institution acts as both an employer and a provider of health care. Employees may receive treatment related to occupational injuries or illnesses through the emergency room or the employee health service.

The health care environment provides significant occupational risk exposures that can result in either occupational injuries or illnesses. In fact, the reported incidence rate of 9.06 for hospitals is greater than the overall average incidence rate for the manufacturing industry (8.05).[1] The incidence rate is determined by the following formula:

$$\text{Incidence rate} = \frac{(\text{No. of OSHA recordable injuries and illnesses}) \times 200{,}000}{\text{Total hours worked by all employees during period covered}}$$

200,000 = base for 100 full-time equivalent workers
(working 40 hours per week, 50 weeks per year)

To determine those rates, the Occupational Safety and Health Administration (OSHA) requires industry, including hospitals, to keep records of employee injuries. Reported workers' compensation data show that nursing aides, orderlies, licensed practical nurses, and registered nurses have an incidence of lower-back injuries similar to that of construction laborers, garbage collectors, and truck drivers.[2] In addition to the exposure to occupational accidents, there are a number of substances used in the health care environment that present occupational risk exposures to employees. This chapter provides an overview of occupational risk exposures to patients and employees and their relation to the overall hospital risk management program.

☐ Joint Commission on Accreditation of Healthcare Organizations Standards

Over the past few years, Joint Commission standards for hospital safety have been strengthened extensively. The 1989 accreditation manual has four Plant Technology and

Safety Management Standards focusing on four areas of safety: safety management, life safety management, equipment management, and utilities management.[3] The new standards provide good guidelines for a general hospital safety program, and the risk manager should study them to make sure the hospital is in compliance.

Standard number one deals with general safety management, including the need for a risk assessment program, functions of the safety officer and safety committee, training requirements, a hazardous materials and waste management program, and comprehensive requirements for emergency preparedness. Standard number two concerns life safety management, based on the 1988 edition of the *Life Safety Code* of the National Fire Protection Association. Standard number three is concerned with equipment management, an important area when considering patient safety issues. This standard focuses on control of clinical and physical risks of fixed and portable equipment used for diagnosis, treatment, monitoring and care of patients, and of other fixed and portable electrically powered equipment. Standard number four, utilities management, describes standards for physical plants.

☐ Accident Prevention

Both employees and patients are at risk of accidental injury in the hospital. Effective prevention of accidents requires that administration and all employees accept the fact that accidents are preventable and that the responsibility for accident prevention is shared throughout all levels of the organization. Safety literature classifies causes of accidents as either unsafe acts or unsafe conditions, with the majority being caused by unsafe acts.[4] However, most safety programs focus on preventing unsafe conditions rather than unsafe acts, because unsafe conditions are more readily identifiable and much easier to correct. Unsafe acts and unsafe conditions occur as a result of system faults in the organizational structure; management can correct those faults if it truly wishes to reduce injuries resulting from accidents. Reducing the number of accidents may be accomplished by identifying and correcting system faults.

☐ Toxic and Hazardous Substances

In performing their normal work duties, health care workers may be exposed to substances that can present occupational health hazards, which may result in occupational illnesses. Employees who suffer an occupational illness receive compensation through their state's workers' compensation system. Because occupational illnesses can result in long-term disability, including large amounts of workers' compensation in addition to medical bills, the risk manager's job is to minimize workers' exposures to these hazards.

The workers' compensation system was originally intended to be an exclusive remedy with fixed limits for payment for employees who suffered injuries or illnesses as a result of their employment. However, some states have allowed employees to sue employers for occupational injury either instead of, or sometimes in addition to, their remedy under the workers' compensation system if the employer's conduct is judged to be in willful disregard of worker safety. Unlike workers' compensation, employers' liability is a tort action without statutory limits.

Third parties are not covered by the workers' compensation system. Third parties include unborn children and family members of workers. The pregnant worker presents a potentially large risk because large levels of mutagenic or teratogenic agents that are safe for the mother may be toxic to her fetus. In addition, the hospital is limited by antidiscrimination law in its ability to restrict the mother's hours or reassign her to another job while she is pregnant. However, when considering reproductive health hazards, hospitals should not discriminate against women, because both men and women are subject to reproductive occupational risk exposures.

According to James L. Griffith, J.D.,[5] lawsuits are increasing because of failure to properly monitor and regulate the use of toxic or hazardous substances in the workplace, and juries have been unsympathetic when hazards are not corrected. The risk manager should ensure that a technically qualified person is coordinating or overseeing a program to provide environmental monitoring where hazardous substances are in use. Monitoring to determine the airborne levels of hazardous substances can be done by a qualified hospital employee, by a consultant, or by a local or state agency that provides this service. In addition, medical surveillance should be conducted on employees who work in areas where toxic or hazardous substances are used. This surveillance can be done by the employee health service, with the active participation of a physician who is knowledgeable in occupational medicine. In addition to establishing a comprehensive environmental monitoring and medical surveillance program for employees who are exposed to hazardous substances, the institution should maintain appropriate health records of employees who are tested under these programs, should questions arise in the future.

OSHA Hazard Communication Standard

On August 24, 1987, OSHA issued the revised Hazard Communication Standard. The revised standard implemented in 1988 expanded compliance with this law beyond the manufacturing industry to cover all employers, including hospitals. State and local "right-to-know" laws, in place in many jurisdictions prior to this standard, are preempted. However, some organizations that do not fall under the jurisdiction of OSHA may still be covered under local "right-to-know" laws. The Hazard Communication Standard requires employers to develop, implement, and maintain a written hazard communication program. Employers must list all hazardous chemicals present in the workplace, evaluate the hazards that these chemicals pose to their employees, and communicate the hazards by, among other means, labeling containers, providing material safety data sheets (MSDSs), and offering training programs.

In addition to the penalties imposed by noncompliance with the law, hospitals may face liability if they are sued by a worker who suffers an occupational exposure. In jurisdictions allowing such suits, noncompliance with the standard can be used to show willful disregard of worker safety. The risk manager should either coordinate compliance or designate a coordinator of federal hazard communication requirements.

Specific Hazardous Substances

Other OSHA standards affecting hospitals include exposure requirements for ethylene oxide and formaldehyde. In addition to those two, there are other hazardous substances for which environmental levels should be monitored, including trace gas anesthesia and solvents in laboratories.

Ethylene Oxide

Ethylene oxide gas and its mixtures are effective sterilants used in hospitals; however, ethylene oxide has been shown (in animal toxicity studies) to be a carcinogen and a mutagen. Health effects in humans that are suspected to be associated with occupational exposure to ethylene oxide include increased incidence of leukemia, adverse reproductive effects, and elevated mutagenic activity.[6] The Occupational Safety and Health Administration has established a permissible exposure limit of one part per million airborne ethylene oxide in the workplace, expressed as a time-weighted average for an eight-hour work shift, and an excursion limit, or short-term exposure limit, of 5 parts per million for a 15-minute exposure period. (The potential adverse effects of exposure to ethylene oxide have prompted some recent activities to lower permissible limits.)

The risk manager, or other person in the facility who is designated to monitor compliance with OSHA standards, should work with line managers and the facility's human resources department to make sure that workers who are exposed to this gas use protective clothing as well as appropriate and safe work practices to minimize exposure. In addition, in order to lower worker exposure levels, it may be possible to make engineering changes to the equipment and the way in which it is installed.

Formaldehyde

Formaldehyde is the most frequently used fixative for tissue specimens and is a sterilant used for dialysis equipment. Formaldehyde has long been known to cause skin irritations, skin disease and skin disorders, and dermal sensitization as a consequence of dermal contact. Long-term inhalation of formaldehyde gas is associated with nasal cancer in experimental animals, and in some studies humans exposed to formaldehyde have demonstrated increased nasal and nasopharyngeal cancer.[7] The current OSHA exposure limit for formaldehyde is 1 part per million as an 8-hour time-weighted average, and 2 parts per million for a 15-minute short-term exposure limit. Laboratory workers can be taught to use protective clothing and to modify work practices where possible to minimize exposure.

Anesthetic Gases

Nitrous oxide, alone or in combination with other agents, such as isoflurane, halothane, or enflurane, has become the most widely used general inhalation anesthetic in the world. Several studies have suggested that some adverse health effects may result from chronic exposure to nitrous oxide. These include irritability, headache, nausea, spontaneous abortion, premature delivery, children with congenital abnormalities, lymphoid malignancies, cancer in females, and hepatic and renal disease.[8] In 1977, the National Institute for Occupational Safety and Health (NIOSH) published a recommended standard,[9] which has been submitted to OSHA. Although this document has not been promulgated formally, it has been used as a standard, and several hospitals have been inspected, cited, and fined (under the general duty clause of the 1970 Occupational Safety and Health Act) in response to employee complaints of inadequate controls of anesthetic gases. The proposed standard is that time-weighted average concentrations of nitrous oxide are not to exceed 25 parts per million in a time-weighted sample obtained during administration of anesthetics in the operating room.[10]

Cytotoxic Agents

The mutagenic, teratogenic, carcinogenic, and local irritant properties of many cytotoxic agents (pharmaceuticals used in chemotherapy) are well established and pose a possible hazard to the health of occupationally exposed individuals.[11] These potential hazards necessitate special attention to the procedures utilized in handling, preparing, and administering these drugs. As with many other hazardous agents, proper disposal of residues and waste products associated with cytotoxic agents is required. Cytotoxic agents should be prepared in a class II biological safety cabinet in an area with minimal traffic and air turbulence. Personnel who prepare such drugs should wear appropriate disposable surgical latex gloves and protective barrier garments. Nurses who administer them should wear gloves and protective barrier garments.[12] Risk managers should work with physicians and nurses to develop safe work practices for handling these drugs, especially in those instances when the physician insists that the drug be mixed at the patient's bedside.

Mercury

Mercury exposure may occur from spills or stains in the histology laboratory, during the repair of biomedical equipment, or from spills from broken thermometers or sphygmomanometers. Mercury vapor can be absorbed through the lungs and skin and can cause transient upper airway irritation, chemical pneumonitis, or dermatitis. Repeated or prolonged exposure to mercury vapor may also affect the central nervous system.[13] Both employees and patients are at risk of mercury exposure, and any spill involving mercury should be cleaned up as soon as possible. Safety personnel should be aware that tiny beads of mercury can lodge in cracks, mix with dust, and penetrate porous material such as floor tiles. Mercury can cling to clothing (especially knit fabrics) and to shoe soles. Liquid mercury collected from spills must be disposed of as a hazardous waste.

Asbestos

Airborne asbestos contamination in buildings is a significant environmental problem. Various diseases have been linked with industrial exposure to airborne asbestos, and the extensive use of asbestos products in buildings has raised concern about exposure to asbestos in nonindustrial settings. The presence of asbestos in a building does not mean that the health of building occupants is necessarily endangered as long as asbestos-containing material remains in good condition and is not disrupted. When building maintenance, repair, renovation, or other activities disturb asbestos-containing material or it is damaged, asbestos fibers are released, creating a potential hazard to building occupants.[14] Current governmental regulation of asbestos poses a serious challenge. Recent federal legislative and regulatory activities indicate that the challenge will heighten, not lessen. In 1986, the Asbestos Hazard Emergency Response Act was signed into law. Among other things, the act directs the Environmental Protection Agency (EPA) to assess the extent of the danger to human health posed by the presence of asbestos in commercial buildings and the means to respond to any such danger. The OSHA regulations adopted in 1986 impose new, more stringent standards upon employers whose employees may be exposed to asbestos-containing materials in the workplace. The legal implications of asbestos-containing materials in commercial buildings is a complex subject that warrants serious attention.[15] The risk manager should determine whether there are any asbestos-containing materials in the hospital and, if so, take action to ensure that programs are in place to prevent exposure of building occupants. An industrial hygienist, available through insurance companies, governmental agencies, or private consulting groups, can be an important resource to the risk manager in this effort.

Other Hazardous Substances

In addition to the substances already mentioned, other materials that present occupational health risks are used in hospitals. These include substances with well-known health effects, such as organic solvents used by laboratory and maintenance workers, and iodine used in physical therapy. New substances, such as therapeutic drugs, also are being introduced into the environment, where there is much uncertainty regarding potential occupational health effects. Ribavirin, for example, is used to treat serious infections resulting from respiratory syncytial virus. Because it is an aerosol, those visiting hospital patients being treated may also be exposed. Such exposure is particularly significant to pregnant women.

As with all hazardous substances, the risk manager should ensure that there are technically competent personnel who are aware of the potential health risks of any substance in use in the hospital and that appropriate programs are in place regarding environmental monitoring, medical surveillance, and worker protection.

☐ Radiation

The risk resulting from radiation exposure remains poorly understood by the average hospital worker. This lack of understanding is complicated further by controversy over assessment of risks associated with chronic low doses.

Although many hospital workers are exposed to radiation, their exposure is often undetectable and usually not greater than the average natural background amount received by the general population. However, there are a number of health care workers involved in diagnostic, therapeutic, and research applications of radioactive materials who are at risk of exposure, and effective monitoring and protection programs should be in place. Monitoring involves requiring radiation workers to wear appropriately placed dosimetry badges to monitor their radiation exposure over time. If recommended exposure levels are exceeded, action should be taken to reduce exposure dose. The Nuclear Regulatory Commission has mandated that any institution using radioactive materials develop a program to obtain exposures that are as low as reasonably achievable (ALARA).[16] Every year, thousands of American workers receive some occupational radiation exposure. Even though only a small fraction of these exposures exceed external and internal dose standards, some radiation workers may either die from or contract some form of cancer during their lifetime. However, the mortality and morbidity rates of radiation workers are the same as those of the general population.[17] In situations involving radiation and other occupational health hazard exposures, it is difficult to prove or disprove that the cause of an occupational illness is an occupational exposure. Therefore, it is in the best interest of the hospital to develop and implement the best possible programs and document the activities of those programs.

☐ Hazardous Waste

Not only must the hospital properly monitor and handle hazardous materials while they are being used in the hospital, it also must dispose of those materials properly. Chemical waste can come from a variety of areas in the health care facility. Laboratories are usually a primary source, but chemicals are also used in such departments and services as housekeeping, food service, maintenance, laundry, and occupational therapy. Chemical waste must be collected at the point of use, segregated, and placed in properly labeled containers to await disposal by a licensed waste disposal contractor. Regulations governing the disposal of hazardous chemical waste are under the Resource Conservation and Recovery Act of 1976 (RCRA). In 1986, hazardous waste regulations were revised to include small-quantity generators, defined as those generating between 100 and 1,000 kilograms per month. Health care facilities should determine which generator classification they fall into.[18] Facilities should also determine whether or not they are bound by federal regulations or if authority has been given by the EPA to local or state agencies to enforce and regulate laws regarding hazardous chemical waste.

At present there are no specific federal regulations governing cytotoxic drug waste. However, several drugs are listed as toxic commercial product wastes by the EPA under the RCRA. Waste products contaminated with cytotoxic drugs should be considered hazardous waste materials. Disposal options depend primarily on state and local regulations or restrictions. Bulk liquid cytotoxic waste should be disposed of as hazardous chemical waste in an EPA-approved landfill or incinerator. Trace-contaminated cytotoxic wastes are best disposed of by on-site incineration at temperatures in excess of 1,000°C with 2-second retention time.[19,20]

Low-level radioactive waste currently is regulated under the requirements of the Low Level Radioactive Waste Policy Act of 1980 as issued by the Nuclear Regulatory Commission either directly or by delegation to approved state plans.[21] In the hospital, radioactive waste may originate from research laboratories, clinical laboratories, the nuclear medicine department, or the radiology department. The radioactive waste management program at the hospital should be under the jurisdiction of the facility's radiation safety officer and radiation safety committee. The radioactive waste management program should include a system for proper identification, collection, segregation, and containment while in storage, and treatment and disposal in accordance with specified regulations.

The RCRA gave the EPA the legal authority to regulate infectious waste. At this time, there are no mandated federal regulations in this area; however, the EPA has issued a publication entitled *Guide for Infectious Waste Management.*[22] Many states have enacted their own regulations regarding the disposal of hazardous infectious waste, and those laws are the regulations that affect the hospital. Hazardous infectious waste includes materials with microorganisms in numbers that may lead to transmission of disease. These materials might include isolation wastes, cultures and stocks of biohazardous agents, human blood and blood products, pathological wastes, contaminated sharps, contaminated animal carcasses, body parts, and bedding.[23] To minimize cost and volume of waste shipped, infectious waste may be treated on-site through proper incineration or steam sterilization.

In general, the facility's hazardous waste management program should include a system for proper categorization of hazardous waste materials, identification of which waste products generated by the facility fall under those categories, a method of proper collection, proper storage facilities, and a method to ensure proper disposal in compliance with all applicable laws and regulations.

□ Emergency Preparedness

The concept of health care emergency preparedness is based on the Civil Defense programs that were developed a number of years ago. Such programs focused on the importance of communitywide planning and preparation and the realization that Civil Defense is merely one aspect of disaster planning for which all health care facilities must ultimately share some responsibility.[24] A comprehensive emergency preparedness program should plan for both internal and external disasters. An internal disaster may include bomb threats, building collapse, fire, or massive utility failure that causes a breakdown in the facility's ability to operate. The hospital's external disaster plan will detail how each department in the hospital will react to a disaster in the community that may precipitate an influx of patients. These may include floods, tornadoes, fires, chemical spills, or a plane crash. In such a situation, the hospital must continue to care properly for its patients and successfully triage and treat a large number of incoming patients.

The development of an effective emergency preparedness program begins with the disaster committee, perhaps the hospital's safety committee or a subcommittee of the safety committee. Membership of the committee should include appropriate representation from hospital departments and services, such as administration, admission, radiology, surgery, laboratory services, engineering, housekeeping, communication, security, emergency services, medical specialties, pharmacy, intensive care, nursing, and auxiliary services. The plan should address alternative sources of essential utilities and the provision of an emergency communication backup system. If portions of the facility become unusable because of an internal disaster, alternative care sites should be identified. Consideration must be given to how the facility would be evacuated should total evacuation become necessary. The external disaster plan should address reassigning use of space to triage incoming patients quickly and reassigning staff to deal with extraordinary demands for supplies, for transporters, and for communicating between assigned disaster areas. In addition, there must be an up-to-date call list readily available at all times in case a disaster happens in the evening, when staffing ratios are low. Effective communication between departments becomes essential in a disaster and is generally the most difficult part of the disaster plan to develop.

An important part of the hospital's external disaster plan will be planning for a disaster that includes spills of nuclear materials. Planning and rehearsing plans for nuclear disaster is necessary in order to dispel the hospital staff's fears about their exposure to such material if they must treat trauma victims who have been contaminated by nuclear materials in a truck, train, or air disaster. The Joint Commission requires that the external disaster plan be rehearsed two times each year.

A fire in a health care institution can be a severe internal disaster. Planning and drilling are important to reduce the potential impact. All staff should be instructed in how to react to a fire. This instruction should stress the hospital's duty to protect patients who may be in immediate danger. At the first sound of an alarm, doors to patients' rooms should be closed to protect them from smoke or other products of combustion. Staff should understand when and how to move patients should a fire become serious. Patients can be moved to other areas within the facility that are separated from the fire site by smoke and fire partitions. The internal disaster plan should address plans for horizontal movement on patient floors and vertical movement if entire floors must be evacuated. The plans developed should be practiced through drills. Internal disaster drills and fire drills are required by Joint Commission standards. The Joint Commission requires each shift to conduct fire drills at least quarterly.

☐ Life Safety Management

The National Fire Protection Association's *Life Safety Code* is not a law or regulation; however, most regulatory standards are based on it, and the requirements of the Joint Commission adopt this code.[25] The intent of life safety management is to ensure that each building in which patients are housed overnight or receive treatment is properly designed and constructed for adequate fire protection and prevention. Buildings should be designed with proper fire detection and suppression systems. This includes appropriate placement and maintenance of smoke detectors, sprinkler systems, and both fixed and portable fire-extinguishing systems. Buildings should also be constructed with time-rated fire walls and smoke partitions, and the integrity of those separations must be maintained in new and renovated areas of the facility. Any penetrations in smoke barriers and fire walls should be properly protected. Exitways should be properly marked, and corridors to exits should be unobstructed. Hospitals should have appropriate fire plans, including plans for evacuating patients, and those plans should be practiced through drills on a regular basis. All staff should receive proper training regarding the institution's fire plan.

☐ Equipment Management

Within the hospital environment, there are a number of pieces of equipment for patient care and nonpatient care that present risk. Risk managers should be aware that recent litigation has focused on medical devices, and hospitals and device manufacturers both have been held accountable for their respective responsibilities regarding that equipment.[26] If a patient injury occurs and hospital equipment is linked to the cause of the injury, the litigation will revolve around whether the incident occurred because the equipment malfunctioned, because of a design defect, or as a result of operator error. The risk manager's investigation must answer this question in cases involving medical equipment.

Written criteria should be developed to determine which pieces of equipment will be included in the hospital's equipment management program. Criteria should include how the equipment will be used, the risks associated with application of the equipment, and what type of maintenance requirements the equipment has. All new equipment entering the institution should be evaluated as to whether it should be included in the equipment management program. All equipment should be checked upon initial receipt by the institution. Testing and preventive maintenance requirements should be specified for each piece of equipment, and appropriate training programs instituted to ensure that all users of the equipment will receive proper training. Thorough documentation should be maintained on the equipment management program, including initial testing, regular preventive maintenance records, and documentation of any reported failures. An appropriate group within the institution should monitor the activities of the equipment management program, including a review of all documentation generated. Within the equipment management program, there should be policies directing staff on handling medical device hazards and recall.

Because hospitals are becoming more involved in home health care, programs also should address the risks associated with devices used away from the hospital. Borrowing and lending of equipment can further add to the risks associated with patient care equipment. Policies also should be in place to deal with patient-owned equipment that might be brought into the hospital. The risk manager should ensure that technically competent personnel are administering and monitoring the equipment management program within the hospital.[27]

□ Emergency Planning for Interruption of Essential Services

Utility systems play an important role in the everyday operation of today's hospital. Without such utilities as air handling, lighting, water, and power for facility equipment, the hospital could not operate. Failure of any utility system presents potential risk that the risk manager should be concerned with. The risk manager, working with the facilities manager, should ensure that there is a backup plan in case of failure of all utilities for life support, infection control, environmental support, and equipment support systems. Typically those components will include such equipment as pumps, motors, control systems, compressors, and air handlers. It should be confirmed that the facility has an adequate emergency power system to provide electricity to designated areas should there be an interruption in the normal electrical power source. The emergency power system should be capable of providing power to critical areas of the facility. Periodic testing should be conducted to ensure that the emergency electrical power system remains adequate to meet the needs of present systems and any new systems that may be added.

The risk manager should ensure that the facility is prepared to manage the failure of any key utility system that supports the patient care environment. Written policies and procedures should be developed to manage utility failures, including emergency electrical systems, plumbing and potable water systems, communication systems, medical gases and vacuum systems, HVAC systems, and other key systems. Facilities administration should develop procedures and establish intervals for appropriate testing and maintenance of all equipment contained in the utilities management program. Those involved in operation and maintenance of utilities systems should be provided with adequate training as needed.[28]

□ The Safety Committee

The institution's safety committee has no operational responsibility or authority. The committee is a policy-making and recommending body that serves as a resource to the safety officer in making the ongoing safety program effective. It identifies safety issues and recommends solutions. All recommendations should be followed up to determine whether the problem was resolved, and the committee's documentation should demonstrate that problems were finally resolved.[29] The membership is made up of representatives of patient care departments and of support services, infection control, human resources, food service, and housekeeping, as well as the facilities manager and the risk manager. It may be chaired by the hospital's designated safety officer, who should be delegated, by board resolution, the authority to act in case of emergency.

Members should receive periodic safety training. In large institutions, the role of the safety committee chairperson and the safety director may be separate. In other hospitals, the same person may fill both roles. The safety director or safety officer must have both the appropriate technical expertise and the time allocated to fulfill the necessary operational responsibilities of the safety program. All members of the committee should have periodic training in some aspect of safety.

The structure of the safety committee may vary widely. A hospital may have one general committee to handle all institutional safety-related matters, or it may set up an umbrella committee with subcommittees that are responsible for designated safety issues. The safety committee may, for example, have a disaster-planning subcommittee, a fire safety subcommittee, and an employee injury subcommittee. To encourage active interest and participation throughout the hospital, members who are not members of the safety committee itself could be appointed to these subcommittees. The risk manager should participate in safety committee activities, and those activities should be communicated to other appropriate committees throughout the institution. The risk manager can assist the safety committee in preparing minutes and reports in such a way that if they are found to be discoverable in a malpractice action, they do not adversely affect the institution.

Standard one of the Joint Commission's Plant Technology and Safety Management standards requires that the committee meet as frequently as required by the chairperson, but not less than every other month. Conclusions, recommendations, and actions of the committee should be reported in writing at least quarterly to administrative, medical, and nursing staff and to others as appropriate in the organization. Written records should verify that appropriate safety-related information is exchanged and that consultation is provided between the safety committee and the members of the various programs or specific departments or services, quality assurance, risk management, the infection control committee, and other appropriate committees and staff members. Written documentation should demonstrate that the conclusions, recommendations, and actions of the safety committee are evaluated by the director of the affected department or service and that proper action is taken and documented in subsequent safety committee minutes. The Joint Commission does not prescribe who should be on the safety committee, but it does require that the safety director or officer serve on the committee and that there be representatives from administration and from clinical and support services.

☐ Conclusion

The Joint Commission recommends that health care institutions take a multidisciplinary approach to hospitalwide quality assurance. Institutions should try to reduce duplication, strengthen organizational linkages, and coordinate complementary monitoring, evaluation, and problem solving among the five review functions of infection control, quality assurance, risk management, safety management, and utilization review. There are opportunities for an efficient team approach if the risk manager and safety director work together in those institutions where the functions are separate. The safety director can serve as a technical resource to the risk manager. Each function should understand fully how the other operates and should share data to encourage joint problem solving.

References

1. National Safety Council. *Accident Facts 1988.* Chicago: NSC, 1988, pp. 44–45.

2. Klein, B. P., Jensen, R. C., and Sanderson, L. M. Assessment of workers' compensation claims for back strains/sprains. *Journal of Occupational Medicine* 26(6):443–48, 1984.

3. National Safety Council. *Supervisor's Safety Manual.* 6th ed. Chicago: NSC, 1985.

4. Joint Commission on Accreditation of Healthcare Organizations. *Accreditation Manual for Hospitals.* Chicago: JCAHO, 1989.

5. Smith, G. M., and Sabin, J. Protecting hospital employees from toxic and hazardous substances in the hospital environment. *Hospital Employee Health,* Special Report, 1986.

6. Elliott, L. J., Ringenburg, V. L., and others. Ethylene oxide exposures in hospitals. *Applied Industrial Hygiene* 3(5):141–45, May 1988.

7. Slavik, N. S. *OSHA/EPA Handling and Disposal of Hazardous Materials.* American Hospital Association Technical Document Series. Chicago: AHA, Dec. 1988.

8. Imbriani, M., Ghittori, S., and others. Nitrous oxide (N_2O) in urine as biological index of exposure in operating room personnel. *Applied Industrial Hygiene* 3(8):223–26, Aug. 1988.

9. National Institute for Occupational Safety and Health. *Criteria for a Recommended Standard: Occupational Exposure to Waste Anesthetic Gases and Vapors.* Pub. no. 77-140. Washington, DC: U.S. Department of Health, Education, and Welfare, 1977.

10. National Institute for Occupational Safety and Health.

11. Jeffrey, L. P. *Recommendations for Handling Cytotoxic Agents.* National Study Commission on Cytotoxic Exposure. Boston: NSCCE, 1987.

12. Jeffrey.

13. Patterson, W. B., Craven, D. E., and others. Occupational hazards to hospital personnel. *Annals of Internal Medicine* 102(5):658–80, May 1985.

14. Price, C. M. *Asbestos in Buildings, Facilities and Industry.* Rockville, MD: Government Institutes, May 1987.

15. U.S. Environmental Protection Agency. *Guidance for Controlling Asbestos-Containing Materials in Buildings.* Washington, DC: U.S. EPA, 1985.

16. U.S. Nuclear Regulatory Commission. *Principles and Practices for Keeping Occupational Radiation Exposures at Medical Institutions as Low as Reasonably Achievable.* NUREG-0267. Washington, DC: U.S. Nuclear Regulatory Commission, 1977.

17. Highlights from the decision of Judge Patrick F. Kelly in the case of *Johnston v. United States. Newsletter of the Health Physics Society* 13(4):1–4, Apr. 1985.

18. Slavik, N. S. *Hazardous Waste Management Strategies for Health Care Facilities.* Chicago: American Hospital Association, 1987.

19. Slavik, *Hazardous Waste Management Strategies for Health Care Facilities.*

20. McLean, A., and Lehmann, R. *Managing Hazardous Wastes and Materials.* Chicago: Joint Commission on Accreditation of Healthcare Organizations, 1986.

21. Findley, E. L. *Achieving Compliance with Hazardous Waste Regulations in 1986: Manual for Hospitals.* Avondale, GA: Findley & Co., 1986.

22. U.S. Environmental Protection Agency. *Guide for Infectious Waste Management.* NTIS PB86-199130, EPA/530-SW-86-014. Washington, DC: U.S. EPA, 1986.

23. Slavik, *Hazardous Waste Management Strategies for Health Care Facilities.*

24. Keil, O., Lipschultz, F., and others. *Plant, Technology, and Safety Management Handbook.* Chicago: Joint Commission on Accreditation of Healthcare Organizations, 1985.

25. National Fire Protection Association. *Life Safety Code.* 1988 ed. (NFPA 101). Quincy, MA: NFPA, 1988.

26. Hyman, W. A. *Risk Management for Medical Equipment and Environmental Safety.* Plant Technology and Safety Management Series. Chicago: Joint Commission on Accreditation of Healthcare Organizations, 1988.

27. Joint Commission on Accreditation of Healthcare Organizations.

28. Joint Commission on Accreditation of Healthcare Organizations.

29. Keil, O. R., Ness, J., and others. *Developing an Effective Safety Program.* Plant Technology and Safety Management Series Update No. 2. Chicago: Joint Commission on Accreditation of Healthcare Organizations, 1985.

Part Four

High-Risk Areas

Highly experienced risk managers often rely on their instincts to decide where risk is most likely to result in financial loss. But most have to play "by the book"—that is, they go with the percentages and devote their attention to those areas where incidents have statistically resulted in the greatest financial loss. This section will help the risk manager who plays the percentages. It describes the areas that are known to be high-risk and suggests ways to manage those risks. The first five chapters in this section deal with specific health services that need careful risk management consideration. Other issues covered in this section include informed consent, infection control, withholding or withdrawing of life support, credentialing and privileging, organ transplantation, institutional review boards and human research, and confidentiality of hospital records.

Chapter 13
Obstetrics

John C. Dronsfield

Several factors combine to make obstetrical and perinatal services an area of focus for the hospital risk manager. The frequency and, more important, the severity of obstetrical claims have consistently been a major concern. Although obstetrical practitioners face the same uncertainties and challenges as health professionals in other clinical areas, the public expects that all mothers should deliver healthy babies. In addition, because birth is a natural process and newborns are resilient, practitioners may ignore variances in the delivery process. Once a claim is made that a damaged infant was delivered, those variances are often identified by experts as "obvious" indicators of fetal distress.

☐ Standards of Care

The American College of Obstetricians and Gynecologists (ACOG) and the Nurse's Association of the American College of Obstetricians and Gynecologists (NAACOG) have worked together to establish integrated guidelines for medical and nursing obstetrical practice. The recommendations, technical bulletins, and joint statements developed by ACOG, NAACOG, and other professional societies frequently are used to establish a national standard of care. When those guidelines are not met, plaintiff's attorneys may use them to demonstrate a lack of compliance with professional standards.

An effective risk management program will ensure that obstetricians, pediatricians, anesthesiologists, nurses, and other clinicians involved in the perinatal process have access to information regarding current and evolving practice guidelines. Policies and procedures should be reviewed to evaluate compliance with those recommendations, and quality assurance/risk management indicators should be developed to monitor compliance with established policies. A familiarity with ACOG/NAACOG recommendations will help the hospital risk manager to ask hospital staff the right questions and will provide the opportunity to modify inappropriate practices or policies.

☐ Electronic Fetal Monitoring

Although much controversy has accompanied the development of electronic fetal monitoring, electronic fetal monitor strips continue to play a pivotal role in obstetrical liability claims. From a risk management perspective, electronic fetal monitoring can provide a continuous, documented record of fetal well-being and may be effective in defending against allegations of negligence. Even a fetal monitor strip that reflects the onset of fetal distress can provide an effective defense to such allegations if nursing staff promptly intervenes. Those potential benefits, however, can quickly disappear if fetal monitoring is not effectively managed and documented.

Common problems with fetal monitoring include the following:

- Improper record retention, resulting in lost or damaged strips
- Nurses' and physicians' lack of training and/or experience in fetal monitor interpretation
- Delays in responding to documented fetal distress
- Documented disagreements regarding the extent or nature of fetal distress present on a particular strip

The risk manager should ensure that the facility retains fetal monitor strips as a permanent part of the medical record. In addition, the risk manager needs to assess procedures for reviewing fetal monitor interpretation skills and practices of nursing and medical staff.

☐ Cesarean Section Capability

The American College of Obstetricians and Gynecologists recommends that any facility that provides delivery services be able to perform an emergency cesarean section within 30 minutes of determining that one is necessary. In addition, certain procedures, such as amniotomies and the administration of pitocin, should be done only when a qualified physician and the other resources required to perform an emergency cesarean are immediately available. Although a review of hospital and medical staff policies may reflect compliance with those guidelines, risk management procedures should be designed to monitor actual practice and permit the review of any cases not meeting those standards.

☐ Perinatal Exposures

The delivery and care of a newborn require a variety of clinical personnel. Nurses, midwives, obstetricians, family practice physicians, pediatricians, residents, laboratory personnel, admission clerks, radiology technicians, and others all may have a role in evaluating or treating patients as they move through the delivery process. Claims alleging a lack of response to fetal distress or delays in treatment often result from a breakdown of communication among members of the perinatal team. For example, a nurse may document fetal distress but *not* document actions taken to communicate that information to the treating physician.

The hospital risk manager should review job descriptions and the responsibilities of each practitioner involved in the perinatal process to ensure that roles are clearly defined. In addition, the qualifications of each individual to perform specific procedures or provide the assigned level of care should be evaluated and documented. Circumstances that require consultation or the presence of a physician or other specialist should also be identified and procedures established to support and monitor compliance with those requirements. Administering pitocin in the absence of a physician qualified to perform a cesarean section or delivering a premature infant without ensuring the presence of appropriate personnel to provide respiratory support are practices that become very difficult to defend if a poor outcome occurs.

Finally, and probably most important, the risk manager needs to help establish an interdisciplinary forum for care givers to address issues of communication and continuity of care. Such a forum should include clinical and administrative representatives from all disciplines involved in the perinatal process and should focus on reviewing the quality and safety of obstetrical and newborn care.

Chapter 14

Emergency Services

John C. Dronsfield

Widespread publicity regarding new emergency medical technology has caused the public to accept medical miracles as commonplace. Emergency practitioners, however, typically meet their patients for the first time during a crisis and, based on limited medical and social history, must make immediate and often critical decisions regarding diagnosis and treatment. Despite the challenges of providing clinical care under those circumstances, patients clearly expect that entrance into an emergency medical system guarantees survival and full recovery.

☐ Regulations and Legal Requirements

As the hospital's "door to society," the emergency department tends to be a focal point for concerns regarding access to health care, patients' rights, child abuse, and other complex issues. Compliance with regulations regarding informed consent, the treatment of minors, patient transfer, duty to warn, denial of treatment, and other requirements can be difficult and, in some circumstances, may interfere with the treatment process.

A review of local regulations and recent legal decisions can assist a risk manager in developing forms and procedures that will document reasonable efforts to comply with established legal requirements. Orienting staff not only to the forms but also to the principles or concepts underlying the use of the forms will help to ensure that procedures are applied in a flexible, reasonable manner. In addition, developing procedures for prompt access to legal and even judicial intervention may be of benefit.

Efforts to address regulations or legal requirements, however, should not overshadow an appropriate focus on patient care. Decisions made solely for legal or financial reasons can set the stage for a lawsuit if it can be demonstrated that patient care was compromised. From a risk management perspective, a decision to provide safe, appropriate patient care is typically the most definable action.

☐ Agency/Contractual Liability

Increasingly, hospitals are being held liable for the quality of medical care provided in their emergency departments regardless of their contractual relationship with the emergency physicians. The legal theory that the emergency physician is the "ostensible agent" of that hospital increases the hospital's exposure for claims in the emergency room (ER). To minimize this exposure, the risk manager can require emergency service physicians or groups to carry adequate insurance. In addition, the risk manager should review the contract with the ER group to ensure that the relationship is that of independent contracting and not employment. Using signs and other statements to inform patients that the physicians are independent practitioners rather than employees of the hospital may defeat the argument that the physician is the hospital's agent. Aggressive medical staff credentialing and privileging activities and ongoing quality monitoring processes, however, continue to provide the most effective response to such medical staff exposures.

☐ Medical Care

More than one physician may be involved in the care of an emergency services patient. Questions regarding who was responsible for the patient at what point in the care can lead to finger pointing and cross-allegations among defendants, which increases the difficulty of defending the claim.

In addressing medical care issues, the risk manager should ensure the following:

- That every patient treated is seen by a physician
- That the physician primarily responsible for the medical management of the patient is clearly identified throughout the patient care process
- That the responsible physician validates patient care decisions made by residents, physician assistants, or other allied health personnel before the patient is discharged
- That emergency department physicians do not write admission orders and that the responsible admitting physician directly evaluates the patient within an appropriate time frame
- That the patient care record documents the preceding steps and demonstrates effective communication of patient status when patient care responsibility is transferred from one physician to another

☐ Admission/Triage

An effective triage, or initial assessment process, is critical to the prompt evaluation and treatment of emergency patients. Allegations of delayed diagnosis or treatment frequently result from processes that permitted an extended waiting period without appropriate patient evaluation.

Each patient who enters the emergency department should be evaluated promptly by a registered nurse or other clinician with appropriate training and experience. The triage process should be designed to:

- Prioritize patient care activities
- Provide immediate intervention for life-threatening conditions
- Establish a relationship with the patient and his or her family and provide the information and support they need to understand that their needs are being addressed

☐ Documentation

A complete, accurate patient care record is critical not only to the provision of safe patient care, but also to the effective defense of liability claims. Records should be reviewed on a regular basis to ensure the following:

- That vital signs are obtained on every patient and rechecked following treatment, during extended stays, or if abnormal
- That patient history is obtained and documented, including medication usage, allergies, last menstrual period, and other significant information
- That times of patient care activities are documented, including both nursing and physician assessments, lab tests, X rays, medication administration, and other treatments or processes
- That the identity of nurses, aides, physicians, and any other individuals assessing or treating the patient is clearly documented
- That any abnormal lab, X-ray, or other test value, including final or late readings, has been addressed
- That discharge instructions have been clearly documented and include an appropriate referral for follow-up care, instructions to return if conditions change, and an acknowledgment of the patient's understanding

☐ High-Risk Clinical Issues

Claims alleging the missed diagnosis of cerebral or spinal injury, myocardial infarction (heart attacks), appendicitis, ectopic pregnancy, and meningitis represent major exposures for emergency department clinicians. Those conditions are particularly difficult to diagnose in the emergency setting. Specific assessment and treatment protocols addressing head injuries, chest pain, abdominal pain, and fever of unknown origin should be developed to address the following:

- Identify specific assessment and diagnostic procedures that should be considered in evaluating each patient in a high-risk category.
- Support the admission of patients with questionable diagnosis.
- Provide detailed, written instructions if patients in these high-risk categories are discharged. The instructions should specify under what conditions and how soon the patient should seek follow-up care.
- Require an appropriate referral for follow-up evaluation and care.
- Establish a patient follow-up or call-back procedure.

☐ Patient Discharge

A well-documented patient discharge process is critical to both high-quality, safe patient care and effective management of potential liability exposures. Risk managers should question any procedure that permits patients to be discharged *without* (1) being seen and evaluated by a physician, (2) documented understanding of follow-up care instructions, (3) a referral for follow-up care, and (4) instructions to return if their condition changes.

☐ Telephone Consultations

Nurses working in emergency departments frequently are asked to respond to telephone inquiries either as a follow-up to a visit by a patient or by people experiencing symptoms who want to be diagnosed without coming in. The risk manager should work with nursing personnel to define how they are to respond to such inquiries. Although in some instances it may be appropriate to answer a question or give advice to someone who was seen recently in the ER, it is not appropriate to discuss symptoms and diagnoses with patients who have not been seen. The best response in all situations is to encourage the patient to be seen by a physician if there is any question about the patient's medical status.

☐ Standards of Care

Although standards for emergency services typically reflect the recommendations of specific specialty areas, the American College of Emergency Physicians (ACEP) and other professional societies are becoming more active in developing practice standards for the provision of emergency medical and nursing care. In addition, ACEP has published an extensive manual addressing liability and risk management issues within emergency medicine. (*Risk Management in Emergency Medicine,* published by the Emergency Medicine Foundation of the American College of Emergency Physicians, Dallas, TX, 1985.)

Chapter 15
Home Health Services

John C. Dronsfield

In response to the aging population, increased consumer demand, and changing patterns of reimbursement, health care organizations have expanded home health programs and activities rapidly over the past 10 years. Although there apparently has not yet been a corresponding growth in malpractice claims from home health, it has created new areas of potential liability.

☐ Employee Safety

Employee safety issues are different in the patient's home than they are in the hospital. Care givers must learn new patient lifting and transfer techniques. They must be taught to be alert to hazards in home environments with which they are not familiar. Patients and family members may respond unpredictably. Security escorts may be necessary for employees to travel through unsafe neighborhoods.

Risk managers may want to review workers' compensation, automobile liability, and other insurance policies to identify gaps in coverage that may result from the expansion of employee activities. Employees should be made aware of the extent of insurance coverage and cautioned that activities outside the scope of the employee's job, such as stopping to do personal shopping while en route to a patient's home, complicate coverage and create increased exposure for both the employee and the hospital.

☐ Incident Reporting/Quality Monitoring

Risk managers may wish to modify procedures for collecting information on incidents that may affect clinical care or the safety and security of patients or staff. Employees may tend not to report occurrences that are out of their control, such as unsafe electrical wiring or angry relatives. The reporting format should facilitate the prompt evaluation and resolution of potential liability exposures. Employee orientation should familiarize home health staff with the types of occurrences they should report.

□ Equipment Management

As home health care relies increasingly on technology, exposures arising from the maintenance and use of medical devices and equipment increase. Wheelchairs, electric beds, and increasingly sophisticated equipment such as respirators and intravenous infusion devices may be part of home health services. Even though the owner of the equipment is primarily liable, the risk manager should address the safety and quality of equipment that program staff use in caring for patients. In addition, documentation that staff have received appropriate training in and orientation to the safe use of equipment can be critical should an accident occur.

□ Staffing

Home health staff are expected to work independently in a variety of environments where they may encounter unpredictable situations and unexpected demands. Such circumstances accentuate the need for effective procedures for selecting, orienting, training, and periodically reevaluating all personnel. Risk managers need to ensure that documentation demonstrates that the qualifications of all staff have been evaluated and that policies permit staff to perform only those functions or procedures for which they have appropriate orientation and training. Policies within home health programs affiliated with a hospital must be consistent with general hospital standards and comply with licensing and other regulatory standards. Staff should not be permitted to perform functions in the home, such as giving injections, taking physician orders, or adjusting intravenous settings, that they would not be qualified to do in the hospital.

□ Patient Education

In the home health environment, patients and members of the patient's family play an active role in patient care. If the patient or family members have not received adequate information about how to provide the services the patient needs and the patient is injured as a result, there may be liability exposure. Patient education should include written instructions or manuals, periodic review and evaluation of the quality of services provided, and procedures for backup phone support for emergencies or to answer questions.

□ Documentation

Documentation is a crucial element in both managing and evaluating patient care. From a risk perspective, effective documentation of discharge planning, patient education, patient care plans, patient services, patient status, and other aspects of patient care activities provides a valuable record and, in some cases, the only record, of program efforts to comply with established standards of safe, high-quality patient care. Risk managers need to ensure that procedures for the periodic centralized review of patient care records are in place. This centralized review facilitates the evaluation of quality and can help to ensure that documented problems are corrected.

□ Fraud and Abuse/Antitrust Issues

A high percentage of home health services and supplies are funded through federal Medicare programs. Medicare regulations prohibit the payment of any remuneration, in cash or in kind, in return for referring a patient who is provided services or supplies under

Medicare programs. Violators may suffer criminal penalties of up to $25,000 and/or imprisonment. In addition, federal antitrust legislation provides severe penalties for unfair competitive practices. Risk managers should make sure that the hospital's attorney has conducted a thorough legal analysis of home health corporate structures and referral arrangements so that program managers do not inadvertently enter into agreements that create a substantial exposure for their institutions.

Chapter 16
Surgery, Anesthesia, and Recovery

John C. Dronsfield

Adverse patient outcomes in surgery most frequently are caused by a breakdown in the continuity of care as the patient moves through the surgical process. The effective management of liability exposures requires a coordinated, integrated surgical process that focuses on providing safe, high-quality patient care. This chapter covers the major areas of concern to the risk manager who is evaluating surgery, anesthesia, and recovery procedures.

☐ Informed Consent

Informed consent is a legal concept that requires that a patient or his or her legal guardian be advised of and understand the risks, benefits, and alternatives prior to agreeing to a procedure or treatment. Informed consent usually is indicated by a signed statement, and it is particularly important when surgery is performed or when anesthesia is induced.

Surgery

It is the physician's responsibility to discuss with the patient the risks, benefits, and possible alternatives of planned surgical procedures. It is the hospital's responsibility to verify that this "informed consent" process has occurred. Rather than focusing on developing the perfect consent form, risk managers should emphasize the benefits of an effective informed consent process, one that builds patient relationships and establishes realistic expectations. Allegations of a lack of informed consent are more easily defended if, in addition to obtaining a signed hospital consent form, physicians document discussions with their patients in progress notes.

Anesthesia

Although no standard practice has been established, some departments have responded to the growing emphasis on the risks of anesthesia by developing a separate anesthesia informed consent form. This separate form may provide some benefit if it documents a more complete process. The risk manager should, however, emphasize the process rather than the form. Providing the patient with information is particularly important in anesthesia, where patients may have only limited contact with the clinician who provides their care.

☐ Surgical Privileges

The hospital, through the medical staff, has a clear responsibility to base the granting of surgical privileges on an evaluation of training and experience that qualifies a physician to safely perform specific procedures. That process requires the medical staff to do the following:

- Determine what surgical procedures the hospital can adequately support with necessary resources and staff
- Establish what level or type of training and experience will adequately qualify a physician to perform the procedure
- Evaluate the training and experience of physicians who are applying to perform the procedure

Although physicians may qualify for privileges in more than one specialty, the same requirements for training and experience should be consistently applied. If the procedure reflects new techniques or the use of new technology, or if no internal resource is available to evaluate a physician's qualifications to perform a particular procedure, outside experts may be needed to evaluate physician qualifications. The risk manager should monitor procedures designed to ensure that appropriate privileges have been granted for all procedures performed in the facility.

☐ Staffing Roles and Responsibilities

In the surgical suite, staff perform roles that are unique to surgical, anesthesia, and recovery activities. Some may be employees, not of the hospital, but of the surgeons. Many perform roles for which there are no licensing or standardized qualifications to demonstrate their competence. Risk managers need to work with the medical staff and hospital personnel to ensure that the responsibilities of surgical assistants, surgical technicians, anesthesia assistants, scrub nurses, postanesthesia recovery nurses, and any other individuals who provide patient care or even observe patients are clearly defined. In addition, either medical staff or hospital procedures should be designed to evaluate and document the qualifications of those staff members to perform assigned functions. Nonhospital personnel should be credentialed through the medical staff credentialing process.

☐ Perisurgical Committee

Although some patient care activities in surgery are assigned to specific individuals, responsibility is shared among care givers for many others. An incorrect consent form, surgery on the wrong leg or wrong patient, incorrect positioning, an inaccurate sponge count, or other similar incidents often lead to major disagreements about who was responsible.

Risk managers need to focus on the staff's shared responsibility to provide safe patient care. An interdisciplinary or "perisurgical" committee that reviews and evaluates all aspects of the surgical/anesthesia/recovery process can provide an effective forum for addressing those interrelated responsibilities. Such a group should include nursing, physician, and administrative representatives from each area. The responsibilities of the committee are to develop policies for safe patient care and to do ongoing monitoring of the quality of patient care.

☐ Intubation

The failure to establish and maintain an adequate airway results in the most severe anesthesia claims. Typically, those cases occur because personnel are not qualified or equipment is unavailable to intubate a difficult or emergency patient. In other instances, the lack of adequate airway results from a displaced or improperly placed endotracheal tube.

In addressing those issues, the risk manager should evaluate anesthesia procedures and resources to ensure the availability of qualified personnel and equipment necessary to respond to the types of patients and conditions cared for in the facility. In assessing surgical patients, care givers must be made aware of any previous problems patients may have had being intubated and if there are any patient characteristics that may cause difficulty in establishing and maintaining the airway. If problems are likely to occur, staff should be appropriately assigned and the patient adequately supervised to provide a safe intubation. The most qualified practitioner available should be notified that problems may develop.

New technologies such as capnography and pulse oximetry have supplemented the traditional "bilateral breath sounds noted/X-ray" approach to verifying endotracheal tube placement. Practitioners should use these monitors to verify that an adequate airway is established and maintained throughout a procedure. The appropriate use of this equipment, the periodic recording of values obtained throughout anesthesia administration and recovery, and the documented response to inadequate or disrupted tube placement contribute to safe patient care and assist the institution in defending allegations of liability.

☐ Extubation

Most patients are extubated prior to being transported to the recovery unit for postanesthesia care. It may be appropriate to evaluate the quality of the anesthesia service if patients frequently are being taken to recovery while still intubated. The facility should have clear procedures for staff to follow when extubating patients. Although patients can be extubated by a qualified nurse, a physician or other staff member qualified to re-intubate the patient should be immediately available.

☐ Equipment Exposures

Advances in technology continue to produce more sophisticated, and more expensive, anesthesia and surgical equipment. Although neither the most sophisticated nor the most expensive equipment is required, an anesthesia service that does not routinely utilize pulse oximetry and capnography in addition to traditional methods of monitoring the patient's status will be very difficult to defend if a poor outcome occurs. To effectively address potential exposures related to the use of equipment, the hospital risk manager needs to do the following:

- Work with anesthesia and surgical staff to ensure that available equipment and monitors meet current standards and are adequate to provide safe anesthesia and surgical services to *all* patients
- Review equipment maintenance contracts, procedures, and documentation of maintenance activities
- Evaluate patient records for documentation of preadministration equipment review (checklist) and for documentation of the use of appropriate monitors (periodic values/monitor readings should also be recorded, even if normal)
- Ensure that procedures for privileging, orientation, and training provide a documented evaluation of each clinician's qualifications to operate available equipment in a safe, efficient manner
- Establish quality review indicators to monitor ongoing compliance with equipment maintenance and operation procedures

☐ Quality Monitoring/Incident Reporting

Staff orientation and training in the functions and purposes of incident reporting and in identifying specific clinical events that must always be reported can assist in the development of efficient surgical incident reporting. In addition, quality monitoring activities can provide the risk manager the opportunity to assist the medical staff and surgical personnel in identifying and reviewing adverse occurrences.

☐ Standards of Care

Several professional organizations have developed practice guidelines and recommendations that relate to both medical and nursing practice throughout the surgical, anesthesia, and recovery process (see bibliography). The American College of Surgeons was one of the first professional organizations to address patient safety; risk managers should be familiar with that organization's *Patient Safety Manual*. The American Society of Anesthesiologists (ASA) also has been aggressive in addressing patient safety issues. The ASA's Patient Safety Foundation publishes a newsletter on safe anesthesia practice and has available a four-part video series on anesthesia patient safety that is a valuable tool for orienting anesthesia and risk management personnel.

☐ Anesthesia Supervision

Current standards permit certified registered nurse anesthetists (CRNAs) to administer anesthesia under the supervision of an anesthesiologist or independently under the direction of a qualified surgeon. Because of this flexibility, a wide range of departmental structures and supervisory relationships are found in hospitals. It is the hospital's responsibility, through the medical staff, to ensure that appropriate, qualified supervision and quality-of-care review processes are established. Risk managers should review departmental practices and question any procedures that (1) appear to assign patients or provide a separate standard of care based on the patient's ability to pay or the time of day, or (2) do not provide patients immediate access, if needed, to a qualified clinician.

☐ Monitoring in the Recovery Unit

Postanesthesia recovery is the final phase of the anesthesia process. Recovery policies should require that recovering patients be accompanied to the recovery unit by anesthesia personnel and that a full, documented patient status report is provided. The use of pulse oximetry and other new technology to support effective patient monitoring during the recovery process should also be addressed in policies, along with procedures for discharging patients from the unit.

☐ Bibliography

American College of Surgeons. *The American College of Surgeons Patient Safety Manual.* Chicago: American College of Surgeons, 1985.

American Society of Anesthesiologists. *The ASA Newsletter.* Park Ridge, IL: ASA, 1989.

Anesthesia Patient Safety Foundation. *The Anesthesia Patient Safety Foundation Newsletter.* Overland Park, KS: APSF, 1989.

Chapter 17
Psychiatry

Virginia P. Johnson

Unlike other areas of the hospital, where reliance on technology is evident, the psychiatric unit generally is devoid of machinery, bright lights, and medical emergencies. The absence of technology, however, does not mean an absence of risk. On the contrary, the fallibility of machinery is replaced by the unpredictability of human beings.

Psychiatric patients are treated in public or private facilities and in general hospitals, not only on the psychiatric unit but on other units as well. In addition, outpatient facilities, substance abuse rehabilitation centers, partial hospitalization programs, and supervised housing all treat the mentally ill.

Most of these outpatient psychiatric facilities are based on the concept that patients can be treated by integrating them into the community rather than by institutionalizing them. Practitioners believe that activities, therapies, and even casual interactions present the opportunity for therapeutic encounters. However, problems arise when there is a mix of diagnoses and behaviors. Patients who are hallucinating, delusional, or paranoid may easily misinterpret their environment and disrupt the milieu. For those patients, the controlled environment of the psychiatric unit plays a significant role in recovery.

Given this diversity of patient behaviors, there is quite a difference between the types of malpractice claims filed in psychiatry and those in other medical areas. Only infrequently are suits based on failure to diagnose or treat or on negligence in treating the patient; they tend instead to focus on a failure to observe, prevent, inform, predict, or protect the patient. The ability to foresee the patient's behavior is the common thread. A frequent psychiatric claim is that the therapist failed to prevent the patient's suicide.[1]

A complicating factor is that patients are expected to participate in their treatment plans and to take active steps in their recovery. This is a generally accepted tenet of almost all mental health professionals. However, mental health patients may not have the ability to do this.[2]

Hospital employees sometimes avoid the psychiatric unit for fear of being injured or seeing others injured or fear of odd or unusual behavior. Nonpsychiatric health care professionals may believe that mental health professionals have magical skills that they themselves lack. There are no mystical techniques, but there are sound therapeutic interventions. A well-trained staff person skilled in a variety of those interventions makes the mysticism tangible, the patients and staff safer, and the risks manageable.

☐ General Guidelines

Three elements that are essential in all areas of risk management but especially in psychiatry are assessment, risk-reduction techniques, and documentation. The risk manager must assess the general scope of psychiatric services, the safety of the physical structure of the unit, the composition and skill level of the staff, specific treatments available, and the adequacy of written policies and procedures. For details of this assessment, refer to figure 17-1.

A strong peer review/quality assurance process is the key to risk reduction. Particular risk strategies will be discussed later as they relate to specific problems; however, certain techniques are common to all services, and those are described in figure 17-2 (p. 168). Although providing care that meets standards of practice is the best defense against malpractice claims, documenting the care provided plays a crucial role in providing evidence that the standard of care was met. Highlighted in figure 17-3 (p. 169) are those areas most important in psychiatry.

☐ Special Problems

The nature of mental illness and the unique therapies used to treat it present a special challenge in risk management. In discussing high-risk areas in psychiatry, it is difficult to separate the psychiatrist's liability from that of the hospital. If the psychiatrist is a private practitioner, the plaintiff may claim that the hospital has a duty to do peer review and oversee the physician's practice. If the psychiatrist is a hospital employee, the duty is clear. In all cases, the psychiatric staff—physicians, nurses, aides, technicians, counselors, psychologists, and social workers—are held responsible for their assessments and treatment. Although as the team leader the psychiatrist is ultimately responsible, he or she depends on information given and observations made by all staff. Such information must be reported appropriately and documented thoroughly.

Psychopharmacology

Drug therapy is a cornerstone of psychiatric treatment, but the drugs may pose serious risks to patients. Malpractice claims relating to psychopharmacology (which includes major and minor tranquilizers and antidepressants, among other drugs) tend to cluster around negligence in prescribing and administering drugs and failure to observe adverse effects.[3] One irreversible adverse effect caused by long-term psychotropic drug use is known as tardive dyskinesia, characterized by involuntary movements, often of the face and tongue. It can also produce severe restlessness. Tardive dyskinesia may occur in as many as 10 to 25 percent of long-term patients.[4]

Two strategies are most effective in minimizing the risks of drug therapy. The first is intensive monitoring of the physicians' prescribing practices to ensure that patients are not receiving excessive doses or prolonged treatment. Monitoring is done through physician peer review and through educating staff in recognizing adverse reactions. The second strategy is getting patients' informed consent. The patient needs to be made aware of the risks and benefits of the drug as well as alternatives to drug treatment. It is the physician's responsibility to prescribe drugs and to ensure an informed consent, with many physicians using a signed form to document this.[5] However, staff members play a significant role in minimizing risks of drug therapy by conscientiously observing patients for signs of adverse reactions and reporting them to the physician and by informing the physician if it is apparent that the patient does not have accurate information about prescribed drugs.

Two other issues surround medications: a patient's refusal to take prescribed drugs and a physician's prescribing dosages that exceed guidelines. Although drugs will

Figure 17-1. General Areas of Assessment

General Scope of Services	Physical Structure of the Unit	Composition and Skill Level of the Staff	Specific Treatments Available	Written Policies and Procedures
Are the following services provided: • Inpatient treatment • Outpatient therapies • Emergency services • Rehabilitation • Long-term care • Partial hospitalization *Is the unit open* (having voluntary patients) *or closed* (having involuntary or committed patients)?	• What shape does the unit have? • What is visible from the nurses' station? • Are there special types of rooms available (i.e., observation or seclusion rooms)? • How visible are activity areas? • How close are the entry doors to the nurses' station? • What doors are kept locked/open? • How are windows secured? • Are there breakaway bars in the tub/shower areas? • How secure is the nurses' station?	• What percentage of the nursing staff are RNs, LPNs, aides? • Are there social workers (Bachelor of Science in Social Work, Master of Science in Social Work) available? • Are there psychologists on staff? • How many activity personnel are on the unit on each shift? • Are there any salaried physicians on staff? • Are there other specialists available (i.e., certified alcoholism counselors)? • What percentage of the staff on each shift is male/female? • How does the ethnic/cultural composition of the staff compare with that of the patients? • What is the experience level of the staff who deal most directly with the patient? • What is the availability of medical consultants?	*Are the following available:* • Psychopharmacology • Individual therapy • Group therapy • Family therapy • Specialized activity therapy • Electroconvulsive therapy (ECT) • Seclusion • Restraints • Drug and alcohol rehabilitation • Adolescent care • Eating disorders treatment • Behavior-modification therapy • Care of the neurologically impaired • Treatment for the mentally retarded • Geriatric psychiatry	*Are there policies for:* • Suicide precautions • Restraints • Management of the violent or assaultive patient • Commitments • AMAs • Smoking rules • Fire plan • Use of seclusion room

Figure 17-2. General Risk-Reduction Techniques

1. Monitor and evaluate accuracy and appropriateness of the treatment planning process as it relates to:

- Diagnosis
- Admission
- Diagnostic assessments (lab results, consultations)
- Actual written treatment plans
- Specific treatments (are they appropriate and properly carried out?)
- Patient responses
- Discharge status and discharge plans after care

2. Perform concurrent monitoring and evaluation of high-risk clinical practices, including:

- Incident reports
- Drug utilization review (poly-pharmacy, dosage adjustments, consent of patients, forcible intramuscular injections)
- Suicides
- ECT

3. Utilize more extensive procedures for evaluating staff

- More specific screening of applicants
- Comprehensive orientation program
- Specific, clear professional privileging process (i.e., which disciplines perform which therapies)

Source: Adapted from Joseph, E. D. Strengthening risk management in psychiatric facilities. *Perspectives in Health Care Risk Management* 8(4):15–18, Fall 1988.

Note: These are general techniques used as part of a departmental quality assurance program.

Figure 17-3. General Documentation Issues

Initial Assessment	Treatment Plan	Consults	Progress Notes
• Thorough history and physical • Clear assessments for suicidal potential and violence potential[a] • Thorough medical evaluation • Mental status assessment • Complete admission notes from psychiatrist and admitting nurse	• Short- and long-term goals • Inclusion of all members of the treatment team	• Informed consent for ECT[a] • Informed consent for psychotropic drugs	• Patient responses to treatment • Current status assessment • Detailed notes whenever the patient's status is changed (i.e., moving from an open to a closed unit; discontinuing or instituting observation; being placed in or out of restraints; pre- and post-passes; pre- and post-ECT, etc.)[a] • Rationale for all treatment changes[a] • Reevaluation of all orders[a] • Complete discharge note with specific aftercare plans

Source: Adapted from Joseph, E. D. Strengthening risk management in psychiatric facilities. *Perspectives in Health Care Risk Management* 8(4):15–18, Fall 1988.

[a]Particular attention should be paid to these items.

stabilize a patient whose behavior is threatening or disruptive, the patient may not realize this and may refuse medication. Clear, situation-specific policies should include direction on dealing with emergency situations and guidelines on managing adult patients who are capable of consenting, adults who are not capable, and minors. Barton's article "Administration of Psychotropic Agents to Patients Who Refuse Such Medications"[6] describes specific policies and action plans for those patients. If the patient's prescribed dose exceeds recommendations, the staff should make sure that the justification for the treatment is documented in the medical record.

Electroconvulsive Therapy

Although not used as frequently as in the past, electroconvulsive therapy (ECT) is still a viable treatment that generally is low-risk. The American Psychiatric Association's *Recommendations Regarding the Use of Electroconvulsant Therapy* is a comprehensive reference. If policies and practice address informed consent, anesthesia requirements, necessary medical workup, emergency management, amount of patient supervision needed, and the credentialing process of all professionals privileged to perform ECT, the risk to the institution from allegations of malpractice is minimized.[7]

Suicide

A frequent malpractice claim in psychiatry is the failure to prevent a patient's suicide. Suicide claims generally include such issues as failure to care appropriately for the obvious suicide risk, improper treatment methods, negligent diagnoses, and failure to warn. Even institutions that do not provide psychiatry service have liability if they assume responsibility for suicidal patients. In hospitals, the most common means of committing suicide are hanging and jumping. Shift change is a particularly high-risk time.[8,9]

Assessment of the Likelihood of Suicide

Many authors have developed rating scales and extensive checklists to assess suicidal potential. However, all of them suggest that the following symptoms may indicate patients at high risk:[10]

- Current suicidal behavior
- History of previous suicide attempts
- Suspicious behavior, such as refusing food or medication, saving medications, talking of death, or checking windows
- Mood changes
- Personality changes
- Patient's inability to promise to control himself or herself
- Recent significant losses
- History of suicide in the family
- Feelings of depersonalization
- Severe and/or chronic illness
- Alcohol or drug abuse
- A developed, lethal, and available plan
- The finalizing of a patient's affairs

Following are also significant times during hospitalization when the patient is at greater risk:[11]

- Upon admission
- When the patient is self-destructive
- When observation has been increased or decreased

- When being considered for or given passes (as many as 75 percent of successful suicides are committed when patients are out on passes)
- Upon discharge

Besides assessing the patient, the staff should make the environment safer, including securing windows and screens, checking the number and length of electrical cords, using breakaway shower rods, minimizing the use of drop ceilings, noting the number and location of emergency exit doors, and ensuring that all doors swing open into the hallways, not into the rooms.[12]

Additional Risk-Reduction Techniques for Suicide

Once a patient is determined to commit suicide, the best preventive strategy is to assign the patient a roommate and a room close to the nurse's station; this increases the staff's ability to make sure that the patient is constantly observed. Policies on suicide prevention must delineate the intensity of observation, how observation strategies are initiated, and how they are discontinued. The roles of the staff must be clearly spelled out. Although the physician is the treatment team leader, other staff members also have responsibility to assess patients' suicide potential. Staff must be taught to distinguish between patients who merely threaten suicide and those who have suicidal intent.

Documentation of Suicide Assessment

Staff must be trained to communicate well with one another and to document suicide assessments thoroughly. Courts are more likely to side with the survivors if documentation is scant. Generally, courts do not hold health care professionals responsible for predicting patient behaviors. As long as practitioners make judgments according to the "reasonable professional" standard and the rationale for treatment decisions is documented, the outcome of litigation is likely to favor the defendants.[13]

Violence by Patients

Violent behavior by patients includes verbal and physical assaults. When patients become assaultive, the institution faces legal, ethical, moral, and patients' rights issues. Psychiatric care givers have several duties. They must maintain a balance between protecting both the violent patient and the potential victim without unduly infringing on their civil liberties, and they must warn potential victims if they know them to be in danger. The difficulty in fulfilling those duties lies in the ability to predict patient behavior. The family's inability to understand the difficulty in predicting violence prompts them to file suit. Again, the standard for assessing negligence is whether the practitioner's judgment was a "reasonable professional" judgment.

The duty to warn arose from a 1974 California decision, *Tarasoff v. Board of Regents of the University of California*, which stated that ". . . when the therapist determines or . . . should determine that his patient presents a serious danger of violence to another, he incurs an obligation to use reasonable care to protect the intended victim against such danger. [The therapist may have to] warn the intended victim or others likely to apprise the intended victim of danger, to notify the police, or take whatever steps are reasonably necessary under the circumstances." Originally, the Tarasoff ruling applied only to an identifiable victim; however, it is possible that this "duty to warn" will extend to threats to property or unnamed third parties as well.[14]

Although the therapist faces the dilemma of balancing the duty to warn with the duty to preserve the patient's trust and maintain confidentiality, judges are likely to focus on how foreseeable the violence was and whether the practitioner could have prevented the outcome.

Assessment of Violent Patients

As with suicide, violence is, for the most part, not predictable. However, there are certain factors that predict the risk. Males between the ages of 15 and 30 who have a history of violence and are drug or alcohol abusers are the most likely to be violent. The health care provider must assess how effectively the patient can control his or her behavior, whether a clear motive for violence exists, and whether the patient has the means to carry out any threats. Particularly in dealing with the assaultive patient, assessment may be hampered by the worker's fear of danger. Staff must be trained to intervene appropriately without fearing injury, and they must have resources available to assist in subduing combative patients. Mental health staff with acute assessment skills may be able to sense impending patient violence. Given the difficulties inherent in predicting behavior, psychiatric staff members can minimize their liability by being well versed in intervention strategies. Clear communication among workers and quick, decisive, and organized action may help to prevent serious harm from violent patients.

Risk-Reduction Techniques for Violent Patients

Psychiatric staff must be specially trained in techniques used to subdue violent patients. The general approach should be nonantagonistic, including allowing the patient space, speaking slowly and clearly, and ensuring enough help, even to the point of a "show of force."

If communicating with the patient fails, restraint, seclusion, and medication may be needed. Organizing resources before confining the patient reduces the chance of injury to both patient and staff. Department policies should specify how staff are to obtain additional assistance when needed. The risk manager must feel confident that staff have developed the skills they need to protect themselves and the patients.

Using restraints and seclusion to subdue patients may be a source of liability. They are restrictive, and they raise issues of incarceration. In addition, both methods may give staff a false sense that the situation is under control, causing them to relax patient monitoring. These interventions should instead prompt more intensive patient observation. Restraints and seclusion are often more effective when coupled with other therapies, such as giving medication or providing verbal and emotional support. Policies for using restraints and seclusion must specify the indications for their use, how to initiate and discontinue restrictive therapies, time limits for using restraints or secluding patients, how often staff should observe patients, and assurances that the patient's environment is free from hazards.

Risk managers can provide education to staff in managing violent patients. The risk manager should also ensure that all serious incidents of violent patient behavior are reviewed by a multidisciplinary team to determine whether patient management was appropriate.

Documentation of Violent Behavior

Descriptions of the patient's behavior, including direct quotes, paint the clearest picture of why restrictive interventions were warranted.

The patient's behavior should continue to be documented throughout the acute phase of agitation, as well as when the decision is made to remove restrictions. Observation checks must be carried out and documented at intervals specified by policy. Insurance representatives who handle psychiatric claims indicate that claims relating to restraints and seclusion center on the staff's failure to observe the isolated patient. Failure to document observations will be construed as failure to observe.

Documentation of violent patients is equally important at the time of discharge. Notes stating the staff's conclusions regarding the likelihood of violence, the proposed course of action, why this action is most likely to be effective, and what actions were taken to ensure the patient's compliance with discharge plans will present a defensible record.

Violence by Staff

Violent behavior by staff against patients, whether verbal or physical, presents a sensitive problem. Reported incidents should be investigated objectively, and confidentiality should be maintained to protect the patient and the staff member. The investigation should be quick and thorough, and the investigator must try to determine whether the staff member or the patient is telling the truth. If necessary, the staff member may be removed from the unit pending the outcome of the investigation.[15] Proper screening of all staff members before hiring them may prevent staff abuse.

Confidentiality

Confidentiality of patient information is a primary risk management concern. It is particularly acute in psychiatry, where there are federal laws governing the release of information on drug and alcohol patients.

In addition, most states have laws governing release of information on psychiatric patients. The risk manager should be well versed in these laws and should seek advice from the hospital's counsel in order to provide a resource to psychiatric staff. To ensure the patient's trust in the therapist, patients should be assured that their therapists will maintain confidentiality unless patients present a threat to themselves or others, or unless the therapist must seek family support to monitor the patient.[16]

Patients' Rights

Health care facilities have a responsibility to ensure that the personal freedoms of patients are restricted only as a last resort for the safety of the patient or others. Even if the patient threatens harm, the institution has a duty to use the least restrictive measures to protect patients, staff, and others.

Commitments

State law regarding involuntary confinement of patients differs from state to state. Many allow a patient to be involuntarily detained on the physician's order for three days after the patient has requested discharge in writing if the practitioner determines that the patient is mentally ill and poses a threat of serious harm to self or others. A commitment hearing must be held prior to the expiration of the statutory period. Indiscriminate commitment of patients, however, may make the physician and hospital liable for negligence, assault, battery, and false imprisonment.[17] When the practitioner weighs the risks and benefits of commitment against the risk that the discharged patient may harm someone, many practitioners believe it may be more prudent to err on the side of commitment.

Risk managers should advise practitioners that involuntarily committing the patient does not give authority to treat the patient if the patient is unwilling to be treated. A separate judicial hearing may be required to compel treatment. The risk manager must be thoroughly familiar with the commitment laws in effect in the state. Specifically, the risk manager must know who may order a commitment, how long the patient may be held for a hearing, and what liability the hospital has while the patient is detained pending a commitment.

AMAs

When a patient is unwilling to accept treatment yet does not meet state commitment criteria, the physician may allow the patient to sign out "against medical advice" (AMA). Staff should attempt to dissuade the patient from leaving and should inform the physician of the patient's intent. In order to diminish the health care facility's potential liability, documentation should specify that the patient was not exhibiting any active violent thoughts or actions but was simply expressing a desire to leave. Unless the physician orders the patient to be held, the patient is requested to sign a release form. If the patient refuses, the staff should document the refusal in the medical record.

Elopements

Occasionally patients will "elope," or escape. A patient escape implies a lack of vigilance by the staff, suggesting that the institution is liable. Staff members and hospitals may be held responsible for acts committed by patients after such escapes.[18]

Informed Consent

Hospital staff members frequently wonder whether mental illness precludes a patient from giving an informed consent for treatment. The risk manager should explain that competent patients of sufficient age must consent before being treated. A psychiatric patient may be declared incompetent through a hearing, but until then, the patient is legally competent unless a physician determines that the patient's clinical state interferes with the ability to comprehend. Hospital staff may intervene in an emergency without consent or, in a life-threatening situation, when the patient opposes intervention.[19]

The physician's assessment of the patient's ability to comprehend risks and benefits will determine whether the patient is able to give an informed consent. Unless there is clear evidence otherwise, psychiatric patients should be considered competent and able to consent for their treatment. The physician's assessment should be documented in the record. In questionable cases, family members may be included in a discussion of the risks and benefits of treatment, or a competency hearing may be initiated. For the protection of the health care professional, all consents, including consent to admit, to leave against medical advice, and to treat with medications, should be treated as informed consents.[20]

Fires, Burns, and Sexual Acting Out

The problems that arise in treating psychiatric patients are as varied as their behavior. Three in particular deserve additional mention: fires, burns, and sexual acting out.

All three problems arise either because of impulsive patient acts or because of inadequate staff supervision. Although there may be few malpractice claims relating to those issues, they do present serious concerns for patient safety. Psychiatric patients often have an impaired sense of reality, may demonstrate little regard for rules, or may not use "common sense." Accordingly, the hospital staff has a greater duty to provide strict surveillance, especially over patients' smoking practices and their sexual activity. Unit rules and regulations should be explained to patients either individually or in a group, with evidence in the record that the rules were explained. Policies specifying the frequency with which staff members are to make rounds, especially at night, and notes to support those rounds will aid in the defense of such claims.

Staff or Visitors as Plaintiffs

Where there is litigation for assaultive behavior, the patient may not always be the plaintiff. Staff or visitors to the unit who are abused or assaulted by patients also may sue either the patient for the assault or the institution for not providing adequate security. If it is determined that the patient knew and understood the consequences of his or her actions, the patient is held to the same standard as someone without a psychiatric diagnosis and may be found civilly liable. If the patient is not responsible, the patient's insurance company has no duty to pay.[21] However, there are different laws and legal precedents in different states, as the following quote describes:

> While mentally ill persons are generally responsible for negligent acts and civil wrongs, the law dealing with employers and insurers is not so clear. The financial liability of an insurer may be determined by whether or not the mental illness impaired the intentional capacity of the defendant. Thus the standards are broader and less clear than those usually spelled out in criminal cases.[22]

References

1. Talbott, J. A. The professional liability crisis: an interview with Joel Klein. *Hospital and Community Psychiatry* 37(10):1012–16, Oct. 1986.

2. Joseph, E. D. Strengthening risk management in psychiatric facilities. *Perspectives in Healthcare Risk Management* 8(4):15–18, Fall 1988.

3. Lieberman, S. Psychiatric risk control. *QRC Advisor: Managing Hospital Quality Risk & Cost* 5(1):1–7, Nov. 1988.

4. Applebaum, P. S., and others. Responsibility and compensation for tardive dyskinesia. *American Journal of Psychiatry* 142(7):806–10, July 1985.

5. Talbott, p. 1015.

6. Barton, E. Administration of psychotropic agents to patients who refuse such medication. *Perspectives in Healthcare Risk Management* 8(4):13–14, Fall 1988.

7. Lieberman, p. 4.

8. Perr, I. N. Suicide litigation and risk management: a review of 32 cases. *Bulletin of the American Academy of Psychiatry Law* 13(3):209–19, 1985.

9. Watzer, H. Malpractice liability in a patient's suicide. *American Journal of Psychotherapy* 34(1):89–98, Jan. 1980.

10. Watzer, pp. 89–98.

11. Prevent patient suicides with early identification strategy. (A summary of a presentation by Nathan Farberow). *Hospital Risk Management* 4(12):157–60, Dec. 1982.

12. Lieberman, p. 3.

13. Bartels, S. J. The aftermath of suicide on the psychiatric inpatient unit. *General Hospital Psychiatry* 9(3):189–97, May 1987.

14. Beck, J. C. The potentially violent patient: legal duties, clinical practice and risk management. *Psychiatric Annals* 17(10):695–99, Oct. 1987.

15. Magazine, C. J. Investigating staff abuse of patients in a psychiatric setting. *Perspectives in Healthcare Risk Management* 8(4):19–22, Fall 1988.

16. Talbott, p. 1013.

17. Psychiatric emergencies. *Emergency Nurse Legal Bulletin* [MedLaw Publishers, Inc.], 1978, pp. 2–8.

18. Psychiatric emergencies, pp. 2–8.

19. Perr, I. N. Legal problems in inpatient psychiatry. *Psychiatric Medicine* 4(4):455–67, 1986.

20. Hostetler, D. Mental health section meeting focuses on quality. *Journal of the American Medical Record Association* 57(5):21–23, May 1986.

21. Perr, I. N. Liability of the mentally ill and their insurers in negligence and other civil actions. *American Journal of Psychiatry* 142(12):1414–18, Dec. 1985.

22. Perr, pp. 1417–18.

☐ Bibliography

Bartels, S. J. The aftermath of suicide on the psychiatric inpatient unit. *General Hospital Psychiatry* 9(3):189–97, May 1987.

Brizer, D. A., and others. A rating scale for reporting violence on psychiatric wards. *Hospital and Community Psychiatry* 38(7):769–70, July 1987.

Calfee, B. E. Are you restraining your patient's rights? *Nursing '88* 18(5):148–49, May 1988.

Develop strong RM program in psychiatric unit to cut risks. *Hospital Risk Management*, May 1988, pp. 66–68.

Farberow, N. L. Guidelines for suicide prevention in the hospital. *Hospital and Community Psychiatry* 32(2):99–104, Feb. 1981.

Kroll, J., and Mackenzie, T. B. When psychiatrists are liable: risk management and violent patients. *Hospital and Community Psychiatry* 34(1):29–36, Jan. 1983.

Levenson, J. Dealing with the violent patient. *Postgraduate Medicine* 78(5):329–35, Oct. 1985.

Northrop, C. E. Nursing actions in litigation. *Quality Review Bulletin* 13(10):343–47, Oct. 1987.

Tan, M. W. Suicide and violence to others: loss prevention strategies. *Perspectives in Healthcare Risk Management* 8(4):9–12, Fall 1988.

Chapter 18
Informed Consent

Fay A. Rozovsky

Consent to treatment is often misunderstood to be an administrative form or document. In fact, consent is a communications process that culminates in the patient's agreeing to certain tests or procedures to be performed by the care giver.[1] The fact that care givers often overlook the process and concentrate on the forms raises significant concerns for risk managers. Unauthorized surgeries, undisclosed risks, and undisclosed treatment options can lead to adverse outcomes and litigation.

This section of the chapter concentrates on the basic requirements for a valid consent, the exceptions to the rules, the right to refuse treatment, pertinent legislative requirements, and problem situations, including those in which children require care. Other sections of the chapter discuss important policy considerations surrounding such issues as death and dying (do not resuscitate/do not hospitalize orders and withdrawal of life support) and the requirements for organ procurement and retrieval.

☐ General Requirements for Valid Consent

For a consent to treatment to be valid, care givers must follow certain well-recognized steps. These steps should be followed in the absence of specific state requirements or exceptional circumstances that trigger the rules governing consent in unusual situations (see "Exceptions to the Rules for Consent," later in this chapter).

Consent Obtained by the Care Giver

The person carrying out the procedure should obtain consent. The best way to ensure a valid consent is to insist that the care giver obtain the patient's consent. "Caregiver" refers to the person who is actually carrying out the diagnostic or therapeutic intervention. It is his or her task to obtain pertinent patient history information, to disclose relevant information, and to answer patient questions. Although a ward clerk or a nurse might be asked to perform the administrative task of getting the patient to sign a so-called "consent" form, it is the care giver's responsibility to complete the actual consent process.

The rationale for this rule is simple. Because it is the care giver who best understands the history, needs, and desires of the patient, it is that individual who should disclose pertinent information and answer relevant questions. This means that the surgeon who is to operate on the patient should inform the patient; it is a function that should not be delegated to a medical resident or fourth-year medical student. By the same token, a nonmedical intervention—such as physiotherapy—obliges the nonmedical practitioner to obtain consent. Although a family practitioner may refer a patient for physiotherapy, it is up to the physiotherapist to secure the patient's authorization for the actual therapy to be employed.

Legal and Mental Capability

The patient must be legally and mentally capable of giving consent. The law presumes that every person is both legally and mentally capable of giving consent to treatment. In the case of legal capacity, this means that the person is not under any court order or statutory impediment that would preclude the ability to authorize care. The fact that a person is under a civil commitment order for psychiatric care does not automatically remove the right to authorize treatment. Instead, the impact of a civil commitment order depends on the specific requirements of state law. However, if the person is under a guardianship or conservatorship of another person, which includes matters of health care, legal capacity to consent has been removed.

The fact that a patient is 16 or even 12 years of age does not mean that he or she is legally incapable of giving consent. In the absence of a state law mandating an age of consent or a court order appointing a guardian of the patient, a minor is considered legally capable of giving consent.

Mental capacity refers to a person's ability to synthesize information and reach a treatment choice. Mental capacity may be permanently impaired, as through an anesthetic accident or severe mental retardation, or compromised on a temporary basis, through alcohol or drug intoxication. Severe pain, shock/trauma, or emotional insult can also lead to transient episodes of mental incapacity. Care givers must exercise judgment to determine whether patients possess the ability to synthesize information and reach treatment choices.

These judgments can be particularly difficult with patients who experience episodes of incoherence or who are sporadically lucid. Equally difficult are situations involving minors, who may be able to appreciate the nature and consequences of certain treatment choices but not others. Thus, an 11-year-old girl who has undergone long-term chemotherapy and repeated bone marrow transplants may be capable of consenting to or refusing consent to a new series of related treatments, but not to therapy for a different ailment. Mental capability is a matter best determined on the facts and information available for each patient.

Lack of Influence or Coercion

Patients must make their decisions about consent free of undue influence or coercion. They should never be confronted with "take it or leave it" choices or threats of reprisals. Because health care facilities are intimidating institutions to many consumers, staff members should be trained to identify patients' anxiety associated with institutional care, which, if not dealt with, can present impediments to a valid consent.

Test or Treatment Specificity

Consent must be given for a specific test or treatment. Authorizations for treatment should be testor treatment-specific. For example, if a care giver is to perform a breast biopsy, the authorization is limited to that intervention. Consent to breast biopsy is not a license to proceed further with a radical mastectomy. However, if an intervention is a "staged" procedure, involving a biopsy and possible removal of a breast, the patient can consent if the physician explains beforehand that more extensive treatment may be necessary, depending on the results of the biopsy. A consent is valid only to the extent that it includes all agreed-upon tests or treatments.

Understanding of Patient History

Consents must be premised on solid history taking. For a care giver to obtain a valid consent necessarily implies a solid understanding of the patient's history. Risk factors, complications, allergies, intolerances, and the like can come to light only through a thorough patient history. Talking with the patient also permits the care giver to determine the patient's needs and desires. A patient may want cataract surgery, but the impending marriage of a favorite grandchild may motivate the individual to postpone the operation to a more convenient time. The family social engagement and the fact that the procedure is elective are factors that should be taken into consideration.

Adequate Disclosure of Information

Disclosure of information must be adequate. There is no fixed rule governing how much information to give the patient. In some states, disclosure is gauged by what the care giver deems appropriate;[2] in other jurisdictions, it is gauged by what a reasonable or prudent person in the patient's position would want to know in the same or similar circumstances. A more traditional approach bases disclosure on what the *actual patient* would want to know.[3] A check of state law will reveal what is the appropriate standard.

Despite the differing disclosure yardsticks, there is general agreement on the categories of information, which include the following:

- The nature and purpose of the proposed test or treatment
- The probable risks and probable benefits of the proposed intervention
- Alternate or reasonable alternate form(s) of care
- The probable risks and probable benefits of the alternate form(s) of care
- Remote or unusual risks that involve severe injury or disability or death
- The risks of refusing care or diagnostic tests

Information should be disclosed in language that is understandable to the patient. The degree of sophistication of the disclosure should be tailored to the patient's ability to comprehend.

Opportunity to Pose Questions

Patients must be given a reasonable opportunity to synthesize the information disclosed by the care giver. Distraught or anxious patients may require more time than those with greater composure. The time required may also vary with the complexity of the recommended intervention and the individual's capacity to process detailed information.

Although patients should not be pressured into decision making, it is reasonable for the care giver to ask if there is any confusion about the recommended intervention or if there is a need for further information. To some extent, this makes it easier for patients to admit concern or lack of understanding. It is a welcomed gesture that can facilitate the care giver–patient relationship.

Questions should be addressed in a clear, frank manner. Absent the need to use the therapeutic privilege exception (discussed below), care givers should not withhold information deemed necessary for the decision-making process.

All Required Elements Obtained

All the elements must be in place for a consent to be valid. From the risk manager's perspective, it is important to monitor the consent processes used in the health facility to make certain that all the required elements of a consent are met. This may require concurrent monitoring of consent processes. It may also require fine-tuning of incident reports to flag inappropriate patient consents.

The risk manager can take a highly visible, positive role in consent matters. By working with the inservice coordinator and medical staff, by sitting on key hospital committees, and by being available to answer staff questions on consent requirements and to help draft or review policies, the risk manager can influence the way in which the facility meets the required elements of consent.

☐ Consent to Research on Human Subjects

Standards governing disclosure in human research are considerably different from those in the therapeutic setting. Federal regulations[4] and some state laws[5] outline specific requirements for consent to human research. Risk managers in hospitals that conduct human research should familiarize themselves with applicable laws. As a general rule of thumb, however, risk managers should realize that the scope of disclosure is greater under human research legislation and regulations.

☐ Exceptions to the Rules for Consent

There are a number of recognized exceptions to the requirements for a valid consent to treatment. Some have been carved out by the courts, whereas others are the product of legislative and regulatory action. It is incumbent upon the risk manager to determine what constitutes the recognized consent exception in his or her state. Legal counsel for the health care facility should be able to supply pertinent information.

The more widely recognized exceptions include medicolegal emergencies, therapeutic privilege, compulsory treatment, and the patient's refusal to be informed.

Medicolegal Emergency

The medicolegal emergency exception is based on the notion that the average person would readily agree to treatment if confronted with a life- or health-threatening event.[6] When such a person is unable to do so because of the severity of injury, the law "implies" consent to such care.

Such an emergency exists when all the following elements are present:

1. The patient has a life- or health-threatening condition requiring immediate care
2. The patient is incapable of participating in the consent process
3. There is no time to obtain consent from a duly authorized representative

When all these elements are present, care givers can proceed with reasonable treatment. What is "reasonable" is determined on a case-by-case basis. For example, suppose an unconscious patient arrives at the emergency department having suffered extensive head wounds and a severe leg injury in a car accident. Without prompt surgery, the patient could die. There is no time to secure consent from a duly authorized legal representative.

At surgery, it is determined that the badly injured leg must be amputated at the knee. Does the medicolegal exception to the rules for consent authorize the amputation? The answer is yes, assuming that the amputation is necessary to eliminate the life- or health-threatening episode. However, the removal of a suspicious mole on the thigh of the same leg would not be authorized. Although the mole may be a source of concern, it is not of the same degree of urgency to warrant treatment without consent.

All the elements of the medicolegal emergency must be present to proceed under the exception. The failure to meet the appropriate standards can easily lead to litigation based on unauthorized treatment.

Therapeutic Privilege

This exception is for patients who may suffer significant emotional or physical harm if they are given disturbing information.[7] To avoid such harm, the law permits care givers to withhold such information. However, the exception is narrowly drawn, and care givers are still obliged to provide patients with other pertinent information. From a risk management perspective it is important to follow an established procedure for using this exception, including the specifics of documenting therapeutic privilege.

Compulsory Treatment

In some situations, patients must submit to treatment. Compulsory tests or treatments are likely to occur for certain communicable diseases or mental health problems. The scope of such compulsory treatment laws is narrowly drawn to avoid undue infringement upon patients' rights.

Despite the fact that treatment may be compelled, good risk management principles suggest that care givers obtain an accurate history and review of medication needs. For example, if a patient under a compulsory treatment order is suspected of having a sexually transmitted disease, it is reasonable to determine whether the recommended treatment of choice is suitable for the individual. The failure to secure a proper history could lead to inappropriate drug therapy, allergic reactions, or death. That the patient's history was obtained should also be documented in the medical record.

Patient's Refusal to Be Informed

Some patients refuse to be given proper disclosure as a prerequisite to a valid consent. They may have complete trust in members of the treatment team, or they may be so anxious about the "gory details" that they prefer to go into a test or intervention in complete ignorance.

Some state laws recognize the right of patients to refuse to be informed.[8] This stance is the antithesis of the whole movement toward patient awareness and effective communication. Moreover, it reinforces consent practices that ignore the need for sufficient disclosure of information.

A patient who declines to be informed can place tremendous pressure on physicians. In some instances, a doctor may correctly decide not to treat a patient in such circumstances, particularly if the patient must be actively involved in the procedure. The physician who decides not to treat must then refer the patient to someone else who may be willing to provide treatment without the benefit of an adequate disclosure of information.

Where patients balk at being informed, a sound risk management strategy that nurses and physicians can employ is to determine *why* there is such resistance. It may be because of a previous bad experience, a preference to remain in the dark rather than face the hard truth regarding the diagnosis, or any number of reasons. Whatever the reason, care givers should be supportive and offer to inform patients in terms that are designed to minimize anxiety.

If care must proceed without a proper disclosure, the care giver should document all attempts to inform the patient, as well as the patient's response to those attempts.

The notation should describe what information was imparted. In this way, a degree of written evidence is in place should the institution face litigation based on inadequate disclosure.

☐ The Right to Refuse Treatment

It is well accepted that it is the patient who should decide what shall be done to his or her body. Implicit in this concept is the right to either authorize care or refuse consent to treatment. However, the right to refuse care is not absolute and has been the subject of considerable litigation.[9]

Case law suggests that a competent adult can decline life- or health-saving care in certain circumstances—typically, where the patient has strongly held religious beliefs and is not the sole support of any minor children.[10] However, where the state demonstrates sufficient interest in preserving life, the right of the patient to refuse consent may have to give way. This is particularly true if more than one life hangs in the balance (as in a situation involving a pregnant woman) and there is a strong likelihood of successful treatment.[11] On the other hand, when patients are terminally ill, case law suggests that the decision to refuse or withdraw from care may be respected.[12] Despite these broad principles, it must be kept in mind that there is considerable pressure to expand the right to refuse care by abandoning distinctions based on patient condition, religious beliefs, and so on.

The right to refuse care can also be exercised by incompetent patients through a duly authorized legal representative.[13] This could be a legal guardian or a person given a durable power of attorney to make health care decisions.

From a risk management perspective, it is important to determine the legal requirements in the jurisdiction governing the exercise of the right to refuse care. The hospital attorney should be involved proactively to develop appropriate responses to difficult situations involving the right to refuse treatment.

☐ Legislative Requirements

Risk managers should familiarize themselves with the wide variety of state and federal legislative and regulatory requirements on consent to treatment. Within a given jurisdiction, there may be overlapping consent provisions. California, for example, has several different legislative requirements governing minors and consent in different treatment settings.[14] Some state laws on consent deal with the standards for litigation rather than the requirements for a valid consent.[15] However, the applicable elements for consent can be construed from those provisions.

Risk managers should also be aware of highly specific consent requirements found in specialized legislation. For example, the general requirements for consent may be inapplicable for patients in mental health facilities.

Laws and regulations other than those specifically addressing consent should also be reviewed carefully for "hidden" consent requirements. In some states, consent requirements may be found in so-called patients' bills of rights.[16] In Massachusetts, for example, the Board of Registration in Medicine has promulgated regulations on consent, a source not often considered when trying to determine state law on authorizations for treatment.[17]

The fact that state legislation and regulations may be "silent" on the matter of consent does not mean that there is no law on the topic. There may be an abundance of case law that has set down the rules for consent. Risk managers should make it a practice to review state consent law on an annual basis. Changes are bound to occur either in case law or legislation and regulations. Legal counsel can assist the risk manager in determining the scope of state requirements on consent to treatment.

Risk managers also must be familiar with consent requirements under federal law. Two that deserve discussion are the consent provisions found in the human research regulations for the Department of Health and Human Services (HHS)[18] and the Food and Drug Administration (FDA).[19] In each instance, the agency has delineated a number of consent provisions that must be followed for federally sponsored human research. It should be noted, however, that other federal agencies may soon come under similar requirements, particularly if the government adopts a uniform approach to human research trials.

Although sometimes overlooked as an important source of direction, the Joint Commission on Accreditation of Healthcare Organizations' guidelines for accreditation contain important material on consent requirements.[20] Risk managers for accredited facilities should be familiar with the Joint Commission standards.

☐ Problem Cases and Consent to Treatment

Consent to treatment is a subject that will never cease to be of concern to risk managers. As treatments change, so do the demands for disclosure and careful history taking. Nonetheless, there are many common, recurrent consent "problem cases." On an intra-institutional basis, these problem cases can be identified and reasonable responses to them can be made part of the facility's consent policy and procedure. Perhaps the most difficult cases involve minors and incompetent adults.

Minors

The presumptions of legal and mental capacity apply equally to children and adults. The fact that a child is not of the age of majority does not necessarily mean that he or she is legally incapable of giving or refusing consent. Much depends on state law and the facts of each case. Some exceptions have been incorporated into state laws that have carved out "age of consent"[21] requirements by legislation. Others have enacted "emancipated minor" laws,[22] making it possible for children who meet certain criteria to be treated as if they are adults for purposes of consent. Still other states have recognized the principle of the "mature minor,"[23] permitting young people to give consent when they are able to understand and appreciate the nature and consequences of a treatment choice.

On the federal level, the HHS regulations governing consent to human research have carved out a rather unusual consent standard for minors.[24] These rules require particular attention in health facilities in which minors are the subject of human research.

Problems can arise when a child is incapable of giving consent or when there is a conflict between the child's desires and those of his or her parents. Parents are presumed at law to be the natural guardians of their children. However, when the parents act in a way that threatens the child's best interests or well-being, the state, under the legal doctrine of *parens patriae,* can step in to safeguard the child.[25] Thus parents who have refused life-saving blood transfusions or surgery have seen the courts respond quickly to the physicians' or hospital's petition to appoint a guardian to authorize necessary treatment.[26]

A related problem arises when the child's parents are separated or divorced and do not agree on the child's treatment, or if the custodial parent is unavailable and the adult accompanying the child for treatment is the parent with visitation rights. After consulting with legal counsel, the risk manager should address these issues in the hospital's consent policy and should be available to staff for inservice education. In addition, the risk manager should work to resolve consent situations not covered by policy.

Consent of minors to abortion will become an even more troublesome issue since the recent Supreme Court decision allowing the states much greater latitude to enact legislation on the topic.

Incompetent Adults

Another troubling issue involves treatment of incompetent adults who are without a duly authorized legal representative. Working with legal counsel, the risk manager should determine whether, under state law, consent can be given by a spouse or other family member, such as an adult son or daughter, what the order of priority is, and what should be done if there is a dispute among similarly situated family members. Health care facilities can anticipate these consent problems and build solutions into the facility's consent policy.

What is more difficult to address, however, is the tendency on the part of some care givers to label elderly persons "incompetent" because they do not respond rapidly to questions, they seem confused or disoriented, or they reject what care givers deem highly appropriate treatment. The "incompetent person" category can be abused quite easily by paternalistic or insensitive care givers. An elderly person's failure to respond may be attributable to a hearing impairment. Confusion and disorientation may be natural coping mechanisms of elderly people who are suddenly thrust into a strange environment. Standing alone, hearing impairment or confusion does not warrant a finding of incompetency. Neither can patients be determined to be incompetent solely because they reject what care givers consider reasonable treatments. What young clinicians deem "reasonable" may be considered highly intrusive by elderly people.

Risk managers should make certain that hospital personnel understand who is responsible for determining competency to consent to treatment. Typically, this judgment is reserved to physicians. However, doctors who lack experience in working with developmentally disabled or elderly patients may reach inappropriate conclusions. Nurses, social workers, and psychologists may be better able to distinguish between incompetence and lesser disabilities. Therefore, to ensure that appropriate assessments of competency are made, risk managers should work with other members of the health care team to set stringent criteria for determining competency and should delineate the positions of those individuals who are responsible for making such assessments. These criteria should be clear and easily applied. Moreover, they should take into account pertinent state laws and should be the subject of inservice education programs so that all care givers are clear on who may be deemed incompetent to consent to treatment.

Patients Who Are Terminally Ill or in a Persistent Vegetative State

Treatment of those who are dying or in a persistent vegetative state (PVS) requires compassion, understanding, and, especially, an ability to convey difficult information in a way that preserves the autonomy of the terminally ill person. For those patients who no longer possess the ability to consent, care givers must deal with surrogate decision makers who are often ill-equipped emotionally to make critical choices.

Consent to treat dying individuals should be part of well-delineated policies and procedures addressing an overall plan of care for those patients and their families. Rather than "compartmentalizing" treatment of the terminally ill into orders not to resuscitate or orders to withdraw nasogastric tubes, it is far better to view treatment of the terminally ill as part of the larger picture of supportive care for the dying and their families.

Policy choices aside, it is essential for the risk manager to understand that there is no clear-cut rule governing consent to treatment of either the terminally ill or those in a persistent vegetative state. Impending changes through the vehicle of a United States Supreme Court decision may help to clear the air on the topic. However, notwithstanding this clarification, each risk manager should obtain from legal counsel state-specific advice on the following matters:

- Legality of living wills executed in another jurisdiction
- Durable powers of attorney executed in another jurisdiction

- Orders not to resuscitate
- Orders not to hospitalize terminally ill patients who reside at home or in a long-term care facility
- Decisions to withdraw respirators or ventilators
- Decisions to withhold or withdraw nasogastric tubes, gastrotomy tubes, intravenous lines, artificial hydration and nutrition, and antibiotics
- Decisions to withhold life-prolonging treatment from terminally ill neonates, including those with anencephalic syndrome
- Surrogate decision making for incompetent terminally ill patients or those with PVS who are without legal guardians and whose family members cannot agree on appropriate treatment

To provide clear-cut legal guidance in each of these cases, the risk manager should assist inservice educators in disseminating information to staff regarding the health facility's policy on treating terminally ill and PVS patients.

☐ Autopsies

There is a distinction between so-called hospital autopsies and forensic or medicolegal postmortem examinations. Hospital autopsies typically are performed both to validate diagnostic and clinical care provided to the deceased and to do quality assurance studies.

The hospital autopsy requires a valid consent from the person responsible for disposing of the decedent's remains. A check should also be made to determine whether the decedent left specific instructions on the disposal of his or her remains. Some may have executed donor cards authorizing removal of organs or tissue for purposes of transplantation or scientific investigation. Others may have ruled out autopsies. The decedent's instructions should be determined prior to any invasive postmortem investigations.

A medicolegal autopsy is quite different. Authorized under state coroner or medical examiner laws,[27] such autopsies are conducted in cases of unusual or suspicious death or a death occurring within a certain time period of admission to a hospital. Although a coroner or medical examiner might "release" a body without conducting a full autopsy, the opposite might also be true. Hence, much is left to the discretion of the medical examiner or coroner in deciding whether a complete autopsy should be conducted.

Because medicolegal autopsies are authorized by statute, there is no need to secure consent for the procedure. Although family members may object on religious grounds,[28] autopsies will often proceed when deemed necessary.[29]

☐ Consent Documentation

Although some states place great weight on "signed consents" from patients, the form itself should not be viewed as "the" consent. Consent is actually a communications process that requires some type of record to ensure continuity of care and appropriate care. Documentation is also important for purposes of legal defense. A written record can be created by using the consent form or by other documentation.

Many hospitals use a "short form" consent document that states that "the nature and purpose and risks and benefits of this procedure have been explained to me." Such forms do not contain any detailed information; rather, it is left to the care giver to provide this information.

The danger is that, should litigation occur, the care giver may not remember the nature of the information that he or she conveyed years earlier, reducing the consent action to a battle of credibility between the patient and the care giver. There is little certainty of who will prevail in such cases.

Therefore, many facilities use the "long form" consent document, which includes considerable detail about the nature and purpose of the recommended treatment, the probable risks and benefits, and reasonable alternate forms of care. Some argue that the long form offers more protection to care givers because it spells out important details for patients. However, if a patient did not read the form or a care giver downplayed important matters, the long form consent provides little defense in litigation.

It is sometimes recommended that hospitals encourage care givers to write detailed notes in patient records, outlining the consent process. Tailored to the individual patient, the note is likely to be given considerable credibility, particularly because it is not a boilerplate document with filled-in blanks. The detailed note is not without its critics, however. Some claim that care givers can write too short a note, leaving out important details whose omission hampers provision of effective treatment and legal defense. Those problems can be avoided by training staff to write consent notations properly. Through question and answer screening, inappropriate documentation can be pinpointed and rectified through appropriate channels (see figure 18-1 for examples of correct and incorrect documentation).

Aside from consent documentation for elective procedures, historical records also are needed in other treatment contexts. For example, if there is no consent in the emergency department record, there should be some indication of why care givers determined that there was no need for a treatment authorization. If patients leave the emergency department or other units of the facility against medical advice, the departure should be documented. The facility may have a "release form" signed by the patient, or, if not, notations may be made in the health care record.

Parents who place their children in the care of babysitters or who go away for a vacation sometimes provide relatives, health care facilities, or their doctors with "general"

Figure 18-1. Examples of Incorrect and Correct Documentation of Consent in a Medical Record

---

Incorrect Documentation

2/3/89 Discussed risks and rewards of operation with patient. Patient agreed to operation tomorrow at 0815 hours.

   The problem with this note is that it does not meet the basic elements of a valid consent. It does not indicate that the patient gave the consent voluntarily or that he or she was apprised of the "probable risks and benefits" of care. It does not indicate that the patient was told of alternative forms of care and the risks of foregoing treatment.

Correct Documentation

2/3/89 Discussed with Mr. James the need for an appendectomy. I explained to him what are considered the probable risks of the procedure and the benefits of the operation. I told him that he would be unable to resume his job as a heavy-equipment operator until we were satisfied that his wound had healed properly. I also advised him of the risks of postponing the operation and taking a "wait and see" approach, including the risk of the appendix bursting and spreading a serious infection throughout his abdomen. Mr. James had no questions about his operation. Mrs. James and Nurse Fonte were in attendance during this discussion. Throughout our discussion, Mr. James was alert and quite confident about the procedure, which is scheduled for tomorrow at 0815 hours.

   This is good consent documentation because it meets all the key elements of a valid authorization for care. It includes a reference to who was present during the consent process, a factor that may be important if there is subsequent litigation. If the writer of this documentation can be criticized at all, it is for failure to specify *what* probable risks and benefits were explained to the patient. This type of oversight could be important in litigation. It can be addressed as part of inservice education rounds.

---

consents for treatment. Blanket consent forms are of dubious legal value, however. A person cannot sign away the right to either consent to or refuse highly invasive diagnostic or therapeutic measures. A form that attempts to cover everything is not much more than a paper tiger.

Risk managers should encourage their hospitals to avoid general consent forms in favor of procedure-specific consent documentation. By the same token, parents should be requested to designate a surrogate decision maker for those children who are incapable of consent rather than supply a general consent form. In this way, care givers have an interested person with whom to interact in determining appropriate treatment.

Some risk managers encourage staff physicians to use videotaped presentations to provide information to patients concerning particular procedures. After viewing the videotape, the patient has the opportunity to discuss the procedure with the physician and clarify anything he or she does not understand. The patient can then indicate consent by signing a form authorizing the physician to proceed. In some cases, hospitals will rely upon detailed notes in the patient record indicating that the patient viewed the videotape and agreed to the procedure or test. A videotape used as an adjunctive tool has the advantage of presenting complete information to all patients who undergo a particularly complicated procedure. However, it cannot replace the patient–care giver dialogue regarding specific risks, needs, and concerns that are integral parts of the consent process.

Should the issue of consent be litigated, the videotape may be convincing evidence to a jury that a patient had sufficient information. Much depends, however, on the specifics of state law governing the evidentiary use of videotapes.

Consent documentation is an important aspect of solid risk management. Careful consideration should be given to what meets the needs of each facility and the requirements of state law. Legal counsel should assist in developing appropriate documentation strategies. Moreover, hospital insurers should be contacted to make certain that the documentation chosen by the hospital is acceptable to them.

☐ Consent Policy and Procedure

To facilitate good consent practices, risk managers should assist their facilities in developing comprehensive policies and procedures that delineate the following:

- The requirements for a valid consent
- The exceptional cases and the requirements for same
- The requirements for consent to human research
- The procedure to follow when patients refuse treatment
- Recognized "problem" cases and the appropriate response to them
- The requirements for documenting consent.

The consent policy and procedure manual should be reviewed at least annually, making certain that changes in state and federal law are incorporated into the requirements. The practical application of the consent policy and procedure should also be incorporated into orientation and inservice education programs. In this way, a pattern can be established of treating consent as a useful part of total health care and not as a piece of paper routinely signed by patients.

References

1. *See* F. A. Rozovsky, *Consent to Treatment: A Practical Guide.* Boston: Little, Brown & Co., 1984 (annual supplements), §1.0. *See also,* F. A. Rozovsky, *Consent to Treatment: A Practical Guide,* 2nd ed. Boston: Little, Brown & Co., 1990 (annual supplements) §1.0.

2. *See* note 1 above, at p. 41.

3. *See, e.g.,* Harnish v. Children's Hospital Medical Center, 439 N.E.2d 240 (Mass. 1982) and Cobbs v. Grant, 502 P.2d 1 (1972).

4. *See* 45 C.F.R. §§46.116–117 (1981) and 21 C.F.R. §50.25 *et seq.* (1981).

5. *See, e.g.,* N.Y. Pub. Health Law §2440 *et seq.* (McKinney 1975) and Va. Code §37.1-234 *et seq.* (1979).

6. *See* note 1 above, at §2.1.1.

7. *Id.,* at §2.3.1; *see also* Utah Code Ann. §76-14-5 (1976).

8. *See, e.g.,* Utah Code Ann. §76-14-5 (1976) and Vt. Stat. Ann. tit. 12, §1909 (1976).

9. *See, e.g.,* Raleigh Fitkin-Paul Morgan Mem. Hosp. v. Anderson, 201 A.2d 537, *cert. denied,* 377 U.S. 985 (1964) 2 and In re Osborne, 294 A.2d 372 (D.C.App. 1972).

10. *See* In re Osborne, note 9 above; *see also* In re Melideo, 88 Misc.2d 974, 390 N.Y.S.2d 523 (1976).

11. *See* Jefferson v. Griffin Spalding County Hospital, 277 S.E.2d 457 (Ga. 1981).

12. *See, e.g.,* Satz v. Perlmutter, 362 So.2d 359 (Fla. 1980).

13. Severns v. Wilmington Med. Center, 425 A.2d 156 (Del. 1980) and Matter of Quinlan, 348 A.2d 801 (1975).

14. Cal. Civ. Code §25.9 (West 1979) dealing with outpatient mental health services and consent by minors; Cal. Civ. Code §34.10 (West 1977) dealing with consent by minors to treatment of alcoholism; and Cal. Civ. Code §34.9 (West 1977) covering sexually assaulted minors and authorization for treatment.

15. *See, e.g.,* N.H. Rev. Stat. Ann. §507-C:2 (1977) and Utah Code Ann. §78.14.5 (1976).

16. *See* R.I. Gen. Laws §23-17.5-7 (1978), a nursing home residents' bill of rights that discusses consent to participate in human research.

17. *See* 243 Code of Mass. Regs. 1.00 *et seq.*

18. 45 C.F.R. §§46.116–117 (1981).

19. C.F.R. §50.25 *et seq.* (1981).

20. *See* AMH/88 *Accreditation Manual for Hospitals.* Chicago: Joint Commission on Accreditation of Healthcare Organizations, 1987, at pp. xiii, 11, 36, 37, 66, 97, 99, 135, and 187.

21. *See, e.g.,* R.I. Gen. Laws §23-4.6-1 (1979) and S.C. Code §44-45 10 (1972).

22. *See* Alaska Stat. §09.65.100 (1975) and Nev. Rev. Stat. §129.030 (1981).

23. *See* Cardwell v. Bechtol, 724 S.W.2d 739 (Tenn. 1979), for an excellent analysis of the mature minor rule.

24. *See* 45 C.F.R. §46.408 (1983).

25. *See, e.g.,* In re Vasko, 263 N.Y.S. 552 (1933) and Mitchell v. Davis, 205 S.W.2d 812 (Tex.Civ.App. 1947). For a detailed discussion of this matter, *see* §5.16 *et seq.* in *Consent to Treatment: A Practical Guide,* note 1 above.

26. *See, e.g.,* Morrison v. State, 252 S.W.2d 97 (Mo.Ct.App. 1952) and Mitchell v. Davis, 205 S.W.2d 812 (Tex.Civ.App. 1947).

27. *See, e.g.,* Conn. Gen. Stat. Ann. §19-530 (1981) and N.Y. County Law §673 (McKinney 1965).

28. *See* Snyder v. Holy Cross Hospital, 352 A.2d 334 (1976), in which members of an Orthodox Jewish family were unsuccessful in their attempt to block a medicolegal autopsy on the body of their son.

29. It should be noted, however, that on occasion the courts will block medicolegal autopsies that are deemed unnecessary given the circumstances of the decedent's death. *See, e.g.,* Atkins v. Medical Examiner of Westchester County, 418 N.Y.S.2d 839 (Supp. 1979), in which a son blocked an autopsy on his mother, whose death resulted from injuries sustained when she was struck by a car. As the court pointed out, the son's deeply held religious beliefs outweighed the medical examiner's curiosity regarding the cause of death.

☐ Bibliography

Rozovsky, F. A. *Consent to Treatment: A Practical Guide.* Boston: Little, Brown & Co., 1984 (annual supplements).

Rozovsky, F. A. *Consent to Treatment: A Practical Guide.* 2nd ed. Boston: Little, Brown & Co., 1990 (annual supplements).

Rozovsky, F. A., and Rozovsky, L. E. *The Canadian Law of Consent to Treatment.* Toronto: Butterworths Canada, 1990.

Southwick, A. F. *The Law of Hospital and Health Care Administration.* 2nd ed. Ann Arbor, MI: Health Administration Press, 1988.

Chapter 19

Infection Control

Joan S. MacDonald

☐ AIDS and HIV Infections

Hospitals have a legal and moral obligation to protect their employees from occupational hazards, including infections acquired from the hospital's patients. When employees fear that they may become infected with fatal or untreatable diseases, they may refuse to care for infected patients. Failure of the institution to allay fears of infection and/or to provide necessary barrier protection lowers employee morale and ultimately jeopardizes patient care.

Adequate risk management in the treatment of acquired immunodeficiency syndrome (AIDS) and other bloodborne diseases begins with institutionwide education and the development of appropriate policies. Policies that do not incorporate rational infection control practices as well as legal and ethical principles are costly to the hospital and potentially dangerous.

☐ Risk Management Strategies in Treating AIDS

Education is the only tool available to stop the spread of AIDS and to allay both employees' and trustees' fears of occupationally acquiring the human immunodeficiency virus (HIV). The risk manager should work with the human resources department or staff education committee to develop education programs. If employees are given adequate information that dispels irrational fears, they are less likely to react inappropriately when faced with caring for AIDS patients. It is also advantageous to extend AIDS education to the families of employees, because relatives' misperceptions can color employee attitudes.

Initial education should include principles of disease transmission. The human immunodeficiency virus is acquired by sexual contact, by introducing infected blood into another's bloodstream, and perinatally by infants of infected mothers. It is *not* acquired through casual contact. Transmission of HIV in the health care setting is limited to contaminated needle-stick accidents and gross infected blood contamination of broken skin.

The education program can compare the number of deaths of health care workers infected in the workplace by hepatitis (estimated at 200 per year) with the total number of AIDS-infected health care workers in the history of the disease (less than 200). The program should explain precautions that health care workers should take to protect themselves. Those precautions should be taken whether a patient is known to carry HIV or not, because many carriers have yet to be tested for infection. Health care workers should treat all blood and body fluids as if they are infectious, regardless of the patient's diagnosis.

Universal Precautions

Universal Precautions are guidelines developed by the Centers for Disease Control (CDC), Atlanta, to prevent transmission of bloodborne infections.[1] The Occupational Safety and Health Administration (OSHA) enforces the CDC guidelines by invoking its "general duty" clause to protect employees from occupational hazards. Violations, determined by random inspections, carry penalties of up to $10,000 for each violation.[2] The guidelines include the following:

- Handwashing
- Use of appropriate barrier protection, such as gloves, gowns, masks, and goggles
- Environmental decontamination
- Measures to reduce accidental needle-stick injuries, including injunctions against recapping, breaking, or bending used needles
- Use of puncture-resistant containers for sharps disposal
- Evaluation and modification of procedures to accommodate Universal Precautions
- Education aimed at changing old habits

Policy Development

The following issues pertaining to AIDS should be assessed by the risk manager; written policies for them may need to be developed.

Refusal to Work

Under OSHA legislation, workers may refuse to perform tasks that they have reason to believe will jeopardize their health and well-being. However, employees do not have the legal right to refuse once appropriate education and barrier protection have been provided. Moreover, an employee's failure to cooperate with rational protocols established by the employer can be construed to be contributory negligence on the employee's part if the employee is exposed. Exposure to some infections is considered a hazard inherent to health care workers. Employees who refuse to care for AIDS patients may be terminated from employment.

Education of Medical Staff

An even bigger challenge for risk managers in trying to combat hospital employees' irrational fear of AIDS infection is educating the hospital's medical staff about who may be tested for AIDS, under what circumstances they may be tested, and the treating physician's legal responsibilities toward patients whose life-styles put them in high-risk categories. Employees may develop inappropriate behavior that is modeled after physician behavior or get misleading or wrong information from physicians with whom they work. The hospital must impose the same standards for treating hospitalized AIDS patients on physicians as it does on its employees. Influencing employee behavior is made more difficult when employees perceive that physicians are treated differently from other health care workers by hospital administration.

Mandatory Routine Testing

Arguments have been made for mandatory testing of hospital patients to protect public health by identifying and controlling infected people. Protecting employees by screening all patients for infections is a costly practice, may lead to a false sense of security for employees, and invades patients' privacy. Given the discrimination against HIV-infected people, the risks of routine testing to the individual patient outweigh the benefits to the general public. The hospital's policies on AIDS testing should include the provision for testing only when it is necessary to treat the patient and with the patient's consent. The policy should also provide for counseling for those who test positive. Counseling provides emotional support and information on life-style changes that AIDS victims must make to prevent infecting others.

Confidentiality and the Need to Know

Laws governing mandatory testing and the issues of consent and confidentiality of information differ from state to state. Application of the principles stated depends on the law of jurisdiction.

To protect patient privacy, identification of HIV-infected patients should be limited to those who need to know in order to care for the patient. However, because information about patients' health is difficult to limit, particularly because it is transmitted by computer, hospitals must also emphasize, in employee inservices, the importance of maintaining the confidentiality of all patient information.

Human Resources

People with HIV infections can continue to work. However, infected personnel have a moral obligation to disclose their condition, if known, and to take appropriate actions to protect others. Using Universal Precautions offers two-way protection: It protects workers from infected patients and patients from infected care givers. In most situations, patients are not exposed to the blood of health care workers; therefore, the risk of transmission can be considered to be very slight. However, because HIV infections can lead to cognitive impairment, infected employees should be assessed on a case-by-case basis and reassigned as necessary.

☐ Risk Management Strategies in Infection Control

The goals of an infection control program are similar to those of any risk management program: to identify, reduce, or eliminate adverse outcomes. In the area of infection control, one risk to be reduced or eliminated is nosocomial infection. Nosocomial infections are those that the patient acquires in the hospital. They are difficult to prevent because they involve risk factors over which the institution has limited control.

Other benefits to be derived from an active infection control program include defending claims of negligence, preventing human suffering from infection, and complying with state and federal regulations. (Laws on particular infection control regulations may differ from state to state.)

Minimum safety standards require that hospitals have (1) a process to identify, track, evaluate, and correct deficiencies in the control of infections, (2) infection control policies and procedures for patient care practices, (3) protection from environmentally associated infection hazards, and (4) a method to detect and control communicable diseases in patients and staff.

Infection Control Program

To assist the new risk manager in evaluating an existing infection control program or in establishing a new one, the following is a list of the essential components of an effective program:

- *A multidisciplinary committee.* This committee is responsible for reviewing nosocomial infections or clusters of infections, advising on control measures, and reviewing hospitalwide infection control policies. Suggested membership includes a physician with special training or interest in infection control, an OR supervisor, a pharmacist, an infection control practitioner, and representatives from nursing, laboratory services, environmental services, and administration.

- *An infection control practitioner.* The practitioner functions as the coordinator of infection control activities. Certification in infection control is advised as a measure of the professional qualifications of the infection control practitioner.[3]

- *A method of surveillance.* The goals of surveillance are early detection of infectious outbreaks, rapid investigation of probable sources/causes, and institution of timely control measures. *Surveillance* is defined as "the systematic collection of pertinent data, the orderly consolidation and current evaluation of the data, and the prompt dissemination of the data to those who need them."[4]

- *Definitions of infection.* Surveillance begins with precise definitions of infections that are approved and understood by all and systematically applied. The CDC provides guidelines for determining the presence and classification of infections as models for acute care facilities.[5] The definitions should be modified as necessary for application in long-term care, because the patient/resident population may not present with classic infection signs and symptoms.

- *A method for collecting data that is appropriate for the type and size of the institution and risk evaluation.* Surveillance data are used to identify problems by service, area, or procedure. The final step in surveillance is reporting the results to the infection committee, hospital services, and nursing units responsible for instituting risk-reducing or control measures.

- *Education of all hospital staff in their roles in preventing infections in patients and staff.* This type of education is a federally required infection control responsibility. Time allocated to this task varies with the size and mission of the institution (15 percent to 45 percent of infection control activities).[6] Educational activities include orientation and inservices to teach aseptic practice and to resolve problems identified in surveillance.

Policy Development

The following established categories of infection control practice should be incorporated into institutional and departmental policies and procedures.

Patient Care Practices: Medical Asepsis

Medical asepsis refers to practices that reduce the numbers of microorganisms and/or prevent or reduce transmission from one person to another; it is also referred to as "clean technique." The following medical asepsis techniques should be used by all personnel involved in nonsurgical patient care:

- Handwashing (the single most important and cost-effective technique of infection prevention)
- Appropriate use of barriers to reduce microbial transmission from patients to personnel (gloves, gowns, masks, and goggles)
- Environmental sanitation (prompt removal and disinfection of blood or body-fluid spills and splashes)

Patient Care Practices: Surgical Asepsis

Surgical asepsis is designed to render and maintain objects and areas free from microorganisms; it is also referred to as "sterile technique." Such techniques are intended for use in the surgical suite, for performance of all invasive procedures, such as inserting catheters and IV lines and suctioning, and for interactions with high-risk patients, including burned or transplant patients. Surgical asepsis techniques include the following:

- Preoperative and intraoperative reduction of bacteria at and around the operative site through patient skin preparation, hair removal, preoperative hand scrubs, and use of antimicrobials and antiseptics
- Use of barriers such as sterile gloves, gowns, drapes, and appropriate attire to reduce transmission of microorganisms from personnel to patients and to maintain a sterile field
- Environmental sanitation (removal of blood and body-fluid spills and splashes and disinfection of the area)

Therapy

Certain therapeutic measures require review, such as ensuring that blood has been screened for infectious bloodborne diseases, and regularly reviewing the clinical use of antibiotics. The purpose of this review is to identify microbial resistance patterns/trends, and control outbreaks resulting from resistant organisms.

Identification of Patients at Risk of Infection

The risk of acquiring a nosocomial infection is related to patient factors, the underlying disease, and the type of treatment rendered. Following are factors that increase the risk of infection:

- Extremes of age (neonates and the elderly)
- Chronic diseases, such as diabetes or obstructive lung disease
- Immune suppression, malnutrition, chemotherapy, organ transplantation, burns
- Invasive treatments, such as IV lines, urinary catheters, surgery, surgical implants, and dialysis

Preventive measures include the following:

- Screening for risk factors, such as nutritional assessments prior to surgery
- Early identification of infected patients to reduce the probability of cross-infection
- Establishment of stringent isolation or barrier protection to prevent cross-infections

Environmental Factors: Plumbing

Plumbing cross-connections that merge potable and nonpotable water supplies have been responsible for many waterborne disease outbreaks. Prevention of backflow or back pressure includes either removing cross-connections or installing cross-connection control devices.[7]

Examples of installations in which back siphonage or backflow is possible include: (1) a rubber hose submerged in a bedpan washer or laboratory sink; (2) a chemical tank with a submerged inlet, (3) water supply to a dishwasher not protected by a vacuum breaker, and (4) a valve connection between the potable and nonpotable water supply, such as a fire sprinkler.

Legionnaires' Disease

Legionnaires' disease may be the leading cause of nosocomial pneumonia in convalescent patients. The bacterium occurs naturally in water and wet soil and is generally believed to be transmitted by contaminated water droplets.

Preventive strategies include intermittent testing of water for the presence of legionnaires' bacteria and periodic hyperchlorinating or superheating the water.

Special-Purpose Water

National standards regulate the quality of water to be used in dialysis.[8] Water should be treated by reverse osmosis plus deionization to remove chemicals, and an ultrafilter should be used to remove bacterial contaminants.

Hydrotherapy tanks have a great potential for infection transmission, particularly for burn patients. The CDC provides guidelines for hydrotherapy tank disinfection.[9] Control of waterborne organisms and patient microflora in immersion tanks includes: (1) maintaining a free chlorine residual of 15 milligrams per liter, (2) draining the tank after patient use, (3) disinfecting the tank with a germicidal detergent, and (4) circulating chlorine through the agitator for 15 minutes at the end of the day. Control of waterborne organisms in hydrotherapy pools includes continuous filtration and maintenance of free chlorine residuals of 0.4 to 0.6 milligrams per liter.

Air

Transmission of infections through the air is rare and difficult to control. However, the air supply should be as free of contamination as possible. Cross-contamination can be controlled by regulating room atmospheric pressure.

Areas of known or probable contamination, such as isolation rooms and central processing decontamination areas, should be maintained at lower pressure than corridors and other adjoining spaces. Areas where invasive procedures are performed or where vulnerable patients are accommodated, such as operating rooms and intensive care nurseries, should be maintained at a higher pressure than corridors. Filtered air must be provided for operating rooms.

Vectors

Insects and rodents contaminate supplies and aid in the spread of foodborne disease. Prevention includes maintaining buildings and grounds in sanitary condition, eliminating breeding areas, providing barriers to entry, and storing garbage in a sanitary fashion.

Foodborne Disease

There have been many documented serious and even fatal food-related outbreaks of infections in health care institutions. The risk of foodborne disease can be prevented by the following:

- Enforcing personal hygiene
- Excluding infected personnel from food preparation
- Educating staff in their infection control activities
- Ensuring adequate cooking time and temperature
- Maintaining appropriate refrigeration, time, and temperature controls for vulnerable foods
- Maintaining a sanitary environment
- Enforcing cleaning and sanitation procedures
- Establishing temperature checks and preventive maintenance for refrigerators, steam tables, and dishwashers
- Inviting public health/sanitation department inspections to assist in a program of prevention and control

Reprocessing Supplies

Contaminated supplies and equipment can transmit infections. Reusable supplies intended for patient use must be appropriately reprocessed and stored and maintained in the intended condition (clean, decontaminated, disinfected, or sterile) until the moment of use. Reprocessing might also be required for a disposable opened, unused "sterile" device; or selected disposable articles that have been used on patients. However, standards for reprocessing and reusing disposables should be developed and strictly adhered to. Such standards should address the manufacturer's recommendations, the hospital's capacity to follow those recommendations, and the ultimate use to which the item will be put. Reprocessing should *never* be considered if sterilization will change the structure or integrity of the item or cause chemical changes in the material. The policy should indicate that only those disposables for which it can be demonstrated that reprocessing can be safely accomplished will be reused.

Other Ways to Prevent Infection

Providing staff with screening, immunization, prophylaxis, and education is critical in preventing infection and cross-infection.

All hospital employees should be screened for tuberculosis prior to employment. Screening patients for tuberculosis should be based on local data and patient/resident population. The elderly and immunocompromised patients are most at risk of infection or reactivation of infection. Policies are required for management of exposed personnel.[10,11] Only employees with demonstrable immunity to hepatitis B should be assigned to the dialysis unit. Employees who sustain needle-stick injuries from, or broken-skin contamination with blood from, patients with HIV infection should be tested for evidence of HIV infection immediately and at six-week intervals per CDC guidelines. The hospital also should establish screening programs for such high-risk areas as dialysis.

The health care facility should provide an immunization program for personnel at risk of exposure to and transmission of vaccine-preventable diseases.[12] Specifically, vaccination against rubella and hepatitis B is recommended for all personnel at risk. Rubella vaccination is recommended for employees who work in the nursery and in the emergency, outpatient, and pediatrics departments; ideally, however, all staff should be immune to rubella. Hepatitis B vaccination is recommended for employees who are exposed to blood—those in the obstetrics/gynecology, emergency, or outpatient departments, operating room, intensive care unit, and the laboratory. This vaccination program could also be extended to those who work in housekeeping and central processing.[13,14]

The facility should have policies that will allay fears of health care employees who have been exposed to infection.[15] Those policies should include such elements as prophylaxis for employees exposed directly to *Neisseria meningitidis* infection, treatment of personnel who have significant tuberculin reactions after exposure to infected patients, and immunoprophylaxis for hepatitis B or non-A non-B hepatitis after certain needle-stick injuries.

☐ Conclusion

A comprehensive infection control program provides protection from infection for patients and personnel and documentation for defense of claims and litigation; in addition, it promotes rational use of resources. The risk manager will not manage the infection control program, but is responsible for ascertaining that the environmental and procedural risks of infection for patients and staff are identified, assessed, and corrected. The risk manager also reports the infection-related indicators of quality and risk to administration and to the board.

References

1. Centers for Disease Control. *Recommendations for Prevention of HIV Transmission in Health Care Settings.* Atlanta: U.S. Department of Health and Human Services, 1987.

2. U.S. Department of Labor/Department of Health and Human Services. Occupational exposure to hepatitis and human immunodeficiency virus. *Federal Register* (210):41818–22, Oct. 20, 1987.

3. Certification Board of Infection Control. P.O. Box 775, Mundelein, IL 60060.

4. Centers for Disease Control. Proceedings of the First International Conference on Nosocomial Infections, Atlanta, Aug. 3–6, 1970.

5. Centers for Disease Control. *Outline for Surveillance and Control of Nosocomial Infections.* Atlanta: U.S. Department of Health and Human Services, 1972.

6. Soule, B. M., editor. *The APIC Curriculum for Infection Control Practice,* Vol. 2. Dubuque, IA: Kendall/Hunt Publishing Co., 1983.

7. U.S. Environmental Protection Agency. *Cross-Connection Control Manual.* Raleigh, NC: EPA Forms and Publications Center, 1973.

8. Association for Advancement of Medical Instrumentation. *American National Standards for Hemodialysis Systems.* Arlington, VA: AAMI, 1981.

9. Centers for Disease Control. *Disinfection of Hydrotherapy Pools and Tanks.* Atlanta: U.S. Department of Health and Human Services, 1982.

10. Williams, W. W. Guidelines for infection control in hospital personnel. *Infection Control* (4 suppl.):326, July–Aug. 1983.

11. Centers for Disease Control. *Guidelines for Prevention of TB Transmissions in Hospitals.* HHS publication no. (CDC) 82-8371. Atlanta: U.S. Department of Health and Human Services, 1982.

12. Williams.

13. Centers for Disease Control. Recommendations for protection against viral hepatitis. *Morbidity and Mortality Weekly Report* 34:313–24, June 7, 1985.

14. U.S. Department of Labor/Department of Health and Human Services. Occupational exposure to hepatitis and human immunodeficiency virus. *Federal Register* 52:41818–22, Oct. 20, 1987.

15. Williams.

☐ Bibliography

Barrett-Connor, E., Brandt, S., and others. *Epidemiology for the Infection Control Nurse.* St. Louis: C. V. Mosby Co., 1978.

Benenson, A., and others. *Control of Communicable Diseases in Man.* Washington, DC: American Public Health Association, 1985.

Castle, M. *Hospital Infection Control Principle and Practice.* New York City: John Wiley & Sons, 1980.

Jackson, M., and Lynch, P. Isolation practices: a historic perspective. *American Journal of Infection Control* 13(1):21–31, 1985.

Longree, K. *Quantity Food Sanitation.* Toronto: John Wiley & Sons, 1967.

Lynch, P., and Jackson, M. Isolation practices: how much is too much or not enough? *Asepsis* 10(3):12–16, 1988.

Perkins, J. J. *Principles and Methods of Sterilization in Health Sciences.* Springfield, IL: Charles C. Thomas, 1983.

Soule, B. M., editor. *The APIC Curriculum for Infection Control Practice.* Vol. 2. Dubuque, IA: Kendall/Hunt Publishing, Co., 1983.

Chapter 20

Withholding/Withdrawing of Life Support

Megan A. Adams

Although technological advances have made it possible for physicians to prolong the survival of critically and terminally ill patients, in some instances this ability to prolong life may exceed the ability to restore health. It is in those situations that patients, families, and physicians may be forced to make collaborative decisions regarding the withholding or withdrawing of life-prolonging medical treatment. Such decisions can involve various types of medical treatment, such as cardiopulmonary resuscitation, ventilator support, dialysis, chemotherapy, antibiotics, or nutritional support. Hospital administrators and risk managers are concerned about potential civil and criminal liability in the area of withholding or withdrawing treatment. As with any high-risk area, planned and systematic policy and procedure development and implementation help alleviate the risk of liability and provide guidance to the members of the health care team when dealing with these difficult situations. A hospital policy also demonstrates a concerted effort on the part of the hospital and medical staff to respect the rights of patients. This chapter will cover the various issues associated with policy development and implementation.

The law in this highly controversial area is unsettled and varies widely from one jurisdiction to the next. On June 25, 1990, the U.S. Supreme Court ruled on a Missouri case (*Cruzon v. Harmon*) involving a young woman in a persistent vegetative state with a life expectancy of another 30 to 40 years. Her parents had requested permission to discontinue nutritional support. In a five-to-four vote, the high court ruled that individual states can apply procedural safeguards pertaining to the withdrawal of hydrational and nutritional support from comatose patients. Information on consent to withhold or withdraw treatment is given later in this chapter. In this area, more than in any other high-risk area, the risk manager must consult with legal counsel before policies are approved and implemented. In writing and approving policy as well as in resolving difficult situations with patients on a case-by-case basis, legal counsel does not make the decisions. Instead, information and advice supplied by legal counsel should be considered along with all other available information and advice bearing on the issue.

☐ Joint Commission Resuscitative Standards

Although the primary reason for developing policies and procedures related to withholding and withdrawing treatment is to ensure appropriate clinical decision making, hospitals are now required to have a policy to comply with newly developed Joint Commission on Accreditation of Healthcare Organizations standards. The standards require that the hospital's chief executive officer, through the management and administrative staff, develop a "do not resuscitate" (DNR) policy in consultation with the medical staff, nursing staff, and other appropriate bodies (for example, social work and pastoral care). The policy must be adopted by the medical staff and ultimately approved by the governing body. The standards require that the policy do at least the following:

1. Describe the mechanism for reaching decisions about withholding resuscitative treatment from individual patients
2. Describe the mechanism for resolving conflicts in the decision-making process, should they arise
3. Describe the roles of the various personnel involved
4. Ensure that decisions about withholding resuscitative treatment respect the rights of patients
5. Include the requirement that appropriate orders be written and documented in the patient's record if resuscitative treatment is to be withheld

Even though the Joint Commission standards address only withholding resuscitative services, hospitals would be well advised to address also the withdrawal of treatment when revising existing policies or when developing policies for the first time.[1]

☐ Policy Development Process

Risk managers can play a vital part in planned and systematic policy development and implementation, which serve to alleviate potential liability exposures attendant to decisions to withhold or withdraw medical treatment and nutrition. Policies help physicians and other members of the health care team in the decision-making process by providing a sound written procedure, a structure for obtaining the advice of medical consultants, and assistance in resolving problems. A hospital policy also serves to demonstrate a concerted effort on the part of the hospital and medical staff to respect the rights of patients and to provide high-quality care.[2]

Because withholding or withdrawing treatment is an area of great controversy, development of a policy of this nature will most likely require extensive interaction with all constituencies of the institution. The task can be assigned to an existing committee, or a special task force can be formed. At a minimum, the group that takes on this task ought to include representation from the medical staff, nursing services, administration, risk management, and legal affairs. The committee or task force will determine policy scope, perform a literature review, collect sample policies, and review applicable state statutes and court decisions. At an early stage, it is most beneficial to develop a work plan that describes the policy development process, approval process, and implementation requirements and coordination. To ensure support for the process, the work plan should be reviewed and approved by the medical staff leadership and administration.[3]

Some very general policy development considerations include the recognition of state statutes or court decisions that might specify certain policy requirements, restrictions, or limitations. Hospitals can also look to state hospital associations and regional, state, or national medical societies for information on policy recommendations or guidelines. (Figure 20-1 provides a listing of selected resources that institutions may want to review and/or consider as guidelines.) The task force should review the hospital's mission or philosophy to ensure that it does not limit patient autonomy in the area of withholding or withdrawing treatment. The decisions in two recent New Jersey cases suggest that hospitals do the following:

1. Have a written mission statement that clearly states that treatment may not be withheld or withdrawn
2. Have a mechanism to notify all patients about that policy at the time of their admission
3. Develop a mechanism to ensure the safe transfer of a patient to another hospital in the event that the patient has requested that treatment be withheld or withdrawn[4]

☐ Policy Scope

The scope of the policy should be determined at the beginning of the process. Some issues to be considered are:

1. *Treatment modalities:* Will the policy be limited to cardiopulmonary resuscitation, or should other treatment, such as dialysis, antibiotics, or nutrition, be included?
2. *Nutritional support:* Is there a distinction between artificial nutrition and hydration and other treatment modalities?
3. *Withholding versus withdrawal:* Will the policy address only the withholding of treatment, such as an order to not resuscitate a patient, or will it also include the withdrawal of treatment, such as removing a patient from a ventilator?

The policy should clearly state the category of patients to which it applies. The cases being litigated involve either patients who have been medically determined to be terminally ill or, even more troublesome, patients who are not terminally ill but are in a persistent vegetative state. The policy should address those patients and distinguish them from patients who are not terminally ill and not in a persistent vegetative state but who refuse treatment. Some states require consultation with a physician not directly involved in the patient's ongoing treatment and care under certain circumstances. Requiring consultation to confirm diagnosis and prognosis is an excellent way for a physician and hospital to be protected in the event of a dispute at a later date, as the consultation is evidence of good and prudent medical practice.[5]

☐ Decision Making and Treatment Options

A policy needs to specify the decision-making process for the competent adult, as well as how and by whom decisions will be made for the comatose, incompetent, or minor

Figure 20-1.   Selected Resources for Policy Development

- President's Commission for the Study of Ethical Problems in Medicine and Biomedical and Behavioral Research: Deciding to Forego Life-Sustaining Treatment: March 1983
- New Jersey Medical Society Supportive Care Program
- California Hospital Association Guidelines on Life-Support Removal
- American Nurses' Association Committee on Ethics, Guidelines on Withdrawing and Withholding Food and Fluid
- Academy of Neurology, Position on Certain Aspects of the Care and Management of the Persistent Vegetative State Patient
- American Medical Association Council on Ethical and Judicial Affairs, Opinion on Withholding and Withdrawing of Life-Prolonging Medical Treatment, Issued on March 15, 1986
- California Medical Association, Committee on Evolving Trends in Society Affecting Life, Withholding and Withdrawing Life-Sustaining Treatment: Ethical Guidelines for Decision Making in Long-Term Care Facilities
- Hastings Center, *Guidelines on the Termination of Life-Sustaining Treatment and the Care of the Dying;*
- Joint Commission on Accreditation of Healthcare Organizations, *1990 Standards*

patient. In the event that a patient is unable to consent, every effort should be made to determine whether the patient had previously stated what type of treatment he or she would have wanted under the medical circumstances. The patient's wishes can be substantiated through written evidence, such as a living will, health care proxy, or durable power of attorney, or, if written evidence is not available, through oral evidence, including discussions with family members, the legal guardian, or close friends. The controlling factor is determining not what the family members, legal guardian, or friends want but what the patient previously expressed or implied. For those patients who have never had the capacity to make decisions on their own behalf, the only guide the surrogate decision maker and physician have is what is in the best interest of the patient.[6-8]

When treatment decisions must be made, the physician should discuss all treatment options fully and completely with the patient or surrogate decision maker. Physicians should be encouraged to include in those discussions members of the health care team who have been involved with the patient's care; that is, nursing staff, social workers, and/or psychiatric consultants. Prior to initiating orders to withhold or withdraw treatment, physicians should inform the nursing staff and other members of the health care team of treatment decisions to ensure that the decisions are known and understood.[9]

☐ Problem Resolution

There are a number of problem situations that can arise when there is no agreement among family members or among physicians or between family and physicians. It is important that the policy contain a section that outlines a mechanism for agreement. The physicians should be directed to contact administration, risk management, or legal counsel for guidance and assistance. Some examples of problem-solving mechanisms include the following:

- Discussions involving representatives from administration and the patient and/or family
- Referral to a hospital review or ethics committee or an ethical consultation team
- Involvement of legal counsel and/or petition to a court of law
- Transfer of patient to another physician or facility

These mechanisms are provided as examples only, and each hospital's policy should reflect resolution mechanisms that are feasible, effective, and timely for the individual hospital.[10] An example of a policy that describes a problem-solving mechanism (an ethical consultation team) is included in figure 20-2.

☐ Documentation

Proper documentation describes the process by which a decision was reached and the basis for the decision. Documentation requirements include, at a minimum, the following:

- A detailed summary of the medical situation, including the outcomes of consultations
- Statements by all hospital personnel, including nurses, social workers, and the hospital chaplain, summarizing discussions with the patient, family, and/or surrogate decision makers
- Written orders completed and signed by the attending physician

The policy should include requirements for the frequency of renewing orders, who may renew orders, and the circumstances, if any, under which verbal orders can be given.

Figure 20-2.   Administration Policy for an Ethical Consultation Team, The Lutheran Hospital of Fort Wayne, IN

1. **Background and Purpose**

   The hope of The Lutheran Hospital is that those persons in its care experience healing and recovery from illness. Toward that goal, The Lutheran Hospital uses the knowledge and resources of modern medicine. At times, those involved face complex and difficult decisions as they seek to provide appropriate care, decisions which involve moral, legal, social, and personal issues in addition to the medical dimensions. For example, recovery from illness is not possible in all situations. Indeed, there are times when a person's medical prognosis and quality of life raise difficult questions as to the benefit and appropriateness of heroic efforts using all possible resources and techniques. Such efforts can, at times, serve only to prolong a painful, inevitable process of dying for the person rather than sustain or provide a meaningful quality of life.

   It is for these and other dilemmas that Lutheran Hospital provides an advisory, interdisciplinary Ethical Consultation Team to assist physicians, patients, and/or families as they seek to make decisions that are ethical, legal, humane, and appropriate to the patient's desires or circumstances. The Team exists in conjunction with the Ethics Committee of the Board of Directors.

2. **Membership**

   A. The Ethical Consultation Team will be convened by a convenor group consisting of a hospital chaplain, a social worker, and an R.N., all serving on the membership of the Ethics Committee. Members of the convenor group serve to facilitate the work of the Team and to refer questions outside the scope of ethical consultation to the appropriate resource.
   B. While the exact makeup of the Ethical Consultation Team will vary with each specific consultation, the team normally consists of:
      1. Case-specific members:
         • Physician(s) involved in patient's care
         • Patient and/or patient's family or a known close friend of the patient
         • Nurse involved in patient's care
         • Hospital social worker or chaplain involved
      2. Ongoing members
         • Consulting physicians (2) (drawn from a pool of physicians representing various specialties)
         • Administrative representative
         • Members of the convenor group (at least one not involved as a case-specific member)
         • Community clergyperson as appropriate
   C. A specific consultation shall include such members of the Team as are available and/or deemed appropriate by a convenor group in conversation with the person(s) requesting the consultation.
   D. A consultation will not occur without the voluntary participation of the physician(s) caring for the patient.
   E. Ongoing advisory members will be chosen and advised of their duties and provided training by the Ethics Committee. The committee will solicit suggestions and input from medical and hospital staff in its selection process.

3. **Function**

   A. The team shall meet, when requested and appropriate (at the patient's bedside, if necessary) to assist the affected person in assessing:
      • The patient's medical situation and treatment choices available, including: where in the hospital or outside of it those options might be utilized and the personal financial considerations pertaining to options
      • The patient's and/or family's desires about the kind of treatment deemed appropriate
      • The religious and/or ethical values and concerns which pertain to this situation
      • The policy guidelines of Lutheran Hospital and any pertinent legal issues
   B. The team will convene promptly when called (within 24 hours' notice, if necessary). It is recognized that, given short notice, some members of the team may not be able to attend a specific consultation.
   C. Each consultation is intended to facilitate open discussion of all the issues, values, concerns, and options surrounding a specific situation. The purpose is to reach a consensus (a general

(continued on next page)   **203**

Figure 20-2.   (Continued)

> feeling of agreement by all members of the team).
> D. Any physician on the staff may request a consultation. Other staff members, including nurses, social workers, or the chaplain, may discuss their concerns wth the physician(s) caring for the patient. Patients or families might also raise questions relating to ethical dilemmas. In such cases, hospital staff members aware of the situation will bring such concerns to the attention of the attending physician(s). If family concerns persist, hospital staff may contact a member of the convenor group. The convenor will assess the situation and will confer with the attending physician, who will determine the appropriateness of convening the team.
> E. Request for consultation will be channeled to one of the convenors. After discussion with the physician(s), the convenor will schedule the consultation or determine another appropriate way of handling the matter.
> F. The proceedings of a consultation team are confidential. Any consensus reached by the Ethical Consultation Team is advisory only.
>
> 4. **Reporting**
>
> A. If a consensus is reached by the consultation, it may be recorded on the medical record of the patient by a physician member of the team and by the convenor. If not, no medical record entry is necessary or appropriate.
> B. The team will periodically report to the Ethics Committee about the number and kinds of cases in which it has assisted, including any proposed changes in the team's procedures or member ship and any recommendations regarding the needfor additional policy guidelines.

Source: Reprinted, with permission, from The Lutheran Hospital of Indiana, Inc., Fort Wayne, IN. The concept was first developed by St. Luke's Hospital, Maumee, OH.

Some hospitals have developed a special order form for the initiation of orders to withhold or withdraw treatment. An example of an order form is provided in figure 20-3. Under certain circumstances, a signed release by the patient or surrogate decision maker may be appropriate. The policy should address whether such a release would be required in all instances or only at the discretion of administration or legal counsel.[11]

☐ Policy Review and Implementation

The initial draft document should be widely circulated for review and discussion. Some committees to include in this review are ethics, risk management, critical care, patient care, nursing council, and medical executive. Successful policy implementation requires a hospitalwide educational effort targeted at the medical/resident staff, nursing staff, and applicable ancillary departments, such as social work services and respiratory care. In order to ensure that the policy or guideline is being followed, a mechanism to monitor effectiveness and compliance should be in place at the time of implementation.

References

1. Miller, R. D. Hospital policies on resuscitation: the 1986 Joint Commission Standards. *Hospital Law Newsletter* 5(3):1–8, Jan. 1988.

2. Office of Technology Assessment. *Institutional Protocols for Decisions About Life-Sustaining Treatment.* Washington, DC: Congressional Board of the 100th Congress, July 1988.

3. Office of Technology Assessment, pp. 24–25.

4. American Health Consultants. Avoid lawsuits by adopting policy on terminating life support care. *Hospital Risk Management* 8(11):152, Nov. 1986.

5. Office of Technology Assessment, pp. 37–39.

Figure 20-3. Orders to Withhold/Withdraw Treatment Form

Instructions: All orders to withhold or withdraw treatment must be indicated below. Orders may be initiated *only* by an attending physician. Orders must be renewed at least every three days by a resident or attending physician. Please complete this form by checking each row below. If orders are changed, a new form must be initiated by the attending physician.

	Provide as Applicable	Withhold/Do Not Initiate	Withdraw/ Discontinue	Comments
Acute/Chronic Care				
CPR—Specify				
Chest compression				
Defibrillation				
Endotracheal intubation				
Assisted ventilation				
Chemical support				
Surgery				
Dialysis				
ICU-transfer				
Transfusions				
Antibiotics				
IV support				
Nutritional support—specify				
Gastro feeding				
Nasogastric feeding				
IV feeding				
Oral feeding				
Comfort measures				
Specialized Treatment				
Chemotherapy				
Radiation therapy				
Pacemaker				
Other—specify				
Other—specify				
Other—specify				

Initial orders (Signature)_____ Date _____ Ext. _____

Orders renewed:

Signature _____ Date_____ Ext._____ Signature_____ Date_____ Ext. _____

Signature _____ Date_____ Ext._____ Signature_____ Date_____ Ext. _____

Signature _____ Date_____ Ext._____ Signature_____ Date_____ Ext. _____

6. Charlson, M. E., and others. Resuscitation: how do we decide? *Journal of the American Medical Association* 310(15):955–59, Mar. 14, 1984.

7. Areen, J. The legal status of consent obtained from families of adult patients to withhold or withdraw treatment. *Journal of the American Medical Association* 258(2):229–35, July 10, 1987.

8. Lehrer, S. M. *In Re Jane Doe.* Court of Common Pleas, Philadelphia County, July Term, 1987, No. 2560.

9. Schwartz, D., editor. Withholding and withdrawing care: practical strategies for clinical decision making. *Medical Ethics Advisor* Atlanta: American Health Consultants, 1986.

10. Office of Technology Assessment, pp. 40–44.

11. Health Law Center. *Hospital Law Manual.* Vol. 1, *Dying, Death, and·Dead Bodies.* Administrator's Vol. Rockville, MD: Aspen Publishers, 1982.

☐ Bibliography

Do Not Resuscitate Orders. Proposed legislation and report of the New York State Task Force on Life and the Law, Apr. 1986.

The Hastings Center. *Guidelines on the Termination of Life-Sustaining Treatment and the Care of the Dying.* Briarcliff Manor, NY, 1987.

Office of Technology Assessment. *Institutional Protocols for Decisions about Life-Sustaining Treatment.* Washington, DC: Congressional Board of the 100th Congress, July 1988.

Read, W. A. *Hospital's Role in Resuscitative Decisions.* Chicago: The Hospital Research and Educational Trust, 1983.

Ross, J. W., and others. *Handbook for Hospital Ethics Committees.* Chicago: American Hospital Publishing, 1986.

Withholding and withdrawing care: practical strategies for clinical decision making. *Medical Ethics Advisor.* Atlanta: American Health Consultants, 1986.

Chapter 21

Credentialing and Privileging

Edgar A. Zingman and Melissa J. Long

The credentialing and privileging of health care practitioners includes peer review activities, which may raise questions of potential legal liability; it is, therefore, a risk management concern. Although high-quality patient care is the focus of the credentialing and privileging process, members of the public or affected practitioners may challenge the hospital, its governing body, medical staff, and allied health care practitioners as a result of credentialing and peer review activities. Patients may allege injury as a result of the incompetence of a practitioner, and blame the hospital or its health care practitioners if they were in a position to identify the incompetence and prevent harm to patients through credentialing or peer review activities. On the other hand, practitioners whose ability to practice their professions has been curtailed because their staff appointment or privileges have been denied or restricted may bring suit for denial of their constitutional rights, for antitrust violations, or for defamation. The solution to the problem posed in these situations lies in developing objective and reasonable criteria and applying those criteria fairly to all practitioners applying for staff appointment and privileges.

☐ Credentialing

The credentialing of physicians and other health care professionals involves both a governmental and a private function. The most basic type of credentialing is licensing and is performed by the state; private credentialing is conducted by the health care institution and is based on a variety of factors, including information supplied by members of the relevant profession, state law, and the specific needs and goals of the health care institution. Private credentialing procedures generally are set forth in the medical staff bylaws and may pertain to both physician practitioners and nonphysician practitioners, sometimes referred to as allied health professionals. The institution's board of trustees is ultimately responsible for approving the criteria for appointment and credentialing and for approving those who may practice in the institution.

As a component of the initial staff appointment process, credentialing requires gathering information on the qualifications of applicants and comparing their qualifications with the approval criteria established by the health care institution. Credentials evaluations and applicant interviews may be conducted in a confidential manner by a credentials committee or a staff representative, and in some cases by members of the service to which the applicant may be assigned. Initial credentials recommendations are made to the relevant medical staff department or to a committee responsible for making recommendations and are sent to the hospital governing body for approval.

Thereafter, the credentials of each practitioner must be reviewed at least every two years, as required by the Joint Commission on Accreditation of Healthcare Organizations, in a manner that is in keeping with the confidential nature of the information. The purpose of this systematic, ongoing monitoring of performance is to maintain and promote high-quality patient care.

☐ Delineation and Granting of Privileges

Medical staff membership or appointment status of physician practitioners exists separately from the granting of privileges. A practitioner's privileges limit the scope of his or her practice to those procedures that he or she is competent to perform. The delineation of clinical privileges requires departments or specialties to develop criteria against which each practitioner is measured. The criteria can be very broad and can include "all procedures expected to be performed by someone trained in general surgery," or they may list specific procedures, which requires that practitioners specify those that they are trained to do. Criteria are approved by the medical staff and the hospital governing body and are applied to all individuals who practice independently in the hospital, regardless of whether they are staff members.

Criteria for Appointment and Delineation of Clinical Privileges

The medical staff is responsible for establishing and incorporating into its bylaws well-defined criteria for staff appointment and for the delineation of clinical privileges. Such criteria must be reasonably related to promoting patient care and not be arbitrary, unreasonable, or anticompetitive. Comprehensive guidelines to aid in the development of appropriate criteria are set forth in the medical staff chapter of the Joint Commission standards.[1]

Acceptable criteria for appointment and delineation of clinical privileges include current licensure, relevant training and experience, current competence, health status, maintenance of malpractice liability insurance, and geographic location. As a condition of continued membership and privileges, the bylaws should require practitioners to report a revocation or suspension of licensure. Additional permissible criteria include peer recommendations and references. The ability of a practitioner to work with others has also been held to be a legitimate concern in determining competence where a practitioner's behavior disrupts hospital routine or otherwise threatens the quality of patient care.

Criteria that have been held to be unacceptable include requirements that discriminate based on sex, race, creed, or national origin. Requiring either medical society membership or recommendations from current medical staff members has been held to be an inappropriate basis for making appointment decisions.

The criteria adopted by the medical staff for credentialing and privileging practitioners must be applied fairly to all who are eligible for appointment to the medical staff. Fairness may be substantiated by evidence relating to the practitioner's current qualifications and by consistent and unbiased enforcement of pertinent bylaws provisions. Furthermore, caution should be exercised in developing and implementing a hospital's private credentialing scheme to prevent the possibility that practitioners will be excluded unfairly from competing in the health care marketplace. The reasonableness of private credentialing standards is tested by weighing the benefits of the standards against the potential harm to competition. The factors considered in this balancing process are whether the criteria are reasonably related to the hospital's maintenance of high-quality care; whether the activity tends to exclude some persons from practicing in the area; and, in certain cases, whether procedural safeguards are in effect.

Reduction, Suspension, and Termination of Staff Privileges

In addition to making recommendations to the governing body concerning the granting or denial of privileges, the medical staff is responsible for invoking disciplinary proceedings when professional performance or other factors indicate a need for corrective action. The medical staff recommends disciplinary action to the governing body; such action may result in the reduction, suspension, or termination of staff privileges.

Privileges may be reduced either as a result of demonstrated incompetence or because a practitioner has not had the opportunity to perform the procedures applied for and thereby maintain the appropriate level of competence. When the practitioner's privileges are restricted, the practitioner may admit patients and provide treatment within those limitations. Suspension of privileges is a temporary measure taken to provide time so that the medical staff may investigate the practitioner and during which the practitioner may pursue the right to hearing and appeal under the bylaws. Termination of staff privileges occurs when the governing body withdraws staff membership or fails to re-appoint a practitioner. To the extent that privileges are dependent on staff membership, such privileges cease, and the practitioner no longer is allowed to admit or treat patients.

Alternatively, a practitioner may be placed on probation or permitted to practice only under supervision. The board may require a practitioner to be supervised when there is a finding of clinical deficiency. Probation may be imposed either for clinical deficiency or because the practitioner's behavior has not been in the best interest of patients or the institution.

Inadequate or substandard clinical performance is the most common ground for disciplinary action. Where the decision of the medical staff and governing body is found to be reasonable and not arbitrary or capricious, the courts generally refrain from interfering and uphold the action taken.

A practitioner's privileges may also be reduced for nondisciplinary reasons. The medical staff and governing body may change criteria for approval of certain procedures in order to conform to changes made in standards of the medical profession or to improve the quality of care. Any such modification of criteria for privileges should be made in accordance with the staff bylaws and should reflect hospital and community needs rather than an anticompetitive purpose.

The medical staff bylaws should establish fair procedures by which privileges may be reduced, suspended, or terminated. The medical staff and governing body must then comply with the bylaws requirements to ensure that any adverse privileges decision is both fair and accurate. Whether the procedures set forth in the bylaws are sufficiently fair to withstand a court challenge brought by an affected practitioner will vary depending on the type of health care institution. Public hospitals are generally expected to comply with constitutional notions of due process, which means that the affected practitioner should be given notice of the reasons for the proposed action and an opportunity to request a hearing. Although, as a matter of law, nonpublic hospitals may have greater flexibility in establishing procedures for decisions about staff membership and privileges, Joint Commission standards require medical staff bylaws to provide for fair hearings and for appeals. Furthermore, the federal Health Care Quality Improvement Act protects institutions from liability in many lawsuits if fair procedures have been followed, and provides a specific list of procedures—which are essentially those required by due process—that will be considered fair. Summary suspension of privileges does not allow the practitioner an opportunity for a hearing prior to suspension; therefore, such action will not satisfy due process standards unless taken to prevent an immediate threat of harm to patients and followed by a hearing held within a reasonable time after the suspension.

Allied Health Professionals' Credentialing and Privileging

Nonphysician practitioners present unique credentialing and privileging issues. Although the Joint Commission permits hospitals to determine the types of practitioners who may practice in the hospital, the laws of each state define various types of professional health care practices and may define which practitioners may practice in a hospital. Antitrust concerns are minimized where decisions about the types of practitioners who may practice in the hospital are made by the governing body rather than by the medical staff.

Important considerations involving nonphysician practitioners include the following:

- Whether a separate allied staff is desirable
- The type of allied practitioners to whom delineated clinical privileges should be granted, and the scope of such privileges
- Whether allied staff must be supervised, for what procedures, and by whom
- On what basis, by whom, and how allied professions should be credentialed
- Whether it is desirable to establish written protocols governing procedures performed by certain groups of allied practitioners
- How quality assurance and peer review will be done
- Whether allied practitioners will have admitting or coadmitting privileges[2]

□ Liability for Participating in Credentialing and Peer Review

Members of the medical staff, members of the governing body, the hospital, and its officers and directors may be sued for their involvement in the peer review process. Physicians who are denied membership or the privileges they seek may sue on a number of theories. Patients may sue claiming that they suffered injury because the hospital was negligent in credentialing physicians.

Medical Staff Liability to the Patient

Chairmen of medical staff departments or services are responsible for knowing whether practitioners in their departments are competent. The Joint Commission requires that a department chairman's responsibilities be set forth in the medical staff bylaws, rules, and regulations. Department chairmen are required to oversee and account for their departments' professional and administrative activities, to recommend criteria for clinical privileges, to recommend privileges for each member of the department, and to ensure that the quality and appropriateness of patient care provided in the department are continuously monitored and evaluated. When department chairmen are made aware of inappropriate patient care, they have a duty to report such deficiencies to the hospital and the governing body so that corrective action may be taken. Failure to comply with quality-of-care standards such as those specified by the Joint Commission may result in the individual liability of department chairmen to persons injured by practitioners whose incompetence was known.

Where a credentials committee exists, it has the responsibility to conduct effective credentialing and peer review and make recommendations to the medical executive committee. Pursuant to Joint Commission standards, the executive committee recommends individuals for medical staff membership and delineated clinical privileges to the governing body for approval. Although to date no medical executive committee or credentials committee has been held liable to a patient for inappropriate care rendered by a committee-approved practitioner, participants in the credentialing and peer review process, like department chairmen, review and evaluate the competence of practitioners and may be subject to liability for ineffective peer review.

Where a medical staff has been characterized as an independent entity rather than part of the integrated hospital organization, courts have allowed the entire medical staff collectively to be sued, based on the duty of the staff to grant privileges only to qualified and competent practitioners. Although cases recognizing this theory have been criticized, hospitals are advised to treat the medical staff as an integrated hospital service by deleting traditional preamble language from the bylaws, by referring to physicians as appointees rather than members, and by providing the staff with legal counsel rather than allowing it to retain independent counsel.[3]

Governing Body Liability to the Patient

Members of hospital governing bodies who participate in the appointment and reappointment of practitioners to date have not been found liable for the consequences of treatment rendered by incompetent appointees. However, a legal basis for such actions exists. Members of the governing body must exercise good faith and ordinary and reasonable care in appointing and privileging practitioners. The duty of care requires them to seek enough information to make what they believe to be a sound judgment regarding who may practice in the facility and what they are allowed to do.

Hospital Liability to the Patient

Hospitals are ultimately responsible for the foreseeable consequences of the appointment or reappointment of an incompetent practitioner when they know, or in the exercise of reasonable care should know, of an individual's incompetency to practice. Therefore, hospitals have a duty to use reasonable care in the selection, review, continuing evaluation, and retention of staff practitioners. The duty of a hospital to exercise due care in selecting and retaining practitioners cannot be delegated. Therefore, even though a hospital assigns credentialing and peer review responsibilities to the medical staff and relies on the staff's expertise in making recommendations, such delegation generally does not relieve the hospital of liability when an improper appointment decision results in injury to a patient.

Liability to the Aggrieved Practitioner

Credentialing and privileging decisions may result in lawsuits being filed against hospitals and individuals involved in peer review by practitioners who seek redress for denial or reduction of their privileges. Potential legal theories in such lawsuits include violation of medical staff bylaws, economic injury, antitrust and restraint of trade, defamation, and discrimination.

Medical Staff Bylaws
Although most courts have not construed bylaws to be a contract between the medical staff and the hospital, the bylaws may nevertheless create rights for practitioners. In particular, medical staffs have been required to comply with those procedural rights enumerated in their bylaws. Although it may be difficult for a practitioner to hold a hospital or medical staff liable solely because of noncompliance with the procedure required by the bylaws, any procedural deficiency may enhance the appearance that facts establishing liability under other theories—for example, anticompetitive or discriminatory motives—are present.

Economic Injury
Economic injury to a physician's private practice may result in allegations of malicious interference with contract, trade, or business or profession. It is a common condition of employment among private practice groups that new employees become privileged at a certain hospital; obviously, a hospital's denial of privileges prevents the practitioner from joining that group. Frequently, practitioners also claim that the denial or the loss

or curtailment of their privileges results in a loss of patients, either because they need hospital privileges to be introduced to patients or to get referrals, or because their patients elect to be treated by others at the hospital where the practitioner is restricted. Privileges decisions that may cause such results should be based on legitimate needs of the hospital and not on the economic concerns of existing practitioners. Even where a practitioner files a lawsuit on a theory other than malicious interference with professional opportunities, it is likely that those types of economic injuries will be claimed as damages.

Antitrust and Restraint of Trade

When two or more persons act jointly to interfere with another's ability to pursue his or her profession, common law and statutory causes of action for restraint of trade are available. Furthermore, there are state and federal antitrust laws that prohibit anticompetitive conduct—such as inappropriate staff exclusions, expulsions, and suspensions—and other limitations on use of services and facilities.

The principal purpose of antitrust laws is to protect and encourage competition. As health care has evolved into one of the nation's major industries, federal and state antitrust laws increasingly have been applied and enforced. Physician and nonphysician practitioners are relying on antitrust laws to remedy adverse privileges decisions where denials of privileges are competitively motivated or based on exclusive agreements.

The Sherman Act

The Sherman Act is the primary antitrust statute. It prohibits the creation of monopolies and restraint of trade or commerce created by agreements among competitors.

Sherman Act claims have been brought against hospitals to challenge almost every type of credentialing decision, including the exclusion of such groups as osteopaths, podiatrists, chiropractors, and nurse practitioners (or the establishment of rules preventing them from performing certain types of procedures), and the denial or limitation of privileges based on individual qualifications. Such claims tend to be successful only if the offended practitioner can show (1) the existence of an agreement among several persons or entities—for example, among multiple members of the medical staff, between the hospital and the medical staff, or between two or more hospitals—to exclude him or her from economic competition, and (2) that the conspiracy affected competition among practitioners in the area.[4]

The Clayton Act

The Clayton Act and subsequent legislative refinements were enacted to make certain practices illegal to the extent that they substantially lessen competition or tend to create a monopoly. Pertinent to the issue of staff privileges and among the practices that Congress intended to make illegal were certain "tying arrangements." Practitioners sometimes claim that hospitals that enter exclusive contracts with private groups specializing in hospital-based services (such as emergency room care and anesthesiology) are engaged in illegal "tying arrangements" because the hospital's patients do not have freedom to select which practitioners will perform those services for them. These claims often fail because the practitioner cannot prove that patients ordinarily would select a provider for such services independent of selecting the hospital.[5]

The Federal Trade Commission Act

The Federal Trade Commission Act prohibits unfair methods of competition and unfair or disruptive practices where either occurs in or affects commerce. As applied to hospitals' credentialing decisions, its prohibitions overlap with the other antitrust laws. Exclusive enforcement powers are granted to the Federal Trade Commission, pursuant to the act. The act has been applied specifically to for-profit organizations and physicians in private practice. However, recent challenges raised against nonprofit organizations may indicate a broadened application of the act in the future.

State Laws

State antitrust laws have been enacted as a result of the unique local nature of health care delivery. Where federal courts find that there is no jurisdiction to resolve litigation brought by an excluded physician under federal law, state antitrust laws may afford the practitioner a remedy.

Enforcement of the Laws

The Antitrust Division of the United States Justice Department is primarily responsible for enforcing the Sherman and Clayton acts, although responsibility is shared with the Federal Trade Commission for enforcement of the Clayton Act. State attorneys general also may bring antitrust enforcement actions. Because the Federal Trade Commission has exclusive enforcement powers under the Federal Trade Commission Act, no private civil suits are authorized.

Application of the Law to Staff Appointment

Physicians who challenge denials of staff appointment or privileges argue that their exclusion from hospital medical practice by the existing staff and hospital has the effect of reducing competition among physicians and therefore violates antitrust laws. Attempts by physicians to use federal antitrust laws have been barred in the past by the exemption of professionals from antitrust laws and by a requirement that the effect of the activity on interstate commerce be substantial. The professional exemption has since been eliminated, and the requisite effect on interstate commerce is increasingly found based on treatment of out-of-state referrals and purchase of products from out-of-state businesses. With the removal of those barriers to the application of antitrust principles came a tremendous increase in the number of claims challenging staff privileges on antitrust grounds, although few have been successful.

Most federal circuit courts of appeal have held that practitioners have standing under federal antitrust law to challenge denial of staff privileges. Practitioners claiming injury from an anticompetitive practice may, if their action is successful, recover treble damages. Where the claimant shows a threatened or continuing violation of the antitrust laws, an injunction may be issued to prohibit further anticompetitive conduct.

Nonphysician practitioners, including allied health practitioners, also have an interest in an institution's selection of criteria for membership and privileges. Podiatrists, chiropractors, nurse anesthetists, and psychologists are among those practitioners who are licensed to practice in areas that encroach upon physicians' practices and who have been excluded from staff privileges. Historically, the reasons for excluding nonphysicians from staff privileges have been that they cannot provide safe patient care or that their practices compete with physician practices. Today, the laws of some states prohibit hospitals from excluding as a whole certain groups of nonphysician practitioners. In addition, such practitioners challenging exclusionary practices base lawsuits on antitrust laws or, in the case of public hospitals, federal constitutional rights such as equal protection, due process, and free speech. Although the law in this area remains unsettled, criteria based on considerations of quality of care are generally upheld. Exclusion of such practitioners because they pose a competitive threat to the existing medical staff will be found unreasonable and will be struck down, and may result in substantial liability for the hospital and other persons involved in the decision to exclude the practitioners.

Public and private hospitals can best defend against allegations of constitutional rights violations and antitrust violations by developing and adhering to objective standards that are clearly ascertainable and nonarbitrary for granting privileges. For example, the bylaws may require the practitioner to carry a reasonable amount of malpractice coverage[6] and may require that the practitioner live within a reasonable distance of the hospital and be available for emergencies. However, it may not be reasonable to require county residence if the hospital is in an urban area or near the county border.[7] Although it is appropriate to impose educational and training requirements for each type of practitioner, it is inappropriate to impose requirements that few in a given practice can meet.[8] A hospital should not permit unfavorable privileges decisions to be based on a practitioner's abrasive personality or inability to work with others unless the person's behavior seriously impairs hospital operations or creates a threat to the safety of patients. For an exclusion resulting in the elimination of an entire class of practitioners to be upheld, the requirement must be reasonably related to the operations of the hospital.[9] Several courts have held that a hospital's exclusion of podiatrists is permissible where based on the good-faith judgment that patient care is better served by using orthopedic surgeons, who are trained to treat the whole person.

A better approach in avoiding charges of inappropriate exclusionary practices may be to refrain from blanket exclusions of classes of practitioners from activities for which they are licensed. Decisions about granting or denying privileges would then be made on the basis of the individual's abilities as measured against the criteria established by the governing board.

Where a decision is made to exclude an entire class of practitioners and no state law prohibits such exclusion, documentation should demonstrate a patient care rationale rather than economic concerns. State laws and professional standards permit certain allied health practitioners to practice only under supervision of physicians. Although a hospital's inability to arrange for physician supervision of certain allied health groups might justify their exclusion, the hospital should clearly document why such supervision is impractical; such an explanation should not be a pretext for excluding potential competitors to members of the medical staff. The hospital's market share of beds should also be considered before a blanket exclusion is adopted; the greater the market share, the more likely it is that a court will find a classwide exclusion unreasonable.

Legal Analysis

The legal analysis of cases involving staff privileges combines antitrust and due process principles. Staff privilege decisions are reviewed for antitrust implications under one of two approaches. "Per se" violations are those practices that are regarded as plainly anticompetitive and unlawful despite any supporting rationale. A practice that is a per se violation of the antitrust laws is considered unreasonable, and courts are precluded from examining the purpose or impact of the practice.

Practices that are not considered per se violations are assessed under a "rule of reason" standard. Considering the circumstances, the court determines whether the restrictive practice actually imposes an unreasonable restraint on competition. Analysis of a practice under the rule of reason approach allows for consideration of the purpose, operation, and effect of the practice.

Courts have appeared to weigh a defendant's purpose more heavily in reviewing health care antitrust cases than in cases involving other industries. Where health care providers are engaged in activities for the purpose of maintaining high-quality care, subsequent antitrust allegations will most likely be analyzed under the more liberal rule of reason.

Under the rule of reason, the reasonableness of a denial of staff privileges is determined after considering a number of relevant factors. Of primary concern is whether the exclusion of the provider has an anticompetitive purpose or effect. An anticompetitive purpose or effect may be found if the aggrieved practitioner has no other health care facilities in which to practice and if the practice or rule on which the denial was based is not reasonable under the circumstances. A determination of anticompetitive motive may be made where the validity of the rule as it relates to individual qualifications for a specific privilege is questionable or where access is controlled by practitioners who are in direct competition with the applicant. Furthermore, a hospital's market power is an important component of the antitrust analysis. Hospitals that have a major share of beds or facilities in a community must consider the effect on competition when they deny staff privileges and when they enter into exclusive agreements with a physician group.

Generally, exclusive agreements between a hospital and a physician or a group practice are held unlawful only where they cause a substantial foreclosure of the market. The reasonableness of an exclusive contract may be determined by balancing the pro-competitive purposes for the arrangement against any anticompetitive purposes and the harm caused.

It should be noted that in determining whether a practitioner's exclusion was "reasonable," the court looks not just at the substantive grounds for denial but also at such procedural aspects as whether adequate notice was given, whether the practitioner was afforded an evidentiary hearing, and whether the decision-making body was unbiased. Provisions for procedural due process are evidence of the hospital's fair and unbiased discretion in making privileges decisions.

Defamation

Hospital employees, physicians on the medical staff, and members of the governing body may be accused of defamation as a result of the review of applicants for medical staff privileges, appointment, and reappointment. For example, it may be defamatory to inform members of the public or a news reporter that a doctor performs unnecessary surgery or abandons his or her patients, or to report to another hospital where the doctor seeks privileges that a doctor is incompetent.[10] Defamation comprises libel and slander. *Slander* consists of spoken statements that result in injury to reputation; *libel* is usually written but may also include recordings and film and photographs, as well as other media. In order to be actionable, defamatory information must be communicated to a third party; that process is referred to as *publication*. Of course, a statement is defamatory only if it is false.

The participants in the peer review process may effectively protect themselves from allegations of defamation by raising particular defenses. The most basic defense to a charge of defamation is that the statements complained of are true. Also, if a practitioner has consented to the making of otherwise defamatory statements, no cause of action for defamation may be brought. Written consent may be required on the staff application form. A practitioner's agreement to comply with a bylaws procedure whose purpose is to protect peer review communications against claims of defamation has been construed to be consent, as has a practitioner's asking someone to give specific reasons for restricting his or her privileges.

Generally, defamatory remarks made within the scope of peer review activities are privileged; in many states, the privilege is expressed in a peer review statute. A privilege may be either absolute or qualified. An *absolute privilege* provides complete immunity. Courts have found an absolute privilege to apply where the defendant, a physician, filed a grievance with the medical society that raised questions about another physician's competence[11] and where the letter in question was written to the Equal Employment Opportunity Commission in response to the practitioner's grievance.[12] It is more common, however, for courts to find a *qualified privilege*, which arises when the subject matter of the damaging statement is of legitimate interest to both the speaker and the audience, and the speaker reasonably believes the audience is entitled to know about it; obviously, this applies to many peer review proceedings, where those in attendance are concerned with identifying quality-of-care problems.[13] A qualified privilege protects the defendant only if the statements were not made with malice. Where communications are absolutely privileged, the presence of malice is irrelevant. Malice is a complex issue, but may be defined most simply as ill will and intent to harm. Obviously, it is important that malice be avoided in conducting peer review procedures.

Even where a derogatory statement about a practitioner is essentially true and therefore not defamatory, a practitioner may attempt to sue for invasion of privacy. Except for the falsity requirement, defamation and invasion of privacy are analyzed under similar legal principles. Generally, invasion of privacy arises from widespread or public dissemination of information, or from disclosure of personal information to those who have no right to know. Therefore, invasion of privacy claims should not ordinarily arise from the peer review process itself. Like defamation, however, invasion of privacy claims may be a concern if participants in the review imprudently discuss the proceedings or the outcome to outsiders not involved in the proceedings.

Discrimination

A practitioner's sex, race, creed, national origin, or handicap are not appropriate factors for peer review bodies to consider in determining whether to grant or deny clinical privileges. Practitioners may challenge adverse decisions based on violations of constitutional rights and of federal and state statutes that prohibit such discrimination. Although a hospital's practitioners, in most cases, are not considered true employees, federal employment laws are often used to challenge credentialing decisions. These challenges are made on the basis that the hospital exercises control over the practitioner's conduct and provides financial incentives to him or her, and thus has an employment-like relationship sufficient to come under the federal laws,[14] or that the hospital, not itself an employer, has interfered with the practitioner's opportunity for employment with a practice group or with patients.[15]

Limitation of Liability

Appropriately drafted medical staff bylaws may provide immunity from civil liability for participants in the peer review and credentialing process, if the standards and procedures in the bylaws are carefully observed. Similarly, protection may be provided by including a hold harmless clause in the application form. Such a clause requires applicants for staff privileges to execute a grant of immunity to and a release from liability of all participants in the credentialing process. The validity of such clauses varies from jurisdiction to jurisdiction and depends on a variety of factors. Risk managers should consult legal counsel for assistance in drafting language that provides protection.

State Immunity Statutes

Many states have enacted immunity statutes to protect members of the medical staff and review committees from civil liability for activities related to the evaluation of applicants. Individuals providing references and information about applicants, at the request of the medical staff and in good faith, are also given immunity. For the most part, such statutes have been held constitutional. However, courts have tended to narrowly construe such provisions. Therefore, because the nature of those statutes is considered to be procedural and not substantive, hospitals should note that protection is provided to only those individuals specifically named in the statute, that such protection is effective only when a statutorily designated function is being performed, and that no protection may be afforded an individual if there is standing to bring the action in federal court.

☐ Health Care Quality Improvement Act of 1986

The Health Care Quality Improvement Act of 1986 is a federal statute that affects medical staff appointment procedures. The act's purpose is to improve the quality of medical care both by providing limited immunity from liability to those who participate in or supply information in conjunction with peer review activities and by requiring adverse medical staff decisions to be reported to a central information bank. Immunity extends to physicians, participants, and health care entities engaged in peer review proceedings.

For immunity to apply, the review action must have been an evaluation of the physician's competence or professional conduct and must have been taken in the reasonable belief that it was in furtherance of high-quality care. Such action must be initiated after a reasonable effort to obtain the facts and with the reasonable belief that the facts warrant the action taken. The physician must be afforded adequate notice and hearing procedures. Although failure to meet the notice and hearing conditions, as defined in the act, does not automatically constitute a failure to satisfy the notice and hearing requirements, compliance with the procedures is deemed to satisfy the act.

Immunity under the act applies only to professional review of physicians, who are defined to include doctors of medicine, osteopathy, dental surgery, and medical dentistry. The act is silent concerning immunity claims arising from adverse privilege decisions relating to nonphysician practitioners.

The act provides for immunity from damage claims only, not from actions for injunctive or declaratory relief or private damage actions under federal or state civil rights laws. There is no immunity from actions brought by the federal government, including antitrust actions. However, health care facilities complying with the act are protected from private antitrust actions brought by aggrieved individuals.

☐ Conclusion

Risk managers reviewing the potential for liability arising from a hospital's credentialing and privileging decisions may justifiably perceive a no-win situation. There is the potential for liability to patients if a hospital is not rigorous enough in its review of practitioners' credentials, and at the same time there exists the potential for liability to excluded practitioners, who may think the hospital's policies are unfair or too rigorous. Nevertheless, it is possible to minimize both threats if the hospital's governing body, medical staff, and others involved in the review of practitioners' credentials remain true to the goal of providing high-quality patient care.

Provisions of the medical staff bylaws and other hospital policies that affect credentialing decisions should be critically analyzed to determine whether they have a legitimate connection to quality of care issues. The bylaws should provide for regular and earnest review of the credentials of new and established practitioners alike, and the standards for review and procedures for decision making should be uniformly and objectively applied to all practitioners. The facility's governing body and risk manager should be alert to the possibility that existing practitioners involved in making recommendations concerning new applicants may be influenced by their own economic concerns, and should attempt to educate involved practitioners about the inappropriateness of such factors and to minimize the decision-making role of persons who may perceive certain applicants to be potential competitors. New applicants should be required to prove their competence, and the privileges of established practitioners should be regularly reviewed to ensure that they are in line with current levels of competence. The facility's governing body has the ultimate authority to make decisions about practitioners' clinical privileges and staff membership, and should independently review the recommendations of the medical staff. Finally, where the review of a practitioner's credentials results in an adverse privileges decision, the hospital should be prepared to prove that its decision-making process followed the procedures set forth in the medical staff and hospital bylaws and assured the practitioner ample opportunity to address unfavorable findings. Although these basic guidelines can never guarantee that no one will sue the health care facility, its governing body, or members of its medical staff as a result of a perceived flaw in the credentials review process, following them will minimize the likelihood that a plaintiff will succeed in holding the facility or those associated with it liable.

References

1. Joint Commission on Accreditation of Healthcare Organizations. *1990 Accreditation Manual for Hospitals.* Chicago: JCAHO, 1989, pp. 95–116.

2. Proger, P. A. Antitrust and the medical staff. *American Academy of Hospital Attorneys 1988 Manual.* Chicago: American Hospital Association, 1988, pp. 28–30.

3. Bennett, H., and Simpson, H. H. *The Hospital and Its Medical Staff: Working Cooperatively in a Changing Legal Environment.* Proceedings of the 11th annual hospital law seminar of the Health Law Institute, 1988, pp. 1–15.

4. Weiss v. York Hospital, 745 F.2d 786 (1984), *cert. denied,* 470 U.S. 1060 (1985), involving an osteopath, is a good example of a claim brought under the Sherman Act on behalf of a group of excluded practitioners. The jury found the hospital was not liable but that the members of the medical staff had conspired to exclude osteopaths without good reason. *See also* Patrick v. Burget, U.S., 108 S. Ct. 1658 (1988) (upholding jury verdict against physicians for $650,000 where peer review proceeding conducted in bad faith caused practitioner to resign from medical staff); Robinson v. Magovern, 521 F.Supp. 842 (W.D. Pa. 1981) (finding that exclusion of thoracic surgeon from teaching hospital did not violate Sherman Act because surgeon was incompatible with hospital's strategy to further teaching and research). A helpful discussion of antitrust issues involved in peer review is Miles and Philp, *Hospitals Caught in the Antitrust Net: An Overview,* 24 Duquesne L. Rev. 489 (1986), reprinted in part in *Peer Review and the Law,* American Bar Association Forum Committee on Health Law, 1986. Other articles in *Peer Review and the Law* also address risk management issues in the peer review process.

5. Jefferson Parish Hospital District No. 2 v. Hyde, 466 U.S. 2, 104 S. Ct. 1551 (1984).

6. *See* Holmes v. Hoemako Hospital, 573 P.2d 477 (Ariz. 1977).

7. Sams v. Ohio Valley General Hospital, 413 F.2d 826 (4th Cir. 1969).

8. Dooley v. Berberton Citizens Hospital, 11 Ohio 3d 216, 465 N.E.2d 58 (1984) (finding two-year residency requirement for podiatrists unreasonable).

9. Clarke, A. M., and Springer, E. W. Medical staff—current issues and approaches. *American Academy of Hospital Attorneys 1988 Manual.* Chicago: American Hospital Association, 1988, pp. 15–22.

10. *See, e.g.,* DeMeo v. Goodall, 640 F.Supp. 1115 (D.N.H. 1986).

11. Franklin v. Blank, 86 N.M. 585, 525 P.2d 945 (Ct. App. N.M. 1974).

12. Paros v. Hoemako Hospital, 140 Ariz. 335, 681 P.2d 918 (Ariz. App. 1984).

13. Seidenstein v. National Medical Enterprises, Inc., 769 F.2d 1100 (5th Cir. 1985); Hayden v. Foryt, 407 So.2d 535 (Miss. 1982); Mayfield v. Gleichert, 484 S.W.2d 619 (Tex. Civ. App.1972).

14. Mallare v. St. Luke's Hospital of Bethlehem, 699 F. Supp. 1127 (E.D. Pa.1988); Mousavi v. Beebe Hospital of Sussex Co., Inc., 674 F. Supp. 145 (D. Del. 1987), *aff'd,* 853 F.2d 919 (3rd Cir. 1988).

15. Pardazi v. Cullman Medical Center, 838 F.2d 1155 (11th Cir. 1988); Doe v. St. Joseph's Hospital, 688 F.2d 411 (7th Cir. 1986).

☐ Bibliography

Hall, M. A. Institutional control of physician behavior: legal barriers to health care cost containment. *University of Pennsylvania Law Review* 137:431, 1988.

Hospital Law Manual. Attorney's vols. 2 and 2B. Rockville, MD: Aspen Publishers, 1988.

McDonald, M. D., Meyer, K. C., and Essig, B. *Health Care Law: A Practical Guide.* Release no. 3. New York City: Matthew Bender & Co., 1988.

Miller, R. *Problems in Hospital Law.* 5th ed. Rockville, MD: Aspen Publishers, 1986.

Chapter 22

Risk Considerations
in Organ Transplantation

Stephan E. Lawton, Mary Elizabeth Giblin, and Michael D. Smith

Federal and state legislators have responded to recent technological developments that allow transplantation of various human organs by enacting statutes governing the practical, ethical, and legal concerns surrounding those advances. In October 1984, Congress passed the first major federal legislation concerning organ procurement and transplantation, the National Organ Transplant Act.[1] The act prohibits the purchase or sale of human organs where the transfer affects interstate commerce. Reasonable payments associated with the removal, transportation, implantation, processing, preservation, quality control, and storage of a human organ, or the expenses of travel, housing, and lost wages incurred by the organ donor, are excluded from the prohibition. In addition, states have enacted various laws, such as required request, informed consent, and brain death statutes, to govern the donation and procurement of organs.

☐ Federal Laws

Federal laws affecting organ transplantation include the National Organ Transplant Act, requirements for the United Network for Organ Sharing, and Medicare and Medicaid regulations.

National Organ Transplant Act

The National Organ Transplant Act authorized the Secretary of Health and Human Services (HHS) to provide financial assistance to qualified organ procurement organizations (OPOs)[2] and to establish and operate by contract an Organ Procurement and Transplantation Network.[3] A qualified OPO is defined as a nonprofit entity that has the following:

- Accounting and other fiscal procedures, as specified by the Secretary, necessary to assure fiscal stability
- An agreement with the Secretary to be reimbursed under Medicare for the procurement of kidneys

- Procedures to obtain payment for nonrenal organs provided to transplant centers
- A defined service area
- A director and such other staff, including organ donation coordinators and organ procurement specialists, necessary to obtain organs effectively from donors
- A board of directors or an advisory board to recommend policies regarding organ procurement.

The act requires that OPOs have agreements to identify potential donors with hospitals and other health care entities in their service areas, that they arrange for the acquisition, preservation, and tissue typing of donated organs, and that they have a system to allocate donated organs among transplant centers and patients according to established medical criteria.

The network is responsible for establishing a national list of organ recipients and a national system to match organs and individuals in accordance with established medical criteria. Other purposes of the network include:

- Maintaining a 24-hour telephone service to facilitate the matching process
- Assisting OPOs in distributing organs that cannot be placed within their respective service areas
- Establishing standards of quality for acquiring and transporting donated organs
- Coordinating the transportation of organs from OPOs to transplant centers
- Providing information to the medical community regarding organ donation

In September 1986, HHS awarded the contract to provide those services to the United Network for Organ Sharing (UNOS).

UNOS Requirements

In order to receive payment under the Medicare and Medicaid programs, transplant hospitals and OPOs are required to be members of UNOS and to abide by its rules and requirements. The United Network for Organ Sharing has established detailed rules and regulations governing membership, standardized packaging for organs and tissues, and organ procurement and distribution.[4] Risk managers should become intimately familiar with those rules because a hospital or OPO that fails to comply with them may lose all Medicare and Medicaid funds, not merely those payments associated with organ transplants.

In order to qualify for UNOS membership, a transplant program must use a laboratory for histocompatibility testing that meets the standards of the American Society for Histocompatibility and Immunogenetics, have an agreement with an independent organ procurement agency or a hospital-based OPO, and satisfy detailed requirements regarding clinical personnel. All potential organ recipients must be listed on the UNOS computerized waiting list. In addition, UNOS requires that all potential organ donors be tested for human immunodeficiency virus (HIV) antibody (Ab), and that potential recipients be tested, except where the testing would violate state or federal laws and regulations.

Medicare and Medicaid Regulations

The Health Care Financing Administration (HFCA) has issued regulations for hospitals and OPOs that participate in the Medicare and Medicaid programs.[5] Hospitals must have written protocols to ensure that the family of each potential organ donor knows of its option either to donate or decline to donate organs or tissues; to encourage discretion and sensitivity with respect to the circumstances, views, and beliefs of the families of potential donors; and to require that an OPO designated by the Secretary of HHS be notified of potential organ donors. Potential donors are individuals who die at an age and under circumstances that would make at least one of their solid organs suitable for transplantation.

Organ procurement organizations that procure organs for hospitals must be designated by the Secretary. Although the Secretary may designate only one OPO for a given service area, the preamble to the HCFA regulations makes it clear that a hospital may work with any OPO that it chooses.[6] In order to be designated as an OPO, an organization must have documented evidence that (1) it has a working relationship with at least 75 percent of the hospitals that participate in the Medicare and Medicaid programs in its service area that have an operating room and the equipment and personnel for retrieving organs, and (2) it conducts systematic efforts to acquire all usable organs from potential donors. In addition, OPOs must provide or arrange for the transportation of organs to transplant centers, have arrangements to coordinate their activities with transplant centers and to cooperate with tissue banks, maintain data in a format that can be readily used by a successor OPO, and have a procedure for ensuring the confidentiality of patient records. Furthermore, OPOs must meet specific performance standards for the procurement and transplantation of cadaveric kidneys, and they must enter into a working relationship with any hospital or transplant center in their service area that requests them to do so.

Currently, Medicare pays for the costs of kidney and heart transplantation if certain conditions are satisfied.[7] The transplantation of pancreases, adult livers, lungs, or heart–lung combinations is excluded from coverage because HCFA considers those procedures to be experimental. Hospitals that acquire organs from nondesignated OPOs will not be reimbursed by Medicare or Medicaid for those procurement costs. In order to provide kidney transplant services to Medicaid beneficiaries, a number of states pay the coinsurance and deductible amounts associated with the procedure. Some states also pay for transplant services not covered by Medicare, such as heart–lung, pancreas, and liver transplants.

□ State Laws

As noted in the previous sections of this chapter, risk managers in hospitals must be cognizant not only of federal statutes and regulations governing organ transplantation, but also of state laws. Individual state laws govern a variety of topics, ranging from informed consent and required request procedures to definitions of brain death. This section will highlight important state laws affecting organ transplantation.

Uniform Anatomical Gift Act

The Uniform Anatomical Gift Act (UAGA) (1968),[8] which was adopted in various forms by all 50 states and the District of Columbia, regulates donations of body parts, indicates who may execute an anatomical gift or become a donee, and specifies the purpose for which a body part may be donated.[9] The UAGA provides legal protection to physicians who follow the expressed wishes of individuals and families who donate organs for transplantation or research.

The UAGA was amended in 1987,[10] significantly strengthening organ procurement efforts and codifying the required request legislation that has passed in many states. The revised UAGA, which has been adopted by Arkansas, California, Connecticut, Hawaii, Idaho, Montana, Nevada, North Dakota, and Rhode Island,[11] stipulates the following:

- Hospital personnel and rescue workers are required to search for a donor document.

- Coroners or medical examiners may permit the removal of body parts for transplantation or therapy if they have made a reasonable effort to examine the decedent's medical records and inform family members and guardians of the option to make or refuse to make a gift, there are no known objections, and a request is received from a hospital, physician, or procurement organization.
- The witness requirement is eliminated on gift documents signed by donors.
- Consent of the next of kin is not required if the donor has made a valid gift prior to death.
- Hospitals are recognized as entities that can receive donations.
- Hospitals have the same "good faith" immunity under the UAGA that individuals had under the previous version.

(See figure 22-1 for a table of jurisdictions wherein the act has been adopted.) Risk managers must, therefore, determine whether the revised UAGA is currently in effect in their states and carefully follow pending legislation.

Determination of Death

The Uniform Determination of Death Act,[12] adopted by a number of states, provides that a person who has sustained either "irreversible cessation of circulatory and respiratory functions" or "irreversible cessation of all functions of the entire brain, including the brain stem" is dead. Many states that have enacted some version of the Uniform Determination of Death Act have added language that permits death to be declared before artificial life-support systems have been removed, greatly facilitating the procurement of viable organs.

Absent a statutory definition, some physicians are hesitant to declare an individual dead on the basis of brain death. Under the 1968 version of the UAGA, however, physicians are protected from liability for declaring the time of death. The UAGA prohibits the physician who declared death and the physician who becomes the donee from participating in the procedures for removing or transplanting an organ.

Warranties

Many states have taken steps to eliminate liability for hepatitis and AIDS transmitted through blood transfusions and organ transplants. These statutes typically state that those involved in the procurement of blood and organs are rendering a service rather than selling a product. As a result, the implied warranties of merchantability and fitness are inapplicable. Thus, the only avenue for recovery left to those who contract diseases through blood transfusions or organ transplants appears to be a recovery in negligence through which a plaintiff must prove that a standard of care existed, the defendant's conduct fell below that standard, and the conduct was the proximate cause of the plaintiff's injury. The duty of care depends on the standard of medical knowledge available at the time.

AIDS

If an individual is found to have AIDS and is therefore unsuitable as a donor, a question arises as to how procurement coordinators may respond to requests from the family regarding the reason for the unsuitability. Various states have enacted laws and policies governing the confidentiality and disclosure of information relating to AIDS and HIV infection. The House Energy and Commerce Committee has also passed a bill providing grants to states for preventive health services related to AIDS.[13] The bill requires states to ensure that information regarding the receipt of services is maintained confidentially, and specifies that state public health officials carry out a program of partner notification

Figure 22-1.   Table of Jurisdictions wherein Uniform Anatomical Gift Act, 1968, Has Been Adopted

Jurisdiction	Laws	Effective Date	Statutory Citation
Alabama[a]	1969, Sp. Sess. No. 164	5-14-1969[b]	Code 1975, §§22-19-40 to 22-19-47, 22-19-60
Alaska	1972, c. 78	1-1-1973	AS 13.50.010 to13.50.090
Arizona	1970, c.147, §3	8-11-1970	A.R.S. §§36-841 to 36-849
Colorado	1969, c. 239	4-24-1969	C.R.S. 12-34-101 to 12-34-109
Delaware	57 Del. Laws c. 445, §2	5-20-1970	16 Del.C. §§2710 to 2719
District of Columbia	P.L. 91-268, to §§1 to 82-1	5-26-1970	D.C. Code 1981, §§2-1501 511
Florida	1969, c. 69-88	6-14-1969	West's F.S.A. §§732.910 to 732.922
Georgia	1969, No. 82	6-14-1969	O.C.G.A. §§44-5-140 to 44-5-151
Guam	P.L. 12-16		10 G.C.A. §§83101 to 83109
Illinois	P.A. 76-1209	10-1-1969	S.H.A. ch. 110 1/2 ¶¶301to 311
Indiana	1969, c. 166	3-13-1969[b]	West's A.I.C. 29-2-16-1 to 29-2-16-10
Iowa	1969 (63 G.A.) c. 137	7-1-1969	I.C.A. § 142A.1 et seq.
Kansas	1969, c. 301	7-1-1969	K.S.A. 65-3209 to 65-3217
Kentucky	1970, c. 68	6-18-1970	KRS 311.165 to 311.235
Louisiana	1968, No. 651	7-31-1968	LSA-R.S. 17:2351 to 17:2359
Maine	1969, c. 193	10-2-1969	22 M.R.S.A. §§2901 to 2910
Maryland	1968, c. 467	7-1-1968	Code, Estates and Trusts, §§4-501 to 4-512
Massachusetts	1971, c. 653	8-12-1971[b]	M.G.L.A. c. 113, §§7 to 14
Michigan	1969, No. 189	3-20-1970	M.C.L.A. §§333.10101 to 333.10109
Minnesota	1969, c. 79	3-26-1969	M.S.A. §§525.921 to 525.94
Mississippi	1970, c. 413	4-6-1970	Code 1972, §§41-39-11, 41-39-31 to 41-39-53
Missouri	1969, S.B. No. 43	5-28-1969	V.A.M.S. §§194.210 to 194.290
Nebraska	1971, LB 799, § 12	8-27-1971	R.R.S.1943, §§71-4801 to 71-4818
New Hampshire	1969, c. 345	8-29-1969	RSA 291-A:1 to 291-A:9
New Jersey	1969, c. 161	9-9-1969	N.J.S.A. 26:6-57 to 26:6-65
New Mexico	1969, c. 105	3-29-1969	NMSA 1978, §§24-6-1 to 24-6-11
New York	1970, c. 466	5-5-1970	McKinney's Public Health Law §§4300 to 4308
North Carolina	1969, c. 84	10-1-1969	G.S. §§130A-402 to 130A-412.1
Ohio	1969, p. 1796	11-6-1969	R.C. §§2108.01 to 2108.10
Oklahoma	1969, c. 13	7-29-1969	63 Okl.St.Ann. §§2201 to 2209
Oregon	1969, c. 175	8-22-1969	ORS 97.250 to 97.295
Pennsylvania	1972, P.L. 508, No. 164	7-1-1972	20 Pa.C.S.A. §§8601 to 8607
South Carolina	1969, No. 356	7-1-1969	Code 1976, §§44-43-310 to 44-43-400
South Dakota	1969, c. 111	3-14-1969	SDCL 34-26-20 to 34-26-41
Tennessee	1969, c. 35	3-25-1969	T.C.A. §§68-30-101 to 68-30-111
Texas	1969, c. 375	5-29-1969	V.T.C.A. Health & Safety Code, §§692.001 to 692.016

(continued on next page)

Figure 22-1. (Continued)

Jurisdiction	Laws	Effective Date	Statutory Citation
Utah	1969, c. 64	5-13-1969	U.C.A.1953, 26-28-1 to 26-28-8
Vermont	1969, No. 53	4-10-1969	18 V.S.A. §§5231 to 5237
Virgin Islands	1984, No. 4890	1-19-1984	19 V.I.C. §§401 to 409
Virginia	1970, c. 460	4-3-1970	Code 1950, §§32.1-289 to 32.1-297.1
Washington	1969, c. 80	6-12-1969	West's RCWA 68.50.340 to 68.50.510
West Virginia	1969, c. 62	3-10-1969	Code, 16-19-1 to 16-19-9
Wisconsin	1969, c. 90	7-1-1979	W.S.A. 157.06
Wyoming	1969, c. 80	2-19-1969	W.S.1977, §§35-5-101 to 35-5-112

Source: National Conference of Commissioners of Uniform State Laws.
Note: Arkansas, Idaho, Montana, Nevada, North Dakota, and Rhode Island have adopted the 1987 version of the UAGA.
[a]Section 22-19-60, governing gifts made by the holder of a valid Alabama driver's license or nondriver identification card, is technically not part of the Alabama UAGA.
[b]Date of approval.

in cases of HIV infection. Risk managers should follow pending legislation and become familiar with various state requirements.

Required Request Laws and Informed Consent

A number of states have enacted required request laws, which specify that the family of a patient be asked to make a donation or be informed of the donation option. Hospital personnel are often excused from making such a request if there are contrary indications from the patient or family, conflicting religious beliefs, or medical reasons making a donation unsuitable for use. In most areas of medical practice, the legal definition of informed consent means that a patient be given enough information about the risks and benefits of a procedure to make a rational decision by himself or herself. Both concepts are incorporated in the revised UAGA, which requires that inquiries regarding donor status and information about the option to make or refuse to make a gift be addressed to the patient, rather than to the next-of-kin. The UAGA specifies that on or before admission to a hospital, or as soon as possible thereafter, each patient who is at least 18 years old be asked: "Are you an organ or tissue donor?" If the answer to the question is yes, the hospital administrator or his or her designated representative must ask for an exact copy of the donation document. If the answer is no, and the attending physician consents, the representative must discuss with the patient the option to make or refuse to make a donation. At a minimum, the representative should inform the patient of the benefits of donation and any potential risks. The answer to the donation question, a copy of any document of a gift or a refusal to make a gift, and any other relevant information must then be placed in the patient's medical files.

If, at or near the time of death, there is no medical record indicating that a patient has made or refused to make an organ donation, the representative should discuss the option with the patient's family and request consent. The request should be made with reasonable discretion and sensitivity; a request is not required if the gift would be unsuitable based on accepted medical standards. An entry should thereafter be made in the patient's medical record indicating the name and affiliation of the person making the request and the name, response, and relationship to the patient of the person to whom the request was addressed.

References

1. National Organ Transplant Act, Pub. L. No. 98-507, 98 Stat. 2339 (1984).

2. National Organ Transplant Act, Pub. L. No. 98-507, §371, 98 Stat. 2339, 2342-44 (1984).

3. National Organ Transplant Act, Pub. L. No. 98-507, §372, 98 Stat. 2339, 2344-45 (1984).

4. *See* UNOS Policies, Articles of Incorporation, and By-Laws. Copies of these materials may be obtained by contacting UNOS, 3001 Hungary Spring Rd., P.O. Box 28010, Richmond, VA 23228.

5. *See* 42 C.F.R. §§482.12(c)(5), 485.301–308.

6. *See* 53 Fed. Reg. 6525.

7. *See* 42 C.F.R. §§405.2100–2184 (conditions for coverage of suppliers of end-stage renal disease services); HCFAR 87-1, 52 Fed. Reg. 10935 (1987) (criteria for Medicare coverage of heart transplants).

8. Unif. Anatomical Gift Act, 8A U.L.A. 30 (1968).

9. See figure 22-1 for a table of jurisdictions wherein the 1968 version of the UAGA has been adopted, reproduced from Unif. Anatomical Gift Act, 8A U.L.A. 28–29 (1968) (Supp. 1990).

10. Unif. Anatomical Gift Act, 8A U.L.A. 7 (1987) (Supp. 1990).

11. Unif. Anatomical Gift Act, 8A U.L.A. 2 (1987) (Supp. 1990).

12. Unif. Determination of Death Act, 12 U.L.A. 322 (1980) (Supp. 1990).

13. H.R. 4785, 101st Cong., 2d Sess. (1990).

☐ Bibliography

Cover, B., and Overcast, T., editors. *Organ Procurement and Transplantation Manual.* Owings Mills, MD: National Health Publishing, 1987. Updated periodically.

Chapter 23

Institutional Review Boards and Human Research Issues

Myra C. Selby

Biomedical investigational research involving human subjects is an activity that must be subject to oversight and review. The body that typically performs this function in hospitals is called the institutional review board (IRB). The IRB is a board, committee, or other group authorized by an institution to review, approve, and conduct continuing review of research activities involving human subjects. The primary purpose of such review ensures the protection of the rights and welfare of the human subjects. In addition, IRB review ensures that risks to subjects are minimized, that risks to subjects are reasonable in relation to anticipated benefits, and that informed consent is sought from each prospective subject.[1]

Federal regulations provide specific requirements for the function and composition of an IRB. The federal agencies responsible for monitoring IRBs and enforcing the regulations concerning investigational research are the Department of Health and Human Services (HHS) and the Food and Drug Administration (FDA).

The federal regulations promulgated by the HHS apply to all research involving human subjects funded in whole or in part by a grant, contract, cooperative agreement, or fellowship with HHS.[2] The federal regulations promulgated by the FDA apply to all clinical investigations regulated by the FDA and clinical investigations that support applications for research or marketing permits for products regulated by the FDA for human use, including, among other things, drugs, medical devices, and biologic products. Federal funds need not be involved in FDA-regulated research.[3] Investigational research activities in the hospital setting generally fall under regulations promulgated by the FDA. A request to conduct research involving human subjects in a hospital usually is presented by a physician, who is referred to as the *investigator*. The company or entity providing the research drug or device is called the *sponsor*.

☐ Function and Membership of the IRB

An IRB must comprise at least five members; membership must be varied as to sex, race, professional background, and expertise. The IRB must include at least one member whose primary concerns are in nonscientific areas and at least one member who is not otherwise affiliated, directly or indirectly, with the institution. This diversity of membership is described in the regulations:

> The IRB shall be sufficiently qualified through the experience and expertise of its members, and the diversity of the members' backgrounds including consideration of the racial and cultural backgrounds of members and sensitivity to such issues as community attitudes, to promote respect for its advice and counsel in safeguarding the rights and welfare of human subjects.[4]

One IRB member can satisfy more than one membership category. For example, one member who is female and who is not otherwise affiliated with the institution would satisfy two membership requirements. An IRB member may not participate in the review of an investigational research project in which the member has an interest, except to provide information to the IRB. The IRB must approve or disapprove the research by a majority vote of the members present at a meeting, and the members present must include at least one nonscientific IRB member.[5] The exception to this approval process is for expedited review, set forth in a later section.

The IRB must adopt written procedures and comply with those procedures for the review of research, including the following:

- Conduct initial and ongoing IRB review of research
- Report IRB findings and determinations to the investigator and the institution
- Determine frequency of review of approved research projects
- Report to the IRB changes in research activity or unanticipated problems involving risks to human subjects or others
- Retain copies of all information reviewed for at least three years after completion of the research

□ IRB Review of Research

The IRB has authority to approve, require modifications in, or disapprove all research activities covered by the FDA and HHS regulations (see figure 23-1 for a sample monitoring form). As a part of its review process, the IRB is required to:

- Ensure that each subject receives information that satisfies the basic elements of informed consent.
- Require documentation of informed consent.
- Notify investigators and the institution in writing of its decision to approve or disapprove proposed research activity, including required modifications to such activity. A decision to disapprove research activity must include a written statement of reasons for that decision and notification to the investigator that he or she shall have an opportunity to respond in person or in writing.
- Conduct continuing review of the research activity at appropriate intervals, but in no case less than one time per year.
- Observe or have a third party observe the consent process and the research activity.[6]

□ Expedited Review

Expedited review is a procedure through which certain kinds of research may be reviewed and approved without convening the full IRB. Federal regulations permit, but do not require, an IRB to review certain categories of research through an expedited procedure if the research involves no more than minimal risk. The list of categories of research that

Figure 23-1. Monitoring Form for Continuing Review

Title of project: _____

Investigator: _____

Date: _____

Dear Investigator:

The Institutional Review Board is required to provide continuing review of research involving human subjects.

Please answer the following questions:

1. Has there been any revision in your study protocol since submission to the Committee or since previous review?   Yes _____ No _____

   If yes above, has the revision been submitted to the Institutional Review Board?
   Yes _____ No _____

2. Have there been any deviations from your investigational protocol?   Yes _____ No _____

   If yes above, specify the deviations on a separate sheet.

3. Have all subjects of your investigation given informed consent to date?
   Yes _____ No _____

   If no above, report the subjects and circumstances involved.
   _____
   _____
   _____

4. Have there been any changes in the informed consent form?   Yes _____ No _____

5. Attach a copy of the consent form in use.

6. Have there been any unexpected events?   Yes _____ No _____

   If yes, please describe on a separate sheet.

7. Have there been any adverse reactions?   Yes _____ No _____

   If yes, attach a list of the subjects and circumstances on a separate sheet.

8. Has there been any emergency use of test articles?   Yes _____ No _____

   If yes, attach a separate sheet stating the subject involved and circumstances.

9. Have there been any significant new findings?   Yes _____ No _____

   If yes, please attach a statement outlining these findings and state whether or not they have been provided to subjects of your research.

10. List the number of subjects involved from inception to date in your research project.
   _____
   _____

The information on this form and its attachments is a true and accurate reflection of the status of my research project on _____ Signed: _____
                                     (Date)   (Investigator)

may receive expedited review is published in the *Federal Register* and revised through periodic republication. The IRB may also use the expedited review procedure to review minor changes in previously approved research during the period for which approval is authorized.

Under an expedited review procedure, review of research may be carried out by the IRB chairperson or by one or more experienced members of the IRB designated by the chairperson. Reviewers may exercise all the authorities of the IRB, except that they may not disapprove the research; research can be disapproved only after review by the full IRB. The IRB is also required to adopt a method for keeping all members advised of research proposals that have been approved through the expedited review procedure.

☐ Informed Consent

Undoubtedly one of the most important aspects of IRB review research activity is the review and monitoring of informed consent, which ensures the protection of the rights and welfare of human subjects. Accordingly, federal regulations specifically describe the basic elements of informed consent as follows:[7]

1. A statement that the study involves research, an explanation of the purposes of the research and the expected duration of the subject's participation, a description of the procedures to be followed, and identification of any procedures which are experimental
2. A description of any reasonably foreseeable risks or discomforts to the subject
3. A description of any benefits to the subject or to others which may reasonably be expected from the research
4. A disclosure of appropriate alternative procedures or courses of treatment, if any, that might be advantageous to the subject
5. A statement describing the extent, if any, to which confidentiality of records identifying the subject will be maintained and noting the possibility that the Food and Drug Administration may inspect the records
6. For research involving more than minimal risk, an explanation as to whether any compensation and any medical treatments are available if injury occurs and, if so, what they consist of, or where further information may be obtained
7. An explanation of whom to contact for answers to pertinent questions about the research and research subjects' rights, and whom to contact in the event of a research-related injury to the subject
8. A statement that participation is voluntary, that refusal to participate will involve no penalty or loss of benefits to which the subject is otherwise entitled, and that the subject may discontinue participation at any time without penalty or loss of benefits to which the subject is otherwise entitled

In addition to the foregoing required elements of informed consent, the regulations require that the following elements be provided to the subject, when appropriate:[8]

1. A statement that the particular treatment or procedure may involve risks to the subject (or to the embryo or fetus, if the subject is or may become pregnant) which are currently foreseeable
2. Anticipated circumstances under which the subject's participation may be terminated by the investigator without regard to the subject's consent
3. Any additional costs to the subject that may result from participation in the research
4. The consequences of a subject's decision to withdraw from the research and procedures for orderly termination of participation by the subject

5. A statement that significant new findings developed during the course of the research which may relate to the subject's willingness to continue participation will be provided to the subject
6. The approximate number of subjects involved in the study

As part of the review process, the IRB must determine whether the additional elements of informed consent should be disclosed to the research subject. The regulations provide that written documentation of informed consent may be in the form of either a written document that embodies all the elements required under the basic elements of informed consent or a short-form written consent stating that the required basic elements of informed consent have been presented orally to the subject or the subject's legally authorized representative.

If the short-form written consent is used, the IRB must approve a written summary of the oral presentation to the subject. This written summary must be signed by a witness and by the person obtaining consent. The subject must receive a copy of the written consent form, whether it is the regular written consent or the short form; in addition, when the short form is used, the subject must also receive a copy of the summary statement.

As in all instances where patient consent is sought, informed consent to participate in an investigational research project will be a dialogue between the investigator and the proposed subject. The document reviewed by the IRB and signed by the subject is *not* the consent—it merely memorializes the consent process.

☐ Emergency Use of an Investigational Drug, Device, or Biologic

Federal regulations define *emergency use* in this context as the use of an investigational drug, device, or biologic on a human subject in a life-threatening situation in which no standard acceptable treatment is available and there is not sufficient time to obtain IRB approval. Emergency or compassionate use may be exempt from FDA requirements for IRB review provided that the emergency use is reported to the IRB within five working days. The investigator is required to obtain informal consent from the subject. Any subsequent use of the investigational product at the institution is subject to IRB approval.

☐ Potential Liability Issues for IRBs

The most probable area of liability exposure for an IRB relates to the IRB's core function—protecting the rights and welfare of human research subjects. Thus, failure to perform any aspect of this function could well create a liability problem. For example, failing to require documentation of informed consent could give rise to IRB liability where there is an adverse result and the patient alleges lack of informed consent.

A less obvious area of potential liability for an IRB includes breach of confidentiality of patient information as a result of the sharing of scientific data. In many instances, the language in an IRB-approved consent form may include promises or assurances of confidentiality that are so broad as to preclude the sharing of the data beyond the original research project.[9] Thus, the IRB must monitor informed consent forms for confidentiality language that prohibits or restricts sharing data.

In addition, IRBs face research projects that present ethical dilemmas, such as requiring HIV antibody tests as an entry requirement in order to protect research staff from exposure to the human immunodeficiency virus, paying patients to serve as research subjects,[10] recruiting research subjects, and using human fetal tissue in research. Although these and other ethical issues raise the difficult question of research ethics, the IRBs must approach the issues with the primary objective of protecting the rights and welfare of human subjects.

☐ Questions Commonly Encountered by IRBs

Q: Can a hospital IRB review a study that will be conducted outside the hospital?

A: Although a hospital IRB is not required to review studies conducted outside the jurisdiction of its institution, the IRB may choose to do so with the institution's approval.

Q: Does the federal government inspect or review IRBs?

A: Yes. The FDA inspects the operation of IRBs periodically through field investigations.

Q: What happens during an FDA inspection of an IRB?

A: The FDA field investigators interview institutional officials and examine the IRB's records to determine whether the IRB is in conformance with FDA regulations.

Q: Is the unapproved use of an approved, marketed product subject to IRB review?

A: The use of an approved, marketed product in the context of a study to develop information about the safety and efficiency of the product is an investigational use subject to IRB review. This is true of a drug for an unapproved use, at an unapproved dosage, by an unapproved route of administration, or in an altered dosage form. An investigational use should be distinguished from a physician's use of a product in an unapproved manner merely as a part of the practice of medicine and not incident to any study or clinical trial.

Q: Must an institution at which research involving human subjects is conducted establish an IRB?

A: Although IRBs frequently exist in an institution that conducts research involving human subjects, this is not required by federal regulations. Generally, however, institutions engaged in research involving human subjects will have their own IRBs to review research conducted on the premises or elsewhere by the staff of the institution.

References

1. Institutional Review Boards, 21 C.F.R. §56.102(g) (1988).

2. Protection of Human Subjects, 45 C.F.R. §46.101(a) (1988).

3. Protection of Human Subjects, 21 C.F.R. §50.1(a) (1988).

4. 21 C.F.R. §56.107(a).

5. 21 C.F.R. §56.108(b).

6. 21 C.F.R. §56.109.

7. 21 C.F.R. §50.25(a).

8. 21 C.F.R. §50.25(b).

9. Sharing scientific data I: new problems for IRBs. *IRB. A Review of Human Subjects Research* (11)6, Nov.–Dec. 1989.

10. Federal regulations address payment to research subjects and state that payment for participation in research study is considered a benefit. However, the regulations do not address the payment of patients to serve as research subjects. 21 C.F.R. §50.20 (1988).

Chapter 24

Confidentiality of Records Maintained in a Hospital Setting

Jane C. McConnell and Andrea M. Praeger

An important risk management responsibility is to maintain the confidentiality of many types of records kept by health care institutions. The primary focus of this chapter is on hospital records, but the principles discussed are equally applicable to other patient care settings. Questions about the confidentiality of patient medical records arise most often when malpractice litigation is brought against the hospital, its employees, or attending physicians. During litigation, plaintiffs seek discovery of medical records and other documents such as peer review records. In other instances, state regulators or the media may seek confidential hospital records. Because hospitals are involved so frequently in litigation, it is crucial for risk managers to be fully apprised of the hospital's rights and obligations regarding the protection of its records. Risk managers should consult legal counsel about laws regarding confidentiality and privilege in their own states in those instances when the hospital's obligations are not clear.

☐ Medical Records

The Joint Commission on Accreditation of Healthcare Organizations requires that all facilities treating patients maintain adequate medical records to serve as a "basis for planning patient care and for continuity in the evaluation of the patient's condition and treatment."[1] The medical record is where clinical information about the patient is recorded; it is a repository of information and a means for communicating among physicians and other providers involved in the patient's care.

The medical record serves other purposes as well. For example, as important business records of the hospital, medical records are accessed by many departments and personnel not involved in direct patient care. These may include administrative staff performing quality assurance and risk management functions, physicians engaged in peer review, and members of the finance department. Outside the institution, various governmental agencies, government-funded organizations, and accreditation bodies monitor the hospital and individual provider performance by reviewing records; third-party payers review medical records for reimbursement; and, in malpractice cases, the record serves as the principal source of evidence about the care the patient received. The hospital should have a clear policy about who may have access to medical records, whether those records are written, computerized, or otherwise maintained.

Confidentiality versus Privilege

Tension exists, therefore, because the legitimate needs of individuals not involved in the patient's care to have access to patient information conflict with the principle that patient information is confidential. There is both an ethical and a legal basis for confidentiality of medical information. The ethical principle of confidentiality, which is incorporated in the standards of each health profession, originates from the idea that an assurance of confidentiality encourages patients to seek needed medical care and to be candid with their physicians about their condition.[2] Confidentiality also is necessary to protect the patient's inherent privacy interest. People receiving medical care are entitled to privacy about their bodily condition.[3]

The legal basis for confidentiality derives from the physician–patient privilege, set forth by statute in almost all states. This is one of several relationships recognized as special by law. The others are attorney–client, husband–wife, and priest–penitent; in all these, the preservation of confidentiality is viewed as essential to the maintenance of the relationship. This need for confidentiality in the physician–patient relationship gives rise to a legal *privilege,* which means that, absent a patient authorization or waiver or an overriding law or public policy, medical information about a patient is insulated from the process known as *discovery,* through which parties to a lawsuit normally can compel disclosure of relevant evidence.[4]

Although most privileges recognized today existed as English common law, the physician–patient privilege is entirely a creation of statute. Most courts, therefore, will construe the relevant statute strictly to protect only those situations and professionals explicitly described.

Professionals Covered by the Privilege

In certain states, the physician–patient privilege has been extended beyond physicians to protect the patient's relationship to other health care professionals, such as psychologists and social workers. In the absence of a statute, there is no privilege between nurses who have acted independently and patients, but with or without a statute, courts have interpreted the physician–patient privilege to include employed nurses, physician assistants, and other professionals working for a physician.[5] Risk managers should check the law of their jurisdiction to ascertain which health care professionals are specifically covered by the privilege.

Information Covered by the Privilege

Once the privilege is determined to exist, it is consistently found to extend beyond oral communications between physician and patient to cover written entries in the patient's record, as well as X rays, cardiograph strips, lab results, and other information concerning a patient's condition that is kept by the individual provider or health care institution.[6] However, in order for that patient information to be privileged, it must satisfy certain criteria: (1) it must have been communicated in the context of the physician–patient relationship, (2) it must have been given with the expectation that it remain confidential, and (3) it must be necessary for the diagnosis and treatment of the patient. Those requirements mean that, in most jurisdictions, although the patient is legally entitled to confidentiality with respect to his or her medical records concerning diagnosis and treatment, other information, such as the patient's name and address and the fact that he or she is receiving medical treatment, is not privileged.[7]

Assertion of the Privilege

The privilege belongs to the patient because that is the person for whose benefit it exists. Frequently, however, the patient is not available and does not even have knowledge that records concerning his or her treatment have been requested. In such a case, the privilege must be asserted on the patient's behalf by the physician or the institution where the patient received treatment.[8] For instance, a plaintiff alleging negligence during delivery of a baby might seek discovery of the delivery room log or of the actual medical records of other patients who were in the labor and delivery suite on the same day. Similarly, a patient claiming negligence in the performance of a particular procedure might seek a judicial order allowing discovery of the records of other patients who underwent similar surgeries. In those situations, the hospital administrator should raise the issue of privilege for these patients' records. Frequently in such cases, the court will make an *in camera* (in the judge's chambers) inspection of the requested records to determine which materials might be relevant to the lawsuit and can be released without compromising the privilege of the nonparty patients. If records are released, the court may order names and any other identifying details to be removed from copies of the records.[9]

With respect to releasing records of deceased patients, opinion is divided. In some states a surviving beneficiary may assert the privilege for the patient, whereas in others the privilege terminates upon death.[10] Even in those states where a legal responsibility to maintain confidentiality ends with the death of the patient, it is still advisable to obtain authorization from the patient's legal representative to avoid compromising the interests of the family.

Waiver of the Privilege

Unlike assertion of the privilege, a waiver of the privilege may be made only by the patient or, in cases of incompetency, infancy, or death, by the patient's legal representative. Waiver may be either express or implicit. Obviously, a patient may expressly waive the privilege by authorizing the provider to release information to a third party. An example of express waiver occurs when a patient authorizes release of the medical record to an insurance carrier or to an attorney. When a hospital receives a letter from an attorney requesting copies of a patient's medical record, the risk manager should confirm that the letter is accompanied by an authorization from the patient allowing release of the records to the requesting attorney or that the request otherwise complies with state law on release of records.

Implicit waiver of the privilege occurs when a patient brings a personal injury action concerning a medical condition for which he or she was treated, or when the patient otherwise discloses or consents to disclosure of a significant part of the communications previously made to a treating physician. Here, because the patient has placed information about his or her medical condition in issue, he or she may no longer claim the privilege; as one court explained, "the patient–litigant exception precludes one who has placed in issue his physical condition from invoking the privilege on the ground that disclosure of his condition would cause him humiliation. He cannot have his cake and eat it too."[11]

In some instances, defense counsel may seek information on the litigant's medical condition that is not the subject of the suit. For example, to impeach the credibility of the plaintiff's claim about a lasting physical injury,[12] the defense may wish to show that the plaintiff has received psychiatric treatment. In birth injury cases, the defense frequently seeks discovery about the medical condition of the infant's siblings and about other prenatal and labor and delivery records of the mother in an effort to prove a genetic cause for the infant's condition.[13] Court decisions vary from jurisdiction to jurisdiction on whether waiver of the privilege extends to other conditions, and, if it does, how information about them can be obtained from treating physicians who are not parties in the suit.

Courts generally permit liberal discovery of records of subsequent treatment by physicians who have treated the plaintiff for the condition that is the subject of the litigation or is demonstrably related to it. However, even if the defendant is permitted to obtain access to information from the plaintiff's nonparty treating physicians, courts are divided about whether the defendant's risk manager or lawyer may informally discuss the plaintiff's condition with those physicians in the absence of plaintiff's attorney (*ex parte*), or whether they must go through formal discovery proceedings. Most courts have held that, even though there has been a waiver of the physician–patient privilege, the defendant must use formal discovery methods, such as depositions and subpoenas of witnesses or documents. In this way, the legal process retains control of the proceedings and ensures that only relevant, appropriate information is disclosed. Those courts view *ex parte* conferences as a violation of state discovery rules, an unwarranted intrusion upon the physician–patient relationship, and perhaps a breach of the duty of confidentiality.[14] In other jurisdictions, courts have concluded that *ex parte* interviews are not specifically prohibited by applicable discovery rules and are an efficient way of obtaining information that may promote candor and lead to early resolution of claims.[15]

Risk managers sometimes must decide whether a patient who has not yet commenced a lawsuit but has performed some affirmative act, such as sending an "attorney request letter," has waived the privilege, thereby entitling the physician or the hospital to turn over the patient's medical records to its liability insurance carrier. Courts have held that, where a physician has a reasonable basis to believe that a claim for malpractice will be made, the physician and his or her insurer are entitled to investigate and prepare for an anticipated lawsuit, justifying the doctor's disclosure of the medical records to the attorney and/or insurer.[16]

Release of Confidential Information without a Patient Authorization or Waiver

The right of confidentiality and the physician–patient privilege are never absolute. Certain interests of society outweigh the physician's duty to maintain confidentiality of patient records even where there has been no waiver or authorization. Most states have laws mandating physicians and/or hospitals to report communicable diseases, incidences of cancer, cases of suspected child abuse or neglect, gunshot or knife wounds, physician misconduct, and incidents of adverse patient care.[17] The statute or regulation mandating disclosure will usually contain a confidentiality provision restricting the ability of the public to gain access to that information.[18]

Patient authorization is also not a prerequisite to dissemination of information to either internal or external review organizations. This generally accepted rule is reflected in Joint Commission standards, which state that consent is not required for use of the medical record for automated data processing of designated information; use in activities concerned with the monitoring and evaluation of the quality and appropriateness of patient care; departmental review of work performance; official surveys of hospital compliance with accreditation, regulatory, and licensing standards; or educational purposes and research programs.[19]

Increasingly, official agencies such as state health departments and professional review organizations (PROs) are accessing patient records for purposes of quality-of-care reviews. Those agencies, themselves bound to maintain confidentiality of the information they review, must be permitted access to the patient's medical records although no privilege has been waived.

Release of Confidential Patient Care Information to PROs

Professional review organizations are independent organizations, established on a regional basis, that contract with the federal government to perform peer review for purposes of determining the medical necessity and quality of health care services rendered to Medicare beneficiaries. Hospitals are required, under the Peer Review Improvement Act, to enter into contracts with a PRO whereby the PRO reviews pertinent records to ascertain the quality and appropriateness of care provided.[20] Peer review organizations also are charged with reviewing the practice patterns of independent physician providers. The patient care information that the PROs collect cannot be disclosed except in accordance with confidentiality regulations specific to the PRO program.[21]

Essentially, those regulations make confidential all information reviewed by or generated by PROs, other than general summaries or aggregate statistical data, that explicitly or implicitly identifies an individual patient, practitioner, or reviewer. In addition, with respect to sanction reports or quality studies, the name of the institution is confidential. However, the regulations do contain numerous exceptions to the nondisclosure requirements, most of which relate to reporting to state and federal regulatory agencies. In addition, the nondisclosure requirements do not apply to most hearings conducted by the Department of Health and Human Services.

Because the federal regulations for PRO information disclosure are very detailed and specific, a risk manager should consult with counsel about how to proceed when dealing with a special situation.

Release of Information to the National Practitioner Data Bank

The Federal Health Care Quality Improvement Act (HCQIA), passed in 1986, calls for the establishment of a National Practitioner Data Bank (Data Bank), which will contain a centralized source of information on physicians, dentists, and other licensed health care professionals.[22] The act requires that each person or entity, including an insurance company, which makes a medical malpractice payment under an insurance policy, self-insurance, or otherwise, for the benefit of a physician, dentist, or other health practitioner in settlement of, or in satisfaction in whole or in part of, a written claim or judgment against such physician, dentist, or other health care practitioner, must report this information to the Data Bank and to their appropriate state licensing board(s). This act also requires (following due process procedures), (1) state medical and dental boards to report disciplinary actions taken against the license of a physician or dentist, (2) hospitals and other health care entities to report their professional review actions that adversely affect a physician's or dentist's appointment or clinical privileges, and (3) medical and dental societies to report adverse membership actions based on professional competence or conduct.

In addition to the requirement that hospitals must report to the Data Bank via the appropriate state licensing board(s), hospitals must request information directly from the Data Bank on each physician, dentist, or health care practitioner they are considering for appointment and at least every two years on those on their medical staff to whom they have previously granted clinical privileges.

In general, the information reported will be considered confidential and may not be disclosed. It will be disclosed to the physician or practitioner involved and to a hospital or health care entity that needs information concerning a physician, dentist, or other health care practitioner who is on their medical staff or has clinical privileges, or is entering an employment or affiliation relationship with them. With respect to malpractice cases, the plaintiff's attorney may obtain confidential information on a specific physician, dentist, or health care practitioner named in the action or claim upon a showing that the hospital did not, as part of its credentialing and appointment process, obtain information about the individual involved from the National Practitioner Data Bank. The plaintiff's attorney must also agree that the information will be used solely for that specific litigation. Failure to adhere to the confidentiality provisions and its use solely for the purpose requested could result in a $10,000 penalty.

In 1987, when the Medicare and Medicaid Patient and Program Protection Act was passed, certain permissive reporting requirements regarding nonphysician licensed health care professionals were changed to mandatory reporting.[23] These requirements will not be implemented until federal regulations are issued. It is expected that this act's confidentiality provisions, however, will be similar to those under HCQIA, but until federal regulations are promulgated regarding the confidentiality requirements under both the 1986 and 1987 laws, the actual confidentiality procedures to be implemented are not clear.

Physician's Duty to Third Persons in Psychiatric Cases

One of the most difficult areas concerning unauthorized disclosure of privileged patient information arises in psychiatric cases. The guarantee of confidentiality is especially important in the relationship between a patient and psychiatrist. Statutes in many states require institutions to implement special procedures to prevent any disclosure of mental health records.[24] At the same time, situations may arise in which psychiatrists and other mental health professionals treating a potentially violent patient may find a conflict between their fiduciary obligation to maintain confidentiality and their countervailing duty to disclose that a third party may be a potential victim of their patient's violent acts.

First set forth in the landmark case of *Tarasoff v. Regents of the University of California*,[25] a judicial doctrine has developed that has been codified in most states: When a patient is determined to be a danger to others, the treating psychiatrist or therapist has a responsibility to disclose the danger to the extent necessary to protect potential victims. Some state courts have held that the endangered third party must be specifically identified, whereas others have held that a general threat is a sufficient basis for breach of confidentiality.[26]

In most states, the statutes do not set forth an explicit duty to warn, but rather are permissive, allowing psychotherapists to warn and providing statutory immunity for a failure either to warn or not to warn.[27] Even in states where there is no statutory duty to warn, mental health professionals are aware that they may be sued for malpractice if injury is caused to a third person as a result of a health care provider's failure to warn of a risk of harm from a violent patient.[28] However, before developing a policy for the institution or advising affiliated mental health professionals about disclosure to endangered third parties, the risk manager should review any applicable state statutes and consult with counsel. Of course, health care professionals should always consider alternatives to disclosure, such as encouraging patients to disclose themselves or placing patients in preventive detention. *Tarasoff* principles also occasionally are applied in situations in which a physician has knowledge that a third person is in danger of contracting a contagious disease from a patient.[29]

Patient Access to Their Own Medical Records

Although the hospital generally is viewed as the owner of the medical record, the record is maintained for the benefit of the patient, and the patient generally is viewed as having some proprietary rights to the information contained in his or her records. Many states have adopted laws regarding patients' access to their own records. They set forth specific guidelines stating under what circumstances a patient has access to the record, whether access may ever be denied, and whether and how much a hospital may charge for copying records.[30] Even in states that do not have a specific statute, both from a patients' rights and public relations perspective it is advisable to develop a policy that allows patients reasonable access to their hospital records. Such a policy should be communicated to the medical staff.

Release of Patient Information in Civil Litigation

After a lawsuit is commenced, both sides then engage in "discovery," whereby they gain access to factual information about the dispute in the control of their adversary or of persons who are not parties to the suit. (Whether this information will later be "admissible" in a trial is a separate inquiry.) Discovery can take years and is often quite acrimonious.

The breadth of discovery varies from state to state and between federal and state courts. Even within a single jurisdiction, there may be special local rules regulating discovery. In general, federal courts are more liberal in allowing parties to make very general requests for documents, especially from other parties to a case. In contrast, many states require that document demands be very specific.

With respect to parties to the lawsuit, discovery of documents is initiated by serving a notice specifying, with reasonable particularity, the documents sought to be reviewed as well as the time, place, and manner of inspection. In almost all situations, a discovery request to a party must be served on the party's attorney (if the party is represented by an attorney), not on the party itself. It is then the attorney's responsibility to either arrange for production of the documents or go to court and move for a protective order challenging the form or scope of the discovery demand.

Document discovery from nonparties (for example, the hospital where a patient was treated when only the patient's private physician has been sued) is also authorized but is more cumbersome. Usually it involves a two-step process: serving a discovery notice on all other parties to the lawsuit and then serving a subpoena or court order on the nonparty in possession of the documents.

A subpoena is a method by which a witness is subjected to the jurisdiction of the court and required to give relevant information under penalty of contempt for disobedience. Basically, there are two kinds of subpoenas: a *subpoena ad testificandum*, which seeks testimony from the witness, and a *subpoena duces tecum*, which requires production of documents, books, papers, or other records.[31] When documents are sought from a nonparty, it is a common practice to require an individual officer or employee of the nonparty to appear personally at a deposition to verify the authenticity of the documents. That formality can be waived if all parties agree.[32]

It is important to understand that, despite its official-looking appearance, a subpoena is rarely issued by the court itself. A subpoena may be issued by a clerk, by a judge where there is no clerk, by most administrative agencies, by an arbitrator or referee, by any member of a board or commission and, in criminal cases, by a prosecutor. In civil litigation, subpoenas are issued most frequently by the attorney of record of any party to an action. Under the procedural law of most jurisdictions, an attorney, as an officer of the court, has the power to issue such a directive without the court's specific authorization. Therefore, risk managers should carefully scrutinize all subpoenas, including those signed by a judge, and challenge them in appropriate circumstances when the subpoenas request privileged material. In most jurisdictions, it is the hospital's responsibility to assert the physician–patient privilege on behalf of a patient who is not a party to the lawsuit. In addition, many other records maintained by the hospital may be privileged and not subject to discovery by way of a subpoena or otherwise.

Hospitals, as custodians of their patients' medical records, frequently receive subpoenas for records in the context of litigation not involving allegations of medical malpractice. For example, when an acute accident victim sues the other party to the accident, hospital medical records contain information necessary to prosecute the suit. Those records may be subpoenaed by one or both of the parties to the lawsuit.

As a practical matter, a risk manager who believes that a subpoena is requesting privileged materials should contact the attorney issuing the subpoena and request that it be modified or withdrawn. If that is not successful, an application to the court called a "motion to quash" or a "motion for a protective order" is the appropriate and proper method to test the subpoena. In those instances a court may review the dispute *in camera*, after which it will issue an order granting the motion to quash in full or it may order that information that is privileged be removed before the records are produced.[33]

Release of Patient Information to Law Enforcement Agencies

Risk managers frequently ask how they should respond to subpoenas and other less formal requests for patient information received from law enforcement officers, including police officers, district attorneys, and grand juries. In general, without a specific statute compelling disclosure, law enforcement officers have no authority to examine a patient's medical records. This means that test results (for example, blood alcohol levels on a patient brought into the emergency department) should not be disclosed to the police unless required by a statute.[34] Subpoenas and other legal processes issued by law enforcement agencies also should be carefully scrutinized, in consultation with the health care facility's attorney, prior to releasing privileged information.

Special Confidentiality Issues Involving Patient Medical Records

Certain types of medical records contain information perceived as being so sensitive that they are afforded a type of superconfidentiality. Examples are records of patients being treated for alcoholism or drug abuse, records containing AIDS-related information, records containing information concerning abortion and sexually transmitted diseases, and, sometimes, psychiatric records. The following sections discuss the issues surrounding medical records containing information related to alcohol, drug abuse, and AIDS.

Records of Alcohol and Drug Abuse Patients

Special federal rules exist regarding confidentiality of information concerning patients treated or referred for treatment for alcohol and drug abuse.[35] In general, the regulations prohibit any disclosure or release of patient information, whether recorded or not, that would identify the patient as a substance abuser. The regulations were amended in 1987, however, in an attempt to make them clearer and narrow their application with respect to general care hospitals. Under the amendments, a general medical facility is not subject to the regulations unless it has either a distinct substance abuse program or specialized personnel whose primary function is treatment, diagnosis, or referral for treatment of substance abuse patients. Even then, the rules apply only to that special program or unit unless the hospital elects to place the entire facility under the regulations. Therefore, in a situation where a patient who is a substance abuser is being treated for a medical problem other than substance abuse in the general part of the hospital, information concerning that patient will not be covered by the regulations. On the other hand, the records of a patient who is in a substance abuse program are protected, and that patient's records may not be released or transferred, even to another department of the hospital, without a special consent. The regulations require that patients be given a written summary of the confidentiality regulations.

Under the regulations, information may be released *with* the patient's consent if the consent is in writing and contains all of the following elements: the name of the program; the name of the proposed recipient of the information; the name of the patient; the purpose or need for the disclosure; the extent and nature of the information to be disclosed; the signature of the patient or of the person authorized to give consent if the patient is a minor, incompetent, or deceased; the date on which the consent is signed; a statement that the consent is subject to revocation at any time; and the date, event, or condition upon which the consent will expire if not revoked before that time. The regulations contain a sample consent form. Each disclosure made with the patient's written consent must be accompanied by a specific written statement, set forth in the regulations, prohibiting redisclosure.

The regulations permit disclosure without patient consent if the disclosure is to medical personnel to meet any individual's bona fide medical emergency, or to qualified personnel for research, audit, or program evaluation. They also permit disclosure for certain specified purposes, pursuant to a court order, after the court has made a finding that "good cause" exists, that the information is not otherwise available to the requesting party, and that the public interest in disclosure outweighs the potential harm to the patient. The person requesting court-ordered disclosure has the burden of demonstrating its necessity. A subpoena or similar legal document must then be issued in order to compel disclosure.

If a hospital receives a request for disclosure of patient information that does not comply with the regulations, it must respond with a noncommittal answer that will not reveal that a specific patient has been diagnosed or is being treated for substance abuse.

If the request is for treatment information about a patient known to be a substance abuser, the hospital should respond either with the noncommittal answer or by sending a copy of the regulations and an attached statement that the regulations restrict the disclosure of substance abuse records. It is permissible, however, for a hospital to state that a specific person is not and has never been a patient of the program, if such is the case.[36]

Medical Records Containing HIV-Positive or AIDS-Related Information

Because of discrimination against an individual that may result from dissemination of information about that person's positive HIV status, information concerning the HIV antibody status of any individual is highly confidential. States have enacted a variety of laws addressing the confidentiality of HIV test results and of diagnostic and treatment records. Most states make available anonymous HIV testing, but also establish nonanonymous but confidential testing programs under which public health officials have access, under specific conditions, to the names of those testing positive.[37]

Risk managers must review the law in their state and develop written policies that conform their hospital procedures regarding disclosure to the applicable statute. In the absence of such a statute, it may be advisable to model the hospital's policy after the federal drug and alcohol rules so that no HIV or AIDS information is released without a special patient authorization or a special court order.

Recently, there have been a number of legal opinions concerning whether the recipient of a blood transfusion who contracts the AIDS virus may obtain the names of blood donors in order to ascertain the blood bank's compliance with screening protocols. Factors that have influenced the decisions are whether the transfusion took place before effective screening methods were known, whether there is a state AIDS confidentiality law, and whether there is a state law regarding the right to privacy.[38]

☐ Confidentiality of Other Records Maintained by Hospitals

Most states have adopted legislation protecting information generated as part of a hospital's quality assurance activities from discovery or admission into evidence.[39]

Peer Review Privilege

In some states, the so-called peer review privilege is quite narrow, protecting only those proceedings in which physicians review the quality of medical care delivered. More recently, as part of comprehensive tort reform legislation in a large number of states, the privilege has been extended to include all of the hospital's professional committees, such as credentials, utilization review, and quality assurance, as well as to cover other documents that a hospital maintains in connection with programs to monitor and improve the quality of care, regardless of whether they are related to a specific committee performing a medical review function.[40]

Courts have generally recognized, even in the absence of statute, that a guarantee of confidentiality and protection from discovery is necessary to promote an important state interest in effective peer review proceedings. Only a few courts have given greater deference to a plaintiff's need for all relevant information to prove a case.[41]

Some malpractice plaintiff's attorneys have argued that the proceedings and records of peer review committees, physician credentials files, and other quality assurance documents contain relevant evidence about a physician's general qualifications as well as information about the particular case in suit. Sometimes attorneys try to circumvent the privilege relating to those documents by arguing that the applicable statute should be construed to cover only a very narrow category of documents and information. The issue most often arises in lawsuits alleging malpractice by physicians for whom the hospital may have vicarious liability, such as emergency department physicians. With greater frequency, however, it is being raised as part of a claim of corporate negligence on the part of the hospital for negligently credentialing the treating physician.[42]

It is important to emphasize that, even in states with a relatively broad privilege, the applicable statute frequently protects only the review process itself. The statute may cover discussions at committee meetings, as well as records and documents specifically created for a committee, but may not protect documents otherwise available from non-protected sources, such as accident reports made in the ordinary course of business, some patient record information, personnel records, and other administrative records of the hospital, even if they are necessary to the committee's deliberations. In addition, actions taken as a result of the committee's deliberations, such as curtailment of a physician's privileges or other disciplinary action, may not be privileged.[43]

A very significant exception, incorporated into almost every statute, is that the prohibition against discovery does not apply to any statements made by a person at the meeting who subsequently is a party to an action concerning the subject matter reviewed at that meeting.[44] Therefore, if a physician whose practice is being reviewed participates in the meeting, any statements he or she makes may be discoverable in a subsequent malpractice action against the physician and the hospital.

Because of the questionable protection for certain types of information and documents, the hospital's policy concerning peer review materials prepared outside a committee must indicate that they were created to further the work of a committee whose records are privileged under the statute.[45] Some risk managers stamp each such document with a statement that the document has been prepared at the request of a peer review or quality assurance committee and is confidential under the relevant statute.

Other practical suggestions to maximize protection include controlling distribution of and access to peer review committee records; distributing and collecting minutes at meetings rather than mailing them; destroying all copies except the original; prohibiting names of patients and physicians from being recorded in minutes; and inserting provisions in medical staff bylaws that recognize the confidentiality of peer review activities and prohibit unauthorized or voluntary disclosure of peer review information.[46]

How committee minutes are written should also be carefully considered. In order to be privileged under the protective statute (as well as to satisfy outside review organizations), the minutes must show the operation of a legitimate peer review or other quality assurance process that identifies problems and recommends specific corrective action. At the same time, they should be written in such a way that if the minutes do get into the "wrong hands," they will not compromise the hospital's interests. Also to be remembered is that state regulators and accreditation bodies will always have access to those documents, regardless of the discovery statute.

Of course, the summary of discussions at the meeting also must be scrupulously fair, because it may become the basis for discipline against a physician. In the event of litigation against the hospital by a physician whose privileges have been curtailed, the court in all likelihood will permit the physician to review relevant documents, including committee minutes, even if there is a protective statute. In fact, to safeguard the physician's right to due process, most statutes contain an exception that allows a physician access to peer review records when seeking judicial review of an action affecting his or her staff privileges.[47]

The scope of activities, the types of committees, and the specific information and documents that are protected vary widely from state to state. Prior to establishing the hospital's procedures for generating and maintaining records in this area, it is important to become familiar with case law and statutes and regulations of the state. The hospital's bylaws and its quality assurance and risk management plans and practices should be developed to maximize the protection from discovery available in the jurisdiction. In addition, the risk manager, in coordination with legal counsel, should develop systems for reviewing all discovery requests for each type of information to avoid inadvertently releasing a document that may be privileged.

Attorney–Client Privilege

If the state has a very narrow peer review privilege, another privilege that may be available to protect committee minutes and other sensitive documents is the attorney–client privilege. The precise limits of the attorney–client privilege and the extent of protection from discovery afforded to an attorney's work product vary by jurisdiction. In general, where legal advice is sought from a lawyer, the confidential communications between the client and the attorney relating to that advice are protected from disclosure, unless the client waives the privilege.[48] Therefore, when a committee at the hospital discusses a patient care incident and a strong possibility exists that the hospital will be sued, it may be advisable to have outside legal counsel in attendance. The drawback in relying solely on in-house counsel in those circumstances is that some courts have found that in-house counsel function in a dual capacity as administrator/attorney, rendering communications with them not privileged. With outside counsel present, it may be possible to argue that the issues were discussed in anticipation of litigation and are protected from discovery under the attorney–client privilege. If the lawyer keeps the minutes of the meeting and also writes an advisory memo about the committee's deliberations to hospital administration that contains the lawyer's advice and opinions on the matter, those records will probably be protected by the privilege.

Incident/Occurrence Reports

Incident reports can be a source of incriminating evidence if they are made available to persons suing the hospital. Consequently, the discoverability of incident reports has been litigated in many states. If they are protected, protection usually depends on state peer review statutes or statutes creating an attorney–client privilege or insurer–insured privilege.

In many states, incident reports describing occurrences where the hospital has an expectation that it will be sued may be protected under the attorney–client privilege, the attorney work product doctrine, or a similar qualified immunity accorded to reports made to an insurer by an insured in anticipation of or preparation for litigation.[49] However, with respect to minor occurrences that happen very frequently in the hospital, such as patient falls or medication errors, routinely prepared incident reports are more in the nature of accident reports maintained in the ordinary course of business. In most states, such reports are discoverable even if they ultimately are used in connection with litigation of a claim. Discoverability generally will turn on whether the accident report has a "mixed purpose"; it will be protected only if it was prepared exclusively in anticipation of litigation, not if it was prepared also for hospital administrative purposes.[50] In a state with a more comprehensive quality assurance statute, incident reports involving serious occurrences that were prepared both in anticipation of litigation and as part of the hospital's effort to evaluate and improve the quality of health care should be protected.[51]

Unless the risk manager is sure that incident reports are protected by statute or case law, hospital personnel should exercise caution when documenting serious events that may lead to liability. The following guidelines may enhance confidentiality. The event should be reported verbally to the risk manager, who will open a litigation file. That file should contain the risk manager's notes, communications with legal counsel, expert reviews, and other information germane to the case. It can then be argued that those segregated documents are exclusively for purposes of litigation, and so are confidential and protected, rather than for general quality assurance purposes, which may not be protected. If the hospital maintains computerized risk management information systems, those same rules should apply and access should be restricted solely to those with a need to know.

Any incident report should be labeled and treated as confidential, and its distribution should be limited. The risk manager should conduct inservice programs about how to write such a report. Incident reports should contain only a summary of objective facts and should avoid subjective analysis, conclusions, "mea culpas," or finger pointing. They should be addressed to the hospital's lawyer or insurance carrier. Depending on the breadth of state law, the risk manager may consider forwarding a copy of the report to the quality assurance committee.[52]

Even in a state with broad protection, a court may find that the privilege is not absolute and, upon a showing of "exceptional necessity" or "extraordinary circumstances," a plaintiff will be permitted to obtain incident reports generated by the hospital's internal risk management program, as well as related peer review committee documents.[53]

Over the past several years, many hospitals, dissatisfied with the ability of traditional narrative incident reports either to identify many adverse patient occurrences or to serve as a tool for evaluating such occurrences, have developed a variety of more objective reporting forms that can be input for analysis into sophisticated computerized data-collection systems. The risk manager needs to ascertain whether state law shields the documents generated by a hospital's generic reporting or screening program from discovery. In states with some form of quality assurance/risk management privilege, protecting those documents should not be a problem, but in some states with a narrow privilege, generic reporting documents are unlikely to fall either under a peer review privilege or an attorney–client privilege. Therefore, before developing a generic reporting system, a risk manager should review with the hospital's attorney how to maximize available legal protections.[54]

Credentials Files

The Joint Commission requires every hospital to have a process for delineating clinical privileges, as well as for reappointment to the medical staff and reappraising of such clinical privileges. Collection and review of information regarding credentials are also required by most state statutes and are required by the federal Health Care Quality Improvement Act.

Regardless of the extent of protection from discovery accorded to credentials files, they should be maintained with an awareness that, in the future, they might be accessed by a wide variety of third parties, including physicians who have been denied privileges, the Joint Commission, and state and federal regulatory organizations. In addition, there are cases in which malpractice plaintiffs who were treated by private attending physicians have asserted a separate cause of action for negligent credentialing against the hospital. As part of the claim of corporate liability, they have sought discovery of credentialing files. It is unclear at this time how many states will recognize that cause of action, but even in those states that currently grant protection from discovery to credentials files, it cannot be guaranteed that such existing qualified protections will be maintained.[55]

Ironically, regardless of any statutory protection that might exist, if a hospital is sued for negligent credentialing, it may find itself in a Catch-22 situation in which the only way it can defend itself is with the very documents it is seeking to protect. In those states where the statute granting protection does not specifically allow the hospital to use those documents in its defense, some lawyers advise the hospital never to voluntarily disclose peer review or credentialing documents even if, in a particular case where the process was carried out well, they may be helpful to the hospital's defense. Selective disclosure may end up being detrimental in a subsequent case because of the legal precedent that is set.

Some hospitals choose to place only relatively mundane information in individual credential files and "reference" by code the more sensitive information, which is located elsewhere in the hospital, such as the risk management case files, the quality assurance files, or the offices of individual department chairmen. Only at the time of credentials review is all the information brought together for the credentials committee's consideration.

Other hospitals maintain a bifurcated system in which sensitive qualitative information is kept in the credentials files, including information obtained from other institutions, information regarding the physician's history of medical malpractice and professional misconduct, and information about the physician's delivery of medical care obtained through the hospital's quality assurance process. In contrast, the physician's separately maintained personnel file contains objective factual information, such as educational qualifications, date of licensure, salary, and title, but does not include any evaluative comments. The majority of discovery requests can then be satisfied by producing only the personnel file, and the hospital can reserve its confidentiality arguments for the more sensitive credentials files. Whatever system the hospital puts in place for physicians' credentials files should apply to the files of other health care professionals as well.

☐ Conclusion

Each year health care institutions generate increasing numbers and types of records that document the medical care provided to patients as well as a wide variety of ancillary activities that take place in the institution. Most hospital personnel do not understand that every document they create is potentially discoverable in a legal proceeding. Risk managers, therefore, need to inform themselves about the law in their state concerning confidentiality of records maintained by hospitals so that they may educate hospital staff about those issues. As an educator, the risk manager has the dual task of encouraging proper documentation and communication by physicians, nurses, and other personnel while, at the same time, discouraging the practice of some staff to write with excessive detail and to distribute documents beyond those who have a need to know.

It is important, therefore, for the risk manager to be involved in assisting hospital departments to establish policies and procedures concerning the flow of paper and the safeguarding of sensitive information. The risk manager can also promote awareness of confidentiality and discoverability issues among hospital staff by incorporating those issues into inservice programs on medical record documentation, writing of incident reports, and preparation and distribution of materials concerning privileges and credentials. In addition, the risk manager can participate in preparing and making known throughout the institution rules about how to respond to requests for information so that confidential and privileged materials are not inadvertently released. Making hospital personnel knowledgeable about the confidentiality and discoverability of documents is an essential part of every loss-prevention program.

References

1. Joint Commission on Accreditation of Healthcare Organizations. *1990 Accreditation Manual for Hospitals*. Chicago: JCAHO, 1989.

2. *See, e.g.*, The Oath of Hippocrates: "Whatever in connection with my professional practice or not in connection with it I see or hear in the life of men which ought not to be spoken abroad I will not divulge as recommending that all such should be kept secret"; American Medical Association, *Principles of Medical Ethics*, Section 9, adopted by AMA House of Delegates, June 1980: "A physician may not reveal the confidences entrusted to him in the course of medical attendance, or the deficiencies he may observe in the character of patients, unless it becomes necessary in order to protect the welfare of the individual or community"; American Nurses' Association, *Code for Nurses*, No. 2: "The nurse safeguards the client's right to privacy by judiciously protecting information of a confidential nature."

3. States differ about whether there is a legal, as opposed to a moral/ethical, "right to privacy." Under a variety of legal theories, most states protect some type of privacy interest. Some state courts have held that breach of the duty of confidentiality is a tort, and that a cause of action for breach of confidentiality may exist in circumstances where there has been extrajudicial disclosure of confidential information, or in cases, such as custody disputes, where the plaintiff's physical condition is not in issue. *See generally* Annot: Physician's Tort Liability for Unauthorized Disclosure of Confidential Information About Patient, 48 A.L.R.4th 558 (1985); Horne v. Patton, 291 Ala. 701, 287 So.2d 824 (1973) (physician disclosed confidential information to plaintiff's

employer); MacDonald v. Clinger, 84 A.D.2d 482, 446 N.Y.S.2d 801 (1982) (psychiatrist revealed confidential information to patient's wife). Probably a more logical basis for finding liability is that, as part of an implied contract between physician and patient, the physician agrees not to release information about the patient without his or her consent, Hammonds v. Aetna Casualty and Surety Co., 243 F.Supp. 793 (N.D. Ohio 1965). Suits against practitioners for "invasion of privacy" typically allege an unwarranted exploitation of the patient's personality or a publication about his or her private affairs that would cause outrage, mental suffering, shame, or humiliation. *See, e.g.*, Barber v. Time, Inc., 348 Mo. 1199, 159 S.W.2d 291. That type of action might be brought when a photograph or description of the patient is published without the patient's permission. As to whether there is a constitutional right of privacy, although not explicitly stated anywhere in the Constitution, the Supreme Court has held that there is a fundamental right of privacy emanating from various provisions in the Constitution that limit the extent to which the government may interfere with an individual's privacy. Although that principle would not ordinarily result in liability to nongovernmental institutions, it might serve as a limitation on a government-mandated disclosure of individual medical records. *See, e.g.*, Griswold v. Connecticut, 381 U.S. 479 (1965); In re *Search Warrant*, 810 F.2d 57 (3rd Cir.) *cert. denied*, 107 S.Ct. 3233 (1987) (patients have a privacy interest under the Constitution in their medical records in the possession of their physicians; however, the protection afforded by the right to privacy is not absolute and must be balanced against the legitimate interests of the state in securing the information contained therein).

4. The four traditional criteria for a privileged communication are: (1) it originates in confidence that it will not be disclosed, (2) the element of confidentiality is essential to the full maintenance of relationship between the parties, (3) the relationship is one that the community thinks ought to be fostered, and (4) the injury to the relationship that would occur from the disclosing would be greater than the benefit gained by the aid given to the litigation. 8 Wigmore, *Evidence* §2285 at 527 (McNaughton rev. 1961).

5. 8 Wigmore, *Evidence* §2380.

6. Annot.: Physician–Patient Privilege as Extending to Patients' Medical or Hospital Records, 10 A.L.R. 4th 552 (1981).

7. *See, e.g.*, Payne v. Howard, 75 F.R.D. 465 (D.D.C. 1977) (court permitted plaintiff to discover the names and addresses of patients of plaintiff's physician who had received similar treatment so that plaintiff could contact them and determine whether they would be willing to waive the statutory privilege attaching to their records); Hirsh v. Catholic Medical Center, 91 A.D.2d 1033, 458 N.Y.S.2d 625 (2nd Dept. 1983) (disclosure of the name of a nonparty patient who may have witnessed an occurrence would not violate the privilege). *Contra*, Schecket v. Kesten, 126 N.W.2d 718 (Mich. 1964) (names of nonparty patients are protected by physician–patient privilege and are not subject to discovery); N.O. v. Callahan, 110 F.R.D. 637 (D. Mass. 1986) (plaintiffs complaining of inadequate state psychiatric facilities could tour facilities but could not videotape other patients without their consent).

8. *See, e.g.*, Tucson Medical Center, Inc., v. Rowles, 21 Ariz. App. 424, 520 P.2d 518, 523 (1974). ("Our decision . . . that hospital records are covered by the physician–patient privilege mandates that the hospital assert this privilege when neither the patient nor his physician are parties to the proceedings. To hold otherwise would deprive a patient of the confidentiality granted him by [the statute] simply because neither the patient nor his physician are parties to the proceeding." The court then reviewed the record *in camera* to ascertain if there was any relevant nonprivileged information and denied access.)

9. *See, e.g.*, Ziegler v. Superior Court of the County of Pima, 134 Ariz. 390, 656 P.2d 1251 (Ariz. Ct. App. 1982). Other courts have rejected this approach because of the perceived danger that the nonlitigant patient's identity would not remain confidential. Parkson v. Central Du Page Hospital, 105 Ill. App.3d 850, 435 N.E.2d 140 (1982).

10. If there is an executor of the deceased patient's estate, the authorization of the executor usually should be sought before releasing information. If there is no executor, authorization should be obtained from the next of kin. Claim of Gurkin, 434 N.Y.S.2d 607 (N.Y. Sup. Ct. 1980) (wife authorized release); Emmentt v. Eastern Dispensary and Casualty Hospital, 396 F.2d 931, 935 (D.C. App. 1967) (son authorized release; the court stated, "In our view, a son and only child has so vital an identification with any cause of action potentially arising upon his father's

negligently caused demise as would enable him to waive the privilege . . . when there is no personal representative to act in his behalf.") If there is known conflict among next of kin, the authorization of all the nearest kin available should be obtained.

11. In re Lifschutz, 85 Cal. Rptr. 829, 467 P.2d 557 (1970), quoting San Francisco v. Superior Court, 37 Cal.2d 227, 232, 231 P.2d 26 (1951); Hoenig v. Wesphal, 52 N.Y.2d 605, 439 N.Y.S.2d 831 (1981) (by commencing personal injury action, plaintiff waived any privilege he previously had and was required to produce reports of treating physicians).

12. *See, e.g.,* Friedlander v. Morales, 70 A.D.2d 501, 415 N.Y.S.2d 831 (1st Dept. 1979) (court permitted defendant to discover records of plaintiff's treating psychiatrist in case where plaintiff alleged defendant's malpractice caused serious physical injury and emotional sequelae). However, courts will not allow so-called blunderbuss notices for discovery. Although waiver of the physician–patient privilege has occurred, its scope is limited and does not permit discovery information involving unrelated illnesses and treatments.

13. *See, e.g.,* Williams v. Roosevelt Hospital, 66 N.Y.2d 391, 497 N.Y.S.2d 348 (1985). (Infant plaintiff alleged Erb's palsy and brain damage caused by cephalopelvic disproportion and defendant's failure to perform cesarean. Court ruled mother could not refuse to answer questions during her deposition concerning condition of plaintiff's siblings and mother's obstetrical history, although court did not decide, in this case, whether defendant could also gain access to actual medical records of plaintiff's siblings and mother.)

14. Most jurisdictions disapprove of *ex parte* interviews. *See generally* Annot. Discovery: Right to Ex Parte Interview With Injured Party's Treating Physician, 50 A.L.R.4th 714 (1986); *See also* Jordan v. Sinai Hospital of Detroit, Inc., 429 N.W.2d 891 (Mich. App. 1988) (court refused to authorize *ex parte* meetings by hospital's attorneys with nonparty neurologists who treated the patient after she lapsed into a coma because of the defendant's alleged failure to treat her preeclampsia); Petrillo v. Syntex Laboratories, Inc., 148 Ill. App.3d 581, 102 Ill. Dec. 172, 499 N.E.2d 952 (1986) (court held patient's implied consent, in filing suit, was only to release of medical information relevant to suit and must be obtained pursuant to formal rules of discovery); Anker v. Brodnitz, 98 Misc.2d 148, 413 N.Y.S.2d 582 (1979), *aff'd* 73 A.D.2d 589, 422 N.Y.S.2d 887 (2nd Dept. 1979) (court prohibited private interviews with treating physicians during the pretrial discovery phase absent patient's express consent or a court order). *But see* Nielson v. John G. Appison, M.D., P.C., 138 Misc.2d 74, 524 N.Y.S.2d 161 (trial term 1988) (limiting this prohibition to the pretrial discovery stage of litigation and permitting defendants to privately interview plaintiff's treating physicians in anticipation of presenting them for testimony at trial). No court, however, has permitted recovery against a physician for breach of confidentiality under facts such as these.

15. Cases permitting *ex parte* interviews include Doe v. Eli Lilly & Co., 99 F.R.D. 126 (D.D.C. 1983); Langdon v. Champion, 745 P.2d 1371 (Alaska 1987); Cogdell v. Brown, 531 A.2d 1379 (N.J. Super. L. 1987); Moses v. McWilliams, 549 A.2d 950 (Pa. Super. 1988) (interpreted a statutory exception to the privilege for "civil matters brought by the patient" to apply to *ex parte* disclosures by physicians, court noted *"ex parte* interviews are less costly and easier to schedule than depositions, are conducive to candor and spontaneity, are a cost efficient method of eliminating non-essential witnesses . . . and allow both parties to confer with the treating physicians.") (549 A.2d 950, 959).

16. Hammonds v. Aetna Casualty and Surety Co., *supra* note 3; Rea v. Pardo, 132 A.D.2d 442, 552 N.Y.S.2d 393 (4th Dept. 1987).

17. For examples of mandatory reporting statutes, *see, e.g.,* California Penal Code §11160 (injury caused by deadly weapon); Ill Ann. Stat. Ch. 23 §2054 (child abuse); Conn. Gen. Stat. §19a-215 (communicable diseases); Minn. Stat. Ann. 144.34 (abortion).

18. The federal Freedom of Information Act (FOIA), 5 U.S.C. §552-a, sets forth a general rule of disclosure for records in the possession of the executive branch. The statute contains an exception for "personnel and medical files and similar files the disclosure of which would constitute a clearly unwarranted invasion of personal privacy," 5 U.S.C. §552(b) (6). State freedom of information laws contain similar exclusions.

19. Joint Commission on Accreditation of Healthcare Organizations, Standard MR.3.3.1.

20. Title I, Subtitle C, Tax Equity and Fiscal Responsibility Act of 1982, Public L. 97-248.

21. 42 C.F.R. §§476.101–476.143.

22. 42 U.S.C.A. §1111.

23. 42 U.S.C.A. §1320(a) note 7 (West Supp. 1989).

24. Joint Commission on Accreditation of Healthcare Organizations, Standard MR.3.4, recognizes that "When certain portions of the medical record are so confidential that extraordinary means are necessary to preserve their privacy, such as in the treatment of some psychiatric disorders, these portions may be stored separately, provided the complete record is readily available when required for current medical care or follow-up, review functions, or use in quality assurance activities."

25. 131 Cal. Rptr. 14, 551 P.2d 334 (1976).

26. In Tarasoff the victim of the therapist's patient was clearly identified. Subsequently in Thompson v. County of Alameda, 167 Cal. Rptr. 70, 27 Cal.3d 741, 614 P.2d 728 (1980), the California Supreme Court held that the duty to warn depends upon and arises from the existence of a prior threat to a specific identifiable victim. A few courts have gone beyond Tarasoff to hold that psychotherapists will also be liable for their patients' violent acts against persons who are not identifiable in advance but are "foreseeable victims." In those cases, liability arises where the therapist or psychiatric facility negligently releases a potentially dangerous patient who subsequently harms a third party. See, e.g., Leverett v. State of Ohio, 61 Ohio App.2d 35, 399 N.E.2d 106 (1978). ("A hospital may be held liable for the negligent release of a mental patient only when the hospital, in exercising medical judgment, knew or should have known that the patient, upon his release, would be very likely to cause harm to himself or others.")

27. See, e.g., Ill. Stat. Ann. Ch. 91-1/2 §§801 et seq., which provides that confidential records and communications be disclosed "when, and to the extent, a therapist, in his sole discretion, determines that such disclosure is necessary to initiate or continue civil commitment proceedings or to otherwise protect against a clear imminent risk of serious physical or mental injury or death" to the patient or another. Like most statutes, this one allows, but does not require, a psychiatrist to warn.

28. Appelbaum, P. S. Tarasoff and the Clinician: Problems in Fulfilling the Duty to Protect. Am. J. Psychiatry 1985, 142: 425–29.

29. See, e.g., Hoffman v. Blackmon, 241 So.2d 752 (Fla. App. 1970), cert. denied, 245 So.2d 257 (Fla. 1971) (tuberculosis); Skillings v. Allen, 173 N.W. 663 (Minn. 1921). The Tarasoff principle is particularly relevant to the AIDS epidemic, where it is reasonably foreseeable that a patient may spread the virus to a needle sharer or sexual partner.

30. The Uniform Health Care Information Act (1985) has been adopted only in Montana, but many states have passed legislation that accomplishes the same objective. See, e.g., Colo Rev. Stat. tit. 25-1-801; Ill. Ann. Stat. Ch. 110, §8-2001. In states without a statute, courts will sometimes find a common-law right of access.

31. For a discussion of subpoenas in general, see 2A Weinstein, Korn & Miller, New York Civil Practice, ¶¶ 2301.01–2308.11.

32. If the case goes to trial, it is possible that one of the parties may subpoena a hospital employee to testify as a witness. Here, too, the subpoena may require the witness to bring along documents for examination at the trial.

33. Interestingly, a physician–patient privilege may not be asserted to quash a subpoena ad testificandum, on the theory that a witness cannot assert the privilege in advance of the questions being asked. However, the witness can refuse to answer a question seeking privileged material, in which case the questioner could ask a court to determine if the privilege has been raised appropriately and, if not, to order an answer.

34. State v. Copeland, 680 S.W.2d 327 (Mo. App. 1984). A few medical record confidentiality statutes do authorize disclosure of medical records information without patient authorization or a subpoena when necessary to cooperate with law enforcement agencies. See, e.g., S.C. Code §44-23-1090.

35. 42 C.F.R. Part 2.

36. An excellent article explaining the amendments to the alcohol and drug abuse regulations is Kramer, D. V., Confidentiality of Patient Alcohol and Drug Abuse Information, *Kentucky Hospitals* (Spring 1988).

37. George Washington University, Intergovernmental Health Policy Project, State AIDS Policy Center, State AIDS Reports #7, February–March 1989, p. 1.

38. Discovery was allowed in Belle Bonfils Memorial Blood Center v. Denver District Court, 763 P.2d 1003 (Colo. 1988); Tarrant County Hospital District v. Hughes, 734 S.W.2d 675 (Tex. App. 1987) *cert. denied*, 484 U.S. 1065, 108 S. Ct. 1027 (1988); Discovery was denied in Rasmussen v. South Florida Blood Service, Inc., 500 So.2d 533 (Fla. 1987); Krygier v. Airweld, 137 Misc.2d 306, 520 N.Y.S.2d 475 (1987). *See also* Mason v. Regional Medical Center of Hopkins County, 121 F.R.D. 300 (W.D. Ky. 1988) (allowing deposition of blood donor, but entering protective order to limit disclosure of identity).

39. For examples of peer review statutes, *see* Arizona Rev. Stat. Ann. §36.445.01A (West 1989); Cal. Code §1157 (West 1989); Fla. Stat. Ann. §766.101 (West 1989); Ill. Ann. Stat. Ch. 110 §8-2101 (West 1989); N.Y. Public Health §2805-m (McKinneys 1989). Without a statute, courts have refused to create a privilege. Davison v. St. Paul Fire and Marine Ins. Co., 75 Wis.2d 190, 248 N.W.2d 433 (1977) (declining to apply retroactively a subsequently enacted statute granting protection from discovery in malpractice cases and rejecting argument in favor of a common-law peer review privilege).

40. For example, in 1986 the New York law was amended to provide confidentiality protection for all information required to be collected and maintained as part of a hospital's coordinated program of quality assurance and risk management, including records, documentation, committee actions, and incident reports required to be made to the state health department, New York Public Health Law §2805-m (McKinneys 1989). The former peer review statute (which remains in effect) protected a more narrow category of records and proceedings relating to performance of a medical review function, New York Education Law §6527 (McKinneys 1989). The Massachusetts law was similarly amended in 1987 to provide protection for records necessary to comply with risk management and quality assurance programs, Mass. Gen. Laws Ann. Ch. 111, §205(b), *as amended* by H.B. No. 5930 (New Laws 1987).

41. *See, e.g.*, Humana Hospital Desert Valley v. Superior Court County of Maricopa, 154 Ariz. 396, 742 P.2d 1382, 1386 (Ariz. App. 1987) ("If this court were to eliminate the peer review privilege, it would negate an important state interest . . . The confidentiality of peer review committee proceedings is essential to achieve complete investigation and review of medical care. These deliberations would terminate if they were subject to the discovery process."). *See also* Bredice v. Doctors Hospital, 50 F.R.D. 249 (D.D.C. 1970), *aff'd. on reconsid.* 51 F.R.D. 187, *aff'd.* 479 F.2d 920 (D.C. Ct. App. 1973); Willing v. St. Joseph Hospital, 176 Ill. App.3d 737, 531 N.E.2d 824 (Ill. App. 1st Dist. 1988); Caroll v. Nunez, 137 A.D.2d 911, 524 N.Y.S.2d 578 (N.Y. A.D. 3rd Dept 1988). There are far fewer cases holding that peer review information is discoverable. Two such cases, Nazareth Literary & Benevolent Institution v. Stephenson, 503 S.W.2d 177 (Ky. Ct. App. 1973) and Kenny v. Superior Ct., 55 Cal. App.2d 106, 63 Cal. Rptr. 84 (Ct. App. 1967), were subsequently superseded by passage of peer review statutes in those states. *See generally* Annot. Discovery of Hospitals Internal Records or Communications as to Qualifications or Evaluations of Physicians, 81 A.L.R.3rd 944 (1977); Cuneo, M. K., Disclosure v. Confidentiality of Hospital Peer Review Records, *Medical Trial Technique Quarterly* (Wilmette, IL: Callaghan & Co.) pp. 172–83, Fall 1984; Goldberg, B. A., The Peer Review Privilege: A Law in Search of a Valid Policy, 10 Am. J. L. & Med. 151 (1984).

42. In cases alleging corporate negligence of hospitals, most decisions appear to protect against disclosure of peer review records. *See, e.g.*, Terre Haute Regional Hospital, Inc., v. Basden, 524 N.E.2d 1306 (Ind. App. 1988); Humana Hospital Desert Valley v. Superior Court, *supra*; Shelton v. Morehead Memorial Hospital, 318 N.C. 76, 347 S.E.2d 824 (1986); Snell v. Superior Court, 158 Cal. App.3d 44, 204 Cal. Rptr. 200 (1984); Somer v. Johnson, 704 F.2d 1473 (11th Cir. 1983); *contra*, Byork v. Carmer, 109 App. Div.2d 1087, 487 N.Y.S.2d 226 (1985); Greenwood v. Wierdsma, 741 P.2d 1079 (Wyo. 1987).

43. *See, e.g.*, Willing v. St. Joseph Hospital, 176 Ill. App.3d 737, 531 N.E.2d 824 (Ill. App. 1st Dist. 1988). (Interpreting the Illinois Medical Studies Act, the court stated, "Records and documents are protected under the Act if they are utilized as part of the peer review process and not as

a result or consequence thereof . . . the privilege will be accorded only after each document is scrutinized in light of the Act's purpose"); Byork v. Carmer, *supra*, note 41 (upholding but limiting state's peer review statute to the records of the proceedings of peer review committees and not protecting knowledge gained from other sources); Harris Hospital v. Schattman, 734 S.W.2d 759 (Tex. App. 1987) (holding that nondiscoverable records include only those documents generated by committee but not communications between the hospital and physician); Humana Hospital v. Superior Court, *supra*, note 40 (evidence possessed by credentials committee that was not otherwise privileged could be discovered, although credentials committee files themselves were protected); Richter v. Diamond, 108 Ill.2d 265, 483 N.E.2d 1256 (1985) (statutory privilege applies to the peer review process; however, it is not accorded to the imposition of restrictions that may result from the process).

44. *See, e.g.*, Calif. Evid. Code §1157(c): "The prohibition relating to discovery of testimony does not apply to the statements made by any person in attendance at . . . a meeting of any of those committees who is a party to an action or proceeding the subject matter of which was reviewed at that meeting"; Caroll v. Nunez, 137 A.D.2d 911, 524 N.Y.S.2d 578 (1988) (in motion for protective order, court held plaintiff was not entitled to physician's personnel folder or copies of complaints made against him for performing unnecessary surgery, but was to be furnished with any statement made by physician at the hospital's peer review committee proceedings regarding the subject matter of the suit).

45. Jordan v. Court of Appeals, 701 S.W.2d 644 (Tex. 1985) (privilege protects documents prepared by or at direction of hospital committee for committee purposes; does not apply to documents that have been created without committee impetus and purpose).

46. For suggestions about how to protect peer review records *see* Fishman, L. W. Confidentiality of Medical and Peer Review Records. Paper presented at National Health Lawyers Association, 1988 Health Law Update.

47. Many statutes specifically state that the privilege does not apply to proceedings in which a health care provider contests denial or status of staff privileges or authorization to practice. *See, e.g.*, Calif. Evid. Code §1157(c); Kan. Stat. Ann. §65-4915; La. Rev. Stat. Ann. §§44.7 and 13:3715.3. Case law is divided on this question. *See, e.g.*, Roseville Community Hospital v. Superior Court, 70 Cal. App.3d 809, 139 Cal. Rptr. 170 (1977) (statements made by individuals at a committee meeting of the hospital's medical staff are discoverable by persons whose requests for staff privileges were denied); *contra*, Parkview Memorial Hospital v. Pepple, 483 N.E.2d 469 (Ind. App. 1985) (Indiana's peer review confidentiality law applies to civil actions brought by physicians challenging private hospitals' decisions concerning staff privileges as well as to malpractice cases).

48. 8 Wigmore, *Evidence* §2292 (McNaughton rev. 1961).

49. For a discussion of the attorney–client privilege, the insured–insurer privilege, and the work product doctrine, *see generally* Jones, *Evidence* §§19:18–19:19 (1972). Hickman v. Taylor, 329 U.S. 495 (1957) remains the seminal case on the question of the protection afforded to attorney work product. Some statutes, *e.g.*, Florida, specifically provide that incident reports required under a hospital's risk management program "shall be considered to be part of the work papers of the attorney defending the establishment in litigation relating thereto . . . ," making them subject to discovery only upon a showing of undue hardship. Fla. Stat. §395.041 (1987), Fla. R. Civ. P. 1.280(b) (2). Without a privilege, an incident report would represent a contemporaneous statement of fact generated in response to a specific event and would not be protected.

50. Sims v. Knollwood Park Hospital, 511 So.2d 154 (Ala. 1987) (patient, who fractured hip when she fell in hospital, may discover incident report about the fall because it is not a work product protected by the attorney–client privilege; the mere possibility of eventual litigation is not enough to protect the report); *but see* Enke v. Anderson, 733 S.W.2d 462 (Mo. App. 1987) (incident report fell within the attorney–client privilege or the insured–insurer privilege, or if not privileged, was still entitled to the more limited protection available to materials prepared for litigation under the attorney work product doctrine). *See also* Shaffer v. Rogers, 362 N.W.2d 552 (Iowa 1985) (routine internal investigation report was protected even though it might serve a variety of possible future uses; its primary purpose was in anticipation of litigation).

51. *See, e.g.*, Mass Gen. Laws Ann. Ch. 111 §205(b), as amended by H.B. No. 5930 (New Laws 1987), which would provide protection for incident reports as records necessary to comply with

risk management and quality assurance programs; Gallagher v. Detroit Macomb Hospital Association, No. 95084 (Mich. Ct. App. Oct. 3, 1988) (Discovery of an incident report about a patient's fall from bed not permitted; report came within statutory protection afforded to records prepared for hospital quality of care data-collection purposes. Hospital administrator for legal affairs had testified that incident reports on unusual occurrences were routinely forwarded to internal safety and quality assurance committees.)

52. *See generally Hospital Law Manual,* Volume IIA, Rockville, MD: Aspen Publishers, 1986, ¶ 4-5 "Hospital Incident Reports."

53. *E.g.,* the Florida statute specifically provides that discovery of materials protected as work product shall be allowed "upon a showing that the party seeking discovery has need of the material in preparation of his case and that he is unable without undue hardship to obtain the substantial equivalent of the materials by other means." Fla. Stat. §395.041 (1987). But, in application, this is a difficult standard for a plaintiff to meet. Bay Medical Center v. Sapp, 13 FLW 2614, 535 So.2d 308 (Fla. App. 1st Dist. 1988) (Plaintiff was not entitled to production of incident reports in absence of required showing of undue hardship and inability to obtain substantially equivalent materials by other means.)

54. *See* text and note 51, *supra.*

55. *See* discussion *supra,* note 47.

Part Five

Risk Identification and Control

Because health care institutions differ greatly from each other, information specific to each institution must be gathered and analyzed before risk management techniques can be effective. Risk management provides a centralized information-gathering and analysis function. This section describes the specific methods that risk managers use to find out where losses are most likely to occur and how to control and fund the losses that are inevitable no matter how effective loss prevention efforts are.

This section also describes specific techniques that risk managers can use to manage claims and litigation—an important risk management function for which almost all risk managers are responsible. Funding losses is also critical, but it is a skill that many risk managers leave either to the institution's financial managers or to outside insurance brokers and agents. The last two chapters in this section provide instruction on the fundamentals of insurance and some advanced techniques for funding losses through innovative insurance and self-funded programs.

Chapter 25

Systems for Risk Identification

Audrone M. Vanagunas

At the heart of any effective risk management program are systems for identifying both actual loss-producing events and risks of future losses. The identification of potential risks is essential to any risk-prevention program, and the ability to identify and respond to loss-producing events is integral to an effective loss-control program. The means for identifying potential risks and loss-producing events are quite varied; they range from the formal to the informal to the computerized risk-identification system. This chapter will briefly discuss all these systems.

☐ Formal Risk Identification Systems

The purpose of any risk identification system is to identify any incidents or risk situations that may result in loss to the institution. Formal means of identifying these situations include incident reporting and occurrence reporting and screening.

Incident Reporting

The risk identification system that traditionally has been the cornerstone of hospital risk management is incident reporting. The incident report was developed by commercial insurance companies as a means of loss notification in the early 1970s. As such, a form that contained simple information regarding the patient's (or other potential claimant's) name, identifying information, and brief description of the incident was adopted for use in the majority of American hospitals. In fact, many insurance companies still provide the incident report forms to be used by the facility.

An *incident* is generally defined as "any happening which is not consistent with the routine care of a particular patient".[1] This incident, when it occurs, triggers the completion of a report form for transmittal to risk management.

Incident report forms vary in content and structure. Some have only preprinted data elements for check-off, which simplifies computer entry, whereas others have extensive narrative portions. Regardless of the format, some basic information that is contained in most incident reports includes:

- Name, address, and home telephone number of patient, visitor, or employee involved in the incident
- Hospital identifying information, such as admission date, hospital identification number, patient room, admitting diagnosis
- Socioeconomic data about the individual involved in the occurrence, such as age, sex, marital status, employment, and insurance status
- Description of the incident, as well as facts surrounding the event, such as location of the incident; type of incident (e.g., medication error, fall, lost property, elopement); extent of injury incurred; pertinent environmental findings, such as position of bed rails, condition of the floor, physical defects in equipment; and results of any physical examination of the patient, visitor, or employee

The following pertinent facts should be kept in mind regarding the incident report:

- The incident report should be completed at the time of the occurrence by the individual having the most knowledge about the event—that is, the staff member who was involved in the occurrence, who witnessed the occurrence, or to whom the occurrence is reported.
- The report is a confidential document that should be handled expeditiously and in a manner that preserves confidentiality. The original report should be sent to the risk manager immediately upon completion. Copies should not be made. Also, the report must *never* be made part of the medical record.
- In order to ensure appropriate follow-up of reported incidents, a separate follow-up sheet frequently is attached to the incident report form. This form usually is completed by the nursing unit supervisor or other administratively responsible individual who has investigated the occurrence and, when possible, ascertained the cause of the event. It is important to protect the confidentiality of this addendum, as well as the actual incident report.

  If the incident report form requires follow-up information to be entered directly on the form, policies that ensure rapid transmission of necessary information to the risk manager, perhaps by telephone, are essential, because the form usually is not forwarded until it is complete. This delay may mean that the risk manager is unable to do the appropriate follow-up within a day or two of the incident.

  If incident reports are used by the line managers to do quality assurance studies, or if managers insist that they must have the reports for any reason, the risk manager can make the originals available for the line manager's review in the risk manager's office, as long as copies are not made and the originals are not removed from the file.
- If the report is best protected through the assertion of attorney–client privilege, the report should be reviewed by hospital legal counsel and kept in appropriately designated files.

  If protection of the confidentiality of the report is best achieved through statutory protection afforded to quality assurance data, then the reports must be reviewed through the hospital's established quality assurance program. It is best to discuss this with hospital's legal counsel to determine the most appropriate method for preserving confidentiality.
- The incident report is not to be used as a punitive measure in disciplining employees or as a vehicle for airing interpersonal disagreements. It should be a factual account of what happened without finger pointing and accusatory language. If a grievous error was made, an employee may require counseling regarding its potential harm and measures to prevent recurrence; however, the incident report may not be used as evidence against the employee in a disciplinary procedure.
- Incident report data should be collected and analyzed to determine whether there are any trends that represent potential problems in the delivery of care. The results

of this analysis should be distributed and discussed with the individuals and departments involved. The analysis may reveal positive findings, which may be disseminated to employees, as well as problem areas.

Some of the more common problems with traditional incident reporting include the following:[2]

- The absence of a clear definition of what is an "incident." Traditionally, incident reports have been used to report patient slips and falls, medication errors, intravenous infusion problems, and lost valuables. Although those events may occur frequently, claims studies clearly show that they are not the areas of greatest "pay-out" in hospitals.
- The identification of incident reporting as purely a nursing function, thereby discouraging participation by other health care providers, especially physicians.
- The belief that an incident report is a document prepared for the hospital's safety committee, thereby discouraging the reporting of clinically related events.
- Fear on the part of many physicians, nurses, and other health care providers that incident reporting is an admission of negligence that exposes them to liability and could be used against them in court.
- The perception of incident reporting as a routine task or as necessary paperwork with a low priority, with the result that follow-up is too slow or nonexistent.

Some steps that might be taken to improve incident reporting include:

- Clearly defining what is a reportable incident. By indicating—through inservice training, design of the form, and written definitions—what constitutes a reportable incident in the hospital's policies and procedures, the risk manager can expand reporting beyond slips and falls and medication errors.
- Emphasizing the participation of *all* staff members in reporting incidents. Physicians, pharmacists, and laboratory and other ancillary service personnel should be encouraged to participate. Nursing staff are not the only people who should be trained in the use of the incident report form.
- Routing incident reports to appropriate persons. Depending on the routing procedure developed in consultation with hospital legal counsel, the reports should be routed to preserve their confidentiality.
- Providing feedback on results of investigation and problem resolution. By demonstrating to those who use the system the value of incident reporting in identifying problems in patient care and positively addressing those problems, the risk manager can increase the effectiveness of the incident reporting process.

Occurrence Reporting and Screening

In response to the previously mentioned problems with traditional incident reporting, many hospitals have modified their system to ensure the reporting of clinically related adverse patient occurrences. The two basic approaches to accomplish this are focused occurrence reporting and occurrence screening.

Focused Occurrence Reporting

Because one of the primary problems with traditional incident reporting is the lack of a clear definition of what to report, one method for resolving this problem is to clearly define what is a reportable occurrence.

The risk manager needs to educate the staff members about what constitutes a reportable occurrence. Examples of occurrences that need to be reported include:[3]

- Occurrences of missed diagnosis or misdiagnosis that result in patient injury, such as failure to diagnose acute myocardial infarction, fractures, serious head trauma, or appendicitis
- Surgically related occurrences, such as the wrong patient being operated on, the wrong procedure being performed, an incorrect instrument or sponge count, or an unplanned return to the operating room
- Treatment/procedure-related occurrences, such as reactions to contrast material used in a diagnostic procedure, inappropriate exposure to X rays, or burns resulting from improper use of hot packs
- Blood-related occurrences, such as the wrong type of blood given to the patient, transmission of disease via infected blood, or inappropriate use of blood
- Intravenous-related occurrences, such as the wrong solution being administered, infiltration of solution, or an inappropriate infusion rate
- Medication-related occurrences, such as the administration of the wrong medication or dosage, or administration to the wrong patient
- Falls
- Other occurrences that result or may result in injuries to patients or visitors

To further focus the occurrence reporting process, one method adopted in many institutions is the development of specific reportable occurrences in designated clinical areas, such as the emergency department, surgical suite, labor and delivery room, high-risk nursery, and so on. By developing lists of specific adverse outcomes or events in these high-risk areas, the clinical focus of occurrence reporting is addressed, as well as the definition of what needs to be reported (figures 25-1 and 25-2). In this process, the incident report form or a similar form is used to report those occurrences, and the

Figure 25-1.   Operating Room and Recovery Room Occurrences to Be Reported Concurrently to the Hospital's Risk Manager

1. Operation on the wrong patient
2. Wrong procedure performed
3. No written consent for procedure performed or improper consent, except when a physician determines in writing that a consent is not necessary
4. Unplanned removal or repair of an organ or body part, not covered in consent form
5. Patient injury during transfer to/from operating room or recovery room
6. Patient burn resulting from equipment
7. Unplanned disconnection of equipment that has the potential for patient injury
8. Incorrect needle, sponge, or instrument count, or omission of a count required by hospital policy
9. Instrument breakage
10. Foreign object or material found
11. Break in sterile technique except when break was corrected before any patient was exposed to potential contamination
12. Patient operated on for repair of a laceration, perforation, tear, or puncture of an organ subsequent to the performance of an invasive procedure
13. Return to operating room for repair or removal of an organ or body part damaged in surgery
14. Adverse results of anesthesia
15. Intubation resulting in injury (including injury to teeth)
16. Postoperative nerve damage
17. Cardiac arrest except when planned under "cardiac cooling"
18. Respiratory arrest
19. Acute myocardial infarction during or following surgery
20. Death
21. Lack of presurgical consultation for patient required by policy to have consultation
22. Any other untoward patient reactions in the operating room or recovery room

Source: Chicago Hospital Risk Pooling Program.

policies and procedures define what is to be reported. The risk manager receives these reports directly. In most institutions, the data collected through this occurrence reporting process (because of their highly clinical nature) are also reported to the departmental or hospitalwide quality assurance committee for peer review and follow-up. Certainly at least aggregate reports of this information should be reported to quality assurance.

Figure 25-2.   Maternal- and Infant-Related Occurrences to Be Reported to the Hospital's Risk Manager

---

Class I (to be reported within 24 hours)

1. Maternal or infant death, unless fetus weighs less than 500 grams

2. Apgar: Equal to, or less than, 5 at 1 minute

   Equal to, or less than, 7 at 5 minutes

3. Infant injury, e.g., skull fracture, brachial palsy, paralysis, etc.

4. Newborn resuscitation, including intubation and/or instrumentation for the purpose of assisting ventilation, and/or cardiac assistance

5. Transfer of newborn to another hospital's newborn intensive care unit for management of complications

6. Mother transferred to intensive care unit postdelivery

Class II (to be reported prior to patient discharge)

1. Admittance to hospital's newborn intensive care unit or special care unit for management and observation

2. Mother in recovery room for more than two hours for medical complications

3. Mother's unplanned return to the delivery room or surgery

4. Major congenital anomalies of the newborn

Class III (to be incorporated in quality assurance review)

1. High forceps delivery

2. Prolapsed cord

3. Delivery unattended by physician with obstetrical privileges

4. Maternal blood loss resulting in transfusion or an indication for transfusion, e.g., Hgb. 7 grams or less, blood loss greater than 500 cc, or symptomatic patient

5. Maternal injury or complications, e.g., laceration requiring extensive repair, temperature greater than 38°C, retained placenta, etc.

6. Any second stage of labor longer than two hours without direct supervision of physician with obstetrical privileges, or due to complications

7. Minor congenital anomalies of the newborn

8. Recent or ongoing maternal drug abuse during pregnancy

9. Emergency cesarean section that takes more than 30 minutes from decision to delivery

10. Patient in delivery room longer than 30 minutes without documented fetal heart tones

11. No prenatal care prior to admission for labor and delivery

12. Failure to follow American College of Obstetrics and Gynecology standards for monitoring and documenting fetal heart tones during all stages of labor and delivery

---

Source: Chicago Hospital Risk Pooling Program.

Steps that might be taken to avoid the pitfalls in implementing this process include:

- Ensuring that the departmental staff is involved in the development of the list of reportable occurrences so that there is agreement as to the need for reporting.
- Streamlining the reporting process so that the paperwork is not burdensome and so that reporting is encouraged. Because many of the items on the list of reportable occurrences may occur frequently—for example, patients leaving against medical advice from the emergency department—the use of checklists rather than lengthy narrative reports may be more useful.
- Making sure that the results of the reporting are given to the departments involved as quickly as possible for their review and consideration. Emphasize the utility of identifying problems in the quality of patient care rather than the punitive aspect of claims involvement.

Occurrence Screening

Another method that attempts to clearly identify adverse patient occurrences in clinical areas is the occurrence screening process as exemplified by the Medical Management Analysis (MMA) system developed by Joyce Craddick, M.D.[4] This system utilizes a clearly defined list of patient occurrences to screen patient records (figure 25-3).

Using the list of screening criteria, all patient records are reviewed within 48 to 72 hours of admission and every three or four days thereafter until the patient is discharged. The patient chart is also reviewed approximately two weeks after discharge to ensure that compliance with all criteria has been assessed.

An abstract containing patient data and the results of this screening process are prepared for each admission by trained data retrieval personnel. The abstracts are then forwarded to the quality assurance office for follow-up and data collection. Serious occurrences are reported immediately by the patient care reviewers to the appropriate person for action when identified. All occurrences are aggregated to aid in identifying any trends that reflect patient care problems requiring remedial action.

Although occurrence screening is an effective method for identifying adverse occurrences, the implementation of this process in most institutions is done entirely under the quality assurance program. The major pitfall of this system that needs to be addressed is how to ensure appropriate involvement of the risk manager. In some institutions, the risk manager is notified by having the patient care reviewer complete a separate notification form for serious adverse patient occurrences and forward this form to the risk manager. In other instances, the risk manager is part of the quality management team and is apprised of the results of the occurrence screening.

Regardless of the method chosen, in order for this process to be useful to the risk management program, the risk manager should have ready access to these data.

□ Informal Risk Identification Systems

In addition to the more structured systems of risk identification, such as incident reporting, occurrence reporting, and occurrence screening, there are many other sources of information available to the risk manager for identifying actual loss-producing events and potential risks. Some of these sources include:

- Minutes of the meetings of such hospitalwide committees as quality assurance, safety, infection control, and bioethics; and of meetings of such departmental committees as morbidity and mortality, tissue review, pharmacy and therapeutics, and other quality-related committees
- Claims data, including a review of both the hospital's loss experience over a period of time as well as any national or regional trends as reported in various publications

Figure 25-3.   MMA Screening Criteria at a Glance

Criterion 1. Admission for adverse results of outpatient management

a.   Emergency department
b.   Ambulatory surgery/procedure
c.   Hospital-related clinic
d.   Hospital-related service, e.g., home health care
e.   Private office
f.   Other

Exceptions: Specific instructions may be developed by the clinical departments concerning expected admissions for chronic conditions managed in the outpatient setting, e.g., control of a brittle diabetic, chronic severe organ failure disease, multiple metastases of cancer not amenable to definitive treatment.

Criterion 2. Readmission for complications or incomplete management of problems on previous hospitalization

a.   Preexisting complication with deterioration
b.   New complication
c.   Recurrent disease state
d.   Unresolved disease state

Exceptions: Complication or incomplete management that occurred at another hospital not associated with this hospital or involved a practitioner who is not on this medical staff.

Criterion 3. Operative/invasive procedure consent

a.   Incomplete
b.   Missing prior to procedure
c.   Different procedure done from procedure or permit
d.   Different surgeon performed procedure than name on permit
e.   Not signed by patient or legal guardian
f.   No informed consent note
g.   Other

Exceptions: Emergency procedures where the patient was unable and the family or legal guardian unavailable to sign the consent. Life-threatening problems found and addressed during surgery.

Criterion 4. Unplanned removal, injury, or repair of organ or structure during surgery or other invasive procedure, or vaginal delivery

a.   Surgery
b.   Other invasive procedure
c.   Vaginal delivery
d.   Other

Exceptions: None.

Criterion 5. Unplanned return to operating room, delivery room, or other special procedures on this admission

Exceptions: Planned second procedure or second stage of a procedure planned prior to first procedure.

Criterion 6. Surgical and other invasive procedures that do not meet criteria for necessity and appropriateness

a.   Diagnostic tissue-pathology report does not match preoperative diagnosis
b.   Nondiagnostic or normal tissue removed and medical staff criteria for necessity or appropriateness not met
c.   No tissue removed and medical staff criteria for necessity and appropriateness not met
d.   Other

Exceptions: As developed by the medical staff.

(continued on next page)

Figure 25-3. (Continued)

Criterion 7. Blood loss excessive or blood/blood component utilization which is unjustified, excessive, results in patient injury, or is otherwise at variance with professional staff criteria

a. Excessive blood loss occasioned by iatrogenic bleeding or anemia with or without transfusion

Exceptions: As developed by the professional staff.

b. Transfusion of blood or blood components not clinically indicated
c. Transfusion reaction
d. Other

Criterion 8. Nosocomial infection (hospital acquired)

Exceptions: Infection acquired outside the hospital, clinic, or home health care setting that did not involve any member of this medical staff.

Criterion 9. Drug/antibiotic utilization that is unjustified, excessive, inaccurate, results in patient injury, or is otherwise at variance with professional staff criteria

a. Does not meet professional staff criteria for appropriateness

Exceptions: As developed by professional staff.

b. Inadequate/excessive/inappropriate/inaccurate dosage or timing
c. Drug or contrast material reaction/interaction
d. Other

Criterion 10. Cardiac or respiratory arrest/low Apgar score

Exceptions: None.

Criterion 11. Transfer from general care to special care unit

a. Complication necessitating transfer
b. Management problem

Exceptions: Transfer scheduled prior to surgery or other special procedure.

c. Utilization problem
d. Other

Criterion 12. Other patient complications

a. ENT/sensory

Exceptions: None.

b. Cardiac/vascular
c. Pulmonary
d. Gastrointestinal
e. Genitourinary
f. Musculoskeletal
g. Integumentary
h. Endocrine
i. Hematological
j. Emotional/intellectual
k. General/other

Criterion 13. Hospital-incurred patient incident

a. Falls, slips, patient accidents

Exceptions: None.

b. IV problems, such as calculation errors, overloads, or infiltrations
c. Skin problems, such as rash, threatened or new decubitus ulcer
d. Equipment failures/malfunctions

Figure 25-3. (Continued)

e. Other incidents, such as procedural errors, electrical shock or burn, actual or attempted suicide, and lost or damaged property
f. Nursing procedural errors
g. Other

Criterion 14. Abnormal laboratory, X-ray, other test results, or physical findings not addressed by physician

Exceptions: As developed by professional staff.

Criterion 15. Development of neurological deficit that was not present on admission

Exceptions: As developed by the medical staff for expected outcomes, such as deficits following intracranial surgery.

Criterion 16. Transfer to/from another acute care facility

a. Financial reasons
b. Management/procedures not available at this institution
c. Patient option
d. Other

Exceptions: Mandatory transfer for administrative reasons, or transfer for tests not available at this hospital.

Criterion 17. Death

a. Unexpected with surgery
b. Unexpected without surgery
c. Expected disease-related
d. Other

Exceptions: None.

Criterion 18. Subsequent visit to ED or OPD for complications or adverse results related to a previous encounter

a. Hospital admission
b. Ambulatory surgery/procedure
c. Ambulatory clinic/HMO encounter
d. Other

Exceptions: Planned returns for wound checks or suture removal.

Criterion 19. Utilization variations according to medical staff criteria

a. Unjustified admission
b. Concurrent screening guidelines not met
c. Unnecessary days prior to surgery
d. Day/cost outlier
e. Inappropriate resource utilization
f. Inappropriate special care unit utilization
g. Other

Exceptions: As developed by the medical staff.

Criterion 20. Medical record documentation deficiencies—Physician (using monitoring criteria developed by medical staff)

Objective documentation elements:
a–d. Medical record documentation elements that are periodically revised

Exceptions: None.

(continued on next page)

Figure 25-3. (Continued)

Clinical pertinence elements:
e. History and physical
f. Progress notes
g. Physician's orders
h. Consultation
i. Operative report (if applicable)
j. X ray/lab
k. Discharge summary
l. General legibility

Criterion 21. Medical record documentation deficiencies—Nursing (using monitoring criteria developed by nursing QA)

a–d. Medical record elements that are periodically revised   Exceptions: None.

Criterion 22. Departmental or other problem(s)—Ancillary department(s)

Exceptions: None.

Criterion 23. Patient/family dissatisfaction

Exceptions: None.

Criterion 24. Inappropriate discharge planning

a. PRO guidelines not met   Exceptions: Patients who are documented as
b. Referral/response inadequate   not requiring discharge planning.

Source: Reprinted, with permission, from Craddick, J. W., *Improving Quality and Resource Management through Medical Management Analysis*, 1987.

- Survey reports, including those from the Joint Commission on Accreditation of Healthcare Organizations, the state fire marshal, state licensure surveys, and private review organization study results
- Gossip overheard in the employee cafeteria, doctors' lounge, and elevators (although this is a rather casual approach, it is one of the most effective in identifying serious patient or staff problems)
- Floor rounds, in which the risk manager is visible and available to staff members and encourages the sharing of information that may be too sensitive for a written report

Before tackling all these data sources, the risk manager should contact the hospital's legal counsel to determine how to protect the confidentiality of any data the risk manager collects.

☐ Computerized Occurrence Tracking

With the growing availability and use of personal computers in the health care field, there has been concomitant growth in the computerization of risk management data. Although hospitals use many systems that utilize mainframe computers, the growing use of personal computers, with their more reasonable access and generally low cost, has made the computerization of risk management data feasible for most institutions.

There are many commercially available prepackaged software programs designed to track risk management data. There also are many data-based management software programs, such as dBase, Lotus, Metafile, and Paradox, that can be used to customize an individual hospital's management information needs.

The kinds of data that can be tracked utilizing computers include:

- Incident report data
- Occurrence screening information
- Claims data, including professional liability claims, general liability claims, workers' compensation claims, and others, as needed
- Insurance-related data, such as premium costs, contribution rates, and excess-carrier information

The important elements of a computerized system, regardless of the system used or the data input, are as follows:[5]

- Data collection
- Data screening, review, and coding
- Data processing
- Report generation in an easily comprehensible format
- Information analysis and feedback

An effective management information system must have a data-collection form that collects information accurately and quickly and in a manner that allows for easy coding and entry. Incident report forms, as an example, should be either precoded or designed for easy coding to ensure easy and accurate entry and easy retrieval of information. These forms usually contain many check-off boxes and limited narrative description.

The most important element of a successful computerized system is the ability of the program to generate useful and readable reports. Without the capacity to produce aggregate reports and data trends, the utility of a computerized system is minimal. The whole purpose of automating the data is to be able to track information easily and trend the information so as to identify patterns and problems and compare current data with that of last month, last year, and perhaps the past five years.

The kinds of variables related to occurrences that could be analyzed include:[6]

- *Date of the occurrence:* This information is valuable for providing trending information to determine whether the number of occurrences is increasing, decreasing, or remaining stable over time.
- *Type of occurrence:* Looking at the types of occurrences (for example, falls, medication errors, diagnosis-related occurrences, treatment-related occurrences, and so forth) and their frequency is important when trying to identify priorities in loss-prevention activities.
- *Location of the occurrence:* By analyzing where adverse occurrences are most likely to happen, loss-prevention activities can be more readily targeted. Also, this allows for providing profiles to various departments, as requested.
- *Severity of injury:* By focusing on occurrences with the highest likelihood of severe injury (for example, low Apgar scores or anesthesia accidents), one can identify and respond to possible claims with the highest dollar payout.

In addition to those variables, other elements of the occurrence that can be trended include:

- Patient characteristics, such as age, sex, marital status, occupation, method of payment, and admitting diagnosis

- Staff characteristics, such as name, title, employment status (for example, agency versus staff nurse) of all employees involved in the occurrence; or name, department, and specialty of all involved physicians
- Other occurrence-related data, such as time and shift of the occurrence, or physical environment at the time of the occurrence (such as wet floor, inoperative call light, inappropriate bed-rail position)

☐ Conclusion

A meaningful, hospitalwide system that identifies and initiates response to adverse patient occurrences is the backbone of an effective risk management program. It is essential that the hospital's risk manager work on the design and implementation of an effective data-gathering system—whether it is incident reporting, occurrence reporting, or occurrence screening—and that the purposes and value of that system be clearly identified for all members of the health care team.

References

1. Schwegel, K. Physicians join in efforts to reduce risks. *Hospital Medical Staff* 8(11):11, Nov. 1979.

2. Orlikoff, J. E., and Vanagunas, A. M. *Malpractice Prevention and Liability Control for Hospitals.* 2nd ed. Chicago: American Hospital Publishing, 1988.

3. Orlikoff and Vanagunas, pp. 57–58.

4. Craddick, J. *MMA Screening Criteria at a Glance.* Auburn, CA: Medical Management Analysis International, 1987.

5. Kraus, G. P. *Health Care Risk Management, Organization and Claims Administration.* Owings Mills, MD: Rynd Communications, 1986.

6. Orlikoff and Vanagunas, p. 68.

Chapter 26

Claims and Litigation Management*

Ellen L. Barton

Health care entities have a major role to play in addressing the "medical malpractice crisis," not only by ensuring high-quality care but also in managing claims. The health care entity and those individuals who represent it can directly affect the dollars paid in claims by the manner in which they administer those claims. All claims should be handled in a fair and equitable manner, that is, valid claims should be settled promptly and for a reasonable amount, and frivolous or nonmeritorious claims should be vigorously defended. That approach will ensure the entity's reputation for fairness, honesty, and sound judgment. It also will establish a reputation for firmness in resisting nonmeritorious claims.

Settling valid claims as quickly as possible when there is a reasonable demand benefits both the injured party and the health care entity and its affected staff. There are also benefits to be gained from vigorously defending claims that lack merit or involve unreasonable demands. Not only do staff appreciate the recognition of and support for their integrity, but in addition the institution may benefit financially from lower indemnity payments.

The risk manager's role in managing claims will vary, depending on the health care entity's insurance program. If the health care facility is commercially insured, the risk manager's role is to monitor the activities of those with hands-on responsibility for claims management. If the health care facility is self-insured, the risk manager's role is to participate actively in claims management. This chapter sets forth the principles of effective claims management for either case.

☐ Early Identification of Claims

The institution's risk management plan will include a system for reporting actual and potential claims to the hospital risk manager. That reporting can be accomplished through

---

*The introductory section and the sections on pretrial through posttrial procedure have been adapted from Klimon, E. L. The legal process and medical malpractice. *Nursing Economic$* (3)1:44–48, Jan.–Feb. 1985. Sections on the process of testifying through testifying at trial have been adapted from Klimon, E. L. Do you swear to tell the truth? *Nursing Economic$* 3(2):98–102, Mar.–Apr. 1985.

both formal and informal information systems. The hospital risk manager should review incident reports, minutes of hospital committees and conferences, and other similar documents, and follow up where necessary. In addition, the staff should report to the risk manager any complaints from patients or their families about perceived injury or a breach in the quality of care.

It is important that the risk manager have open lines of communication with the medical and nursing staffs, the patient representative, all other ancillary personnel, and administration. The risk manager should make the entire professional staff aware of the need to report dissatisfied patients or potentially compensable events. In furtherance of this goal, the risk manager should provide ongoing education to staff regarding trends in medical malpractice litigation and insurance coverage, reporting of events, release of medical records information, documentation of medical care, discussions with patients and their families, and other related topics.

If any hospital personnel receive letters of representation, demands for damages, or formal legal papers, they should immediately send such notices to the risk manager, who, in turn, should forward them to the appropriate primary and excess insurers, if applicable.

It is the risk manager's responsibility to report actual or potential claims to the health care facility's insurance provider. It is impossible to list all events that should be reported; however, lawsuits, claims, and potentially compensable events generally are considered reportable:

- *Lawsuits:* This category encompasses those cases where formal legal action for damages has been initiated. When a summons or complaint is served at the hospital, the individual receiving it should notify the risk manager immediately by telephone. The risk manager should forward the suit papers to legal counsel or the insurance company (or broker) as soon as possible, noting the date the papers were received. The time periods for the filing of documents will be measured from the date the papers were received. The risk manager should provide any other available information in a cover letter accompanying the suit papers.
- *Claims:* A claim is defined as a formal notification, either orally or in writing, that monetary damages are being sought from the hospital by a third party for an alleged injury. A claim may be made by a patient or by the patient's family, guardian, or attorney. Any hospital personnel receiving such a demand should send copies of all such correspondence and summaries of any other available information to the risk manager as soon as possible.
- *Potentially compensable events:* This category encompasses any incident in which there is neither an active claim nor institution of formal legal action. It includes those cases in which an unexpected event causing injury or potential injury has occurred in the course of a patient's treatment. It also includes those cases where, although there may be no injury, there has been some expression of dissatisfaction or perceived injury, short of an actual claim, by the patient's family.

The risk manager should investigate all incidents and potential claims to the extent necessary to determine whether or not a claim file should be opened. It is this decision that dictates the level of investigation needed and the responsibilities of the involved parties. The risk manager can then evaluate the situation and develop a plan of action to effectively control the loss or potential loss.

☐ The Process of Investigating Claims

The most important aspect of claims handling is the investigation. All claims should be investigated as expeditiously as possible so that valid claims can be settled and nonmeritorious claims can be defended. It is impossible to do either without a thorough investigation of the facts. Once facts are known, the appropriate standard of care may be determined and the potential liability assessed in light of the applicable law. The decision to settle or defend a case should be made only after a full investigation.

Regardless of the risk-financing mechanism chosen to address the professional/general liability exposure, the risk manager plays an important role in the investigative process. In those instances where the risk manager has the major responsibility for claims investigation, he or she should utilize all available resources, such as in-house legal counsel, outside claims adjusters, and the insurance broker, as well as hospital personnel, including nursing and medical staff. However, in all cases, even where the health care facility is commercially insured, the risk manager should direct and maintain control of the investigation. He or she should provide orientation to the investigative process for personnel to be interviewed and should remain present during all interviews by outside adjusters.

Minimum Information Required

The circumstances of each case will determine to a large extent what information should be developed by the person assigned to the investigation. The following investigation checklist sets forth the minimum information required for the investigation of any claim:

1. *Insured parties:* Name, address, phone number, employment or medical staff status, role in the case. Generally, the insured parties include the hospital and its employees who may have been individually named, as well as physicians for whom the hospital has agreed to provide coverage. Hospital employees also may have their own insurance coverage. The hospital's insurer will want to know the coverages provided to named defendants.
2. *Noninsured parties; actual or potential codefendants:* Name, address, phone number, employment or medical staff status, role in the case. Parties not covered by the hospital's insurance usually are physicians and other health care entities who may have provided care and who will have their own coverages.
3. *Dates:* Date of the incident (loss); date the risk manager was notified; date the insurer (commercial, captive, self-insurance trust fund) was notified; date the file was opened; and date the file was closed.
4. *Insurance information:* Limits of liability, primary and excess insurance coverage of all parties, policy numbers, policy periods, potential for third-party actions, other coverage issues.
5. *Claimant information:* Name, date of birth, age, sex, address, phone number, marital status, occupation, annual earnings, dependents.
6. *Claimant's injuries:* Nature and extent of injuries alleged to have occurred, special damages, additional treatment required, subsequent treating physicians.
7. *Current status of case:* Potentially compensable event, claim, or suit; investigation or discovery pending.
8. *Summary of claimant's allegations:* A summary of allegations of improper medical treatment.
9. *Review of the medical records:* Dates of admission and discharge, medical record history number, admitting and discharge diagnoses, treatment provided, summary of nursing notes.
10. *Summaries of interviews:* Summaries of interviews with hospital staff or other parties involved in the incident.
11. *Summary of the facts:* A summary of the facts of the incident as developed by the investigator.
12. *Copies of policies, procedures, and protocols:* Copies of any policies, procedures, and protocols in effect *at the time of the incident* that may have a bearing on the issues.

13. *Copies of the equipment maintenance reports:* If hospital equipment is involved, copies of equipment maintenance reports are needed as well as findings of the clinical engineering department subsequent to the incident; also, copies of any protocols for the maintenance and repair of equipment in question.
14. *Summaries of the results of expert review:* Summaries of any expert reviews conducted on the file.
15. *Evaluation of the legitimacy of damages:* Documents or other material that examine the legitimacy of damages claimed.
16. *Investigator's evaluation of liability:* Recommendations for reserves, and future handling of the claim file.

Sections of the Claim File

As a claim progresses from its initiation to final resolution, documents will be added continually to the claim file. To maintain the information in a logical order, the claim file should be divided into sections such as the following:

- *Correspondence:* This section contains the incident report or first notice of the claim, relevant correspondence pertaining to the claim, and follow-up notations.
- *Expenses:* This section contains documentation for all loss adjustment costs, such as independent adjusters' fees, fees for expert reviews, billings for independent medical examinations, and legal expenses.
- *Legal papers:* This section contains copies of the summons and complaint, interrogatories, transcribed depositions or summaries, and motions.
- *Expert reviews/investigation:* This section contains the analyses of medical experts and experts retained for the purpose of assessing damages. The summaries of the investigation may also be contained in this section.
- *Medical records:* As long as the entire original medical record is easily accessible, only copies of pertinent parts of the medical record need to be kept in the file. In addition, other records, such as computed tomography scans, electroencephalograms, and fetal monitoring strips, should be maintained.

Depending on the case, it may be necessary to create additional sections, such as "Damages" or "Medical Literature," if the nature of the injury is severe and permanent or the basis of liability involves a complex and unusual medical issue.

Diary Review

The risk manager should maintain a diary system to periodically review all claim files. By assigning dates for periodic review, the risk manager can make decisions about handling the case before some new activity mandates action. Each claim file should reflect the next date for review, and there should also be master diaries for all claims files—by date and alphabetically by name. On each review, the following issues should be considered:

- Status of investigation
- Assessment of liability
- Documentation of damages
- Adequacy of reserves
- Availability of expert witnesses

On diary review, the risk manager should examine each case for recent developments and note those developments in the file. Each diary review should include an evaluation of the investigation remaining to be completed and recommendations for future handling of the claim. Because most professional and many general liability claims remain open for two to seven years, it is helpful to summarize the information in an organized fashion so that it can be periodically updated.

The claim status report (figure 26-1, pp. 272–74) provides a format for organizing the facts, the standard of care, the potential liability, and the chronology of legal events.

Investigative Techniques

The investigative process is composed of three steps: (1) discovery of the facts, (2) determination of the applicable standard of care, and (3) assessment of the applicable legal principles. Once those steps have been completed, the risk manager can make a decision to settle or defend the claim. The investigation checklist previously referred to assists in identifying the relevant information. The following techniques facilitate the investigation:

- Interview the involved staff before interviewing the claimant. This allows the information provided by the claimant to be put into perspective. The investigator's questions should not be based on the claimant's side of the story; doing so could put the staff being interviewed on the defensive and hinder open response.
- Do not allow the hospital's attorney to interview the claimant before the claimant is represented by counsel; a premature interview may be used against the health care facility at a later date.
- Always obtain an informal expert review. This review will assist in determining the applicable standard of care. It can also help in formulating questions to ask the claimant or his or her attorney. Most expert reviewers will be physicians; however, if the issue involves nursing care, the expert review should be performed by a qualified *nursing* expert. Often quality assurance department staff can perform such reviews.
- If preliminary information indicates that there is clear liability on the part of the health care facility, offer to arrange a conference for the claimant and his or her representatives to discuss the situation with physicians and other health care professionals; this may defuse the claimant's need to "get even" and so avoid the claim. Many times, the claimant is seeking only an acknowledgment that there was an error, as well as an apology. This conference should be arranged before the claimant has retained legal counsel. Although in most instances it is not appropriate for the risk manager to attend this conference, he or she should have a preliminary meeting with the health care professionals and representatives of administration.
- During the preliminary investigation, do not record interviews with witnesses or request that they write statements; these activities hinder witnesses from giving the interviewer all the relevant information. Informal interviews are far more likely to produce valuable information that will allow the most appropriate decision to be made in handling the claim.
- If preliminary information indicates that there is clear liability on the part of the health care facility, make direct contact with the claimant as soon as is practicable. This may avoid the need for either party to obtain legal counsel and thus eliminate attorneys' fees and reduce the amount of the settlement.
- Verify all information gathered in the investigation process, especially with regard to the claimant's damages. It may be prudent to conduct a *sub rosa* investigation, that is, to get background checks through interviews with neighbors, employers, and coworkers. Such investigations can be enormously time-consuming and should be performed by professional investigators.

Figure 26-1. Claim Status Report

Claimant name: _____ Claim no. _____

Address: _____

Phone: _____ Sex: _____ Marital status: _____

Age (D.O.B.): _____ No. of dependents: _____

Occupation: _____ Income: _____

_____

Date of occurrence: _____
Incident report: Yes _____ No _____
First notice lawsuit: Yes _____ No _____
Date reported to risk manager: _____
Date reported to primary insurer: _____
Date reported to excess insurer: _____

Description of Occurrence:

_____

_____

Named Insured:

_____

Insured Staff:

Name: _____ Department: _____

Position: _____

Noninsured Staff:

Name: _____ Department: _____

Position: _____

Address: _____

Insurance Coverage:

_____

_____

Investigation Completed:

_____

_____

Investigation Remaining:

_____

_____

Figure 26-1.   (Continued)

Evaluation:

_____

_____

Administrative Actions:

Department: _____

Action: _____

Status: _____

_____

Case Evaluation:

Strengths: _____

_____

Weaknesses: _____

_____

Reserve History:

Reserve	Expense/Indemnity	Date
_____	_____	_____
_____	_____	_____
_____	_____	_____

Lawsuit History:

Caption: _____

Court: _____ Docket no.: _____

Date of service: _____ Answer filed: _____

Judge: _____ Trial date: _____

Jury trial: _____ Nonjury trial: _____ Arbitration: _____

Claimant's attorney: _____

Address: _____ Phone no.: _____

Defense attorney: _____

Address: _____ Phone no.: _____

_____

(continued on next page)

Figure 26-1.   (Continued)

Discovery:

Interrogatories:

Propounded to plaintiff, date: _____

Answers received, date: _____

Received from plaintiff, date: _____

Answered, date: _____

Depositions:

Witness: _____ Date: _____

Discussion: _____

_____

Discovery remaining: _____

_____

Motions: _____

_____

Third-party actions: _____

_____

Claimant's expert(s): _____

Specialty: _____

Opinion: _____

Defense expert(s): _____

Specialty: _____

Opinion: _____

Settlement Negotiations:

Medical specials: _____

Lost wages: _____

Other: _____

Demand: _____ Date: _____

Offer: _____ Date: _____

Final outcome and discussion: _____

_____

Source: Neumann Insurance Co., Englewood, CO.

Documentation

In order to make an informed evaluation of the merits of the claim, the claim file should contain the following:

1. Summaries of all investigations by claims personnel, independent adjusters, or risk management personnel.
2. Summaries of any interviews with involved staff or other parties relating to the subject of the claim.
3. Copies of any statements by involved staff that relate to the subject of the claim.
4. Copies of all pertinent medical records and other clinical reports. The original hospital record should be properly secured at the hospital. The risk manager, in conjunction with medical records personnel, should review it periodically to see whether attorneys have reviewed it or requested information from it.
5. Copies of any expert reports, or summaries of expert evaluations, if the expert has not provided a written report.
6. If the claim is in suit, copies of all pleadings.
7. Reports from defense counsel assigned to the case, including status reports or legal research papers prepared by the attorney, as required by developments in the case.
8. Copies of all correspondence with codefendants, their insurers, and excess carriers.
9. Copies of all bills, invoices, and records of payments.
10. Copies of any other correspondence relating to the claim.
11. Copies of all reports required for establishing and processing claim files, including first notice of claim reports, reserve reports, and claim status reports.

Both the claimant and the health care facility are interested in maintaining the confidentiality of the information in the claim file. It should be made available only to parties with a legitimate need for that information.

Depending on the nature of the health care facility's insurance program and the risk manager's role, it is not necessary that the risk manager maintain all the items in the claim file. For example, the risk manager may prefer to file deposition summaries rather than the complete deposition transcript. However, all involved parties should agree on who is responsible for maintaining what documentation.

The risk manager should keep claim files in a secure location with limited access. All original medical records, X rays, tracings, equipment, devices, and supplies that may be necessary to the defense of a claim also should be well protected.

Because medical records must be available in case patients are readmitted, the risk manager must work with the medical records department to have records of patients who have filed claims put in a separate file cabinet. When a lawsuit is filed, the medical records department should "sequester" that patient's medical record (that is, keep it separate, with severely limited access) and label it to indicate its special status. The risk manager should periodically review the need to continue to sequester the record. Radiographs should be treated in the same way.

When the risk manager suspects that a claim may be brought, he or she should immediately have copies of pertinent parts of the medical record made and maintained in the claim file. If someone alters the record, the risk manager will have a copy of the unaltered record and will be in a better position to protect the institution.

☐ Reserving

Reserving, that is, setting aside an amount of money that will be paid out in indemnity and loss adjustment costs by the time the case is settled or resolved, is more art than science. Reserving can be done by the insurance company, by the risk manager, or by an outside claims management firm. Because there is no formula for establishing a reserve for a case, the risk manager should be involved, especially if the entity is commercially insured, to provide information regarding the locality where the incident occurred and any additional facts that might affect damages and costs. In addition, the independent adjuster and defense counsel may be able to provide valuable advice to the insurance company (if the entity is commercially insured) or the risk manager (if it is self-insured).

The proper reserving of claims is critical to the financial soundness of the insurer, the risk pool, or the self-insurance fund. Because reserves must accurately reflect the insurance fund's monetary exposure, the health care facility, with the active participation of the risk manager, should establish guidelines for appropriately reserving claims.

All claims, whether in suit or not, should be reserved as soon as sufficient information is available to assess the liability exposure. Although some cases may have reserves established within 30 days of notification, others may take years. When possible, all cases should be reserved within 90 to 180 days after notification.

Where a health care facility is self-insured, either the risk manager or an independent claims management service should establish reserves for both the actual indemnity costs (the amount paid in damages) and for expenses (the amount paid to investigate and settle or defend the claim). Reserves for expenses should be established to cover the cost of investigation and expert review. However, anticipated legal expenses need not be included unless and until legal process has been initiated. Where an institution is commercially insured, the insurance company is responsible for setting reserves.

As the claim develops, new information from experts, defense counsel, or adjusters may require changing the reserve. Part of the diary review mentioned earlier includes reviewing the reserve to make sure it is still accurate, and adjusting it if necessary. Reserves may be increased or decreased; however, it is important to avoid what is referred to as "stepladdering" reserves. *Stepladdering* is the process of steadily increasing reserves at periodic intervals as each new development comes to light. It is important to avoid stepladdering reserves in order to maintain accuracy of actuarial projections. The best way to avoid stepladdering is to complete a thorough investigation as soon as possible so that the initial reserve is valid for the life of the file.

Just as important as the reserve itself is documentation of the process used and the factors considered in establishing or adjusting a reserve. Factors to consider in establishing a reserve include the following:

1. *Claimant information:* Age, sex, occupation, annual earnings, dependents, and diagnosis.
2. *Information regarding the claimant's injury:* Nature of injury, extent of injury (whether partial, temporary, or permanent), and prospects for rehabilitation.
3. *Facts of the occurrence:* As alleged by claimant, as developed by investigator, documentation in the medical record, and statements of witnesses.
4. *Parties involved:* Identification, levels of education, and evaluation of credibility.
5. *Damages and financial information:* Medical specials, pain and suffering, lost wages, payment status of claimant's counsel, and liens. Medical specials may include hospital, clinic, or nursing home charges; physician or dentist fees; costs for medication or prosthetics; and private-duty nursing care charges.
6. *Expert witnesses:* Reports of expert witnesses, identity and qualifications of experts for claimant and defense, experience of experts with procedure or treatment in question, and experience of experts in litigation. (Note: Experts may include physicians, nurses, pharmacists, economists, or others with expertise in a particular area.)
7. *Verdict and settlement values:* Outcomes for similar injuries in the particular jurisdiction or geographic area.

8. *Information regarding claimant's attorney:* Attorney's experience, both generally and in regard to the type of case in question; plaintiff's attorney's willingness to settle or try the case.

9. *Information on codefendants and possible third-party actions:* Includes availability of additional insurance coverage.

10. *Intangible factors:* Includes appearance and jury appeal of the claimant, physicians, staff, or other witnesses, and the sympathy factor.

11. *Evaluation of liability issues:* Includes both favorable and unfavorable issues.

Figure 26-2 (p. 278) provides a concise method for documenting the reserving process, thereby validating the adequacy of the reserve.

☐ Settlement and Negotiation Techniques

As is true of many other skills, successfully negotiating settlement of a medical malpractice claim is the result of experience. However, the quality of that experience depends in large part on an understanding of the process of negotiation and how various techniques operate within the process.

The filing of a lawsuit initiates an adversarial process involving three parties. The first party justifies its position and attempts to destroy the second party's position. The second party does likewise to the first party. Then a third, uninvolved, party, the judge or jury, makes the decision. Negotiation, on the other hand, should be a collaborative effort between two or more *involved* parties to settle their differences. When settlement negotiations take place after the initiation of a lawsuit, negotiations should not be conducted by defense counsel, because defense counsel is retained to represent its client in an adversarial process and may not always be in the best position to collaborate in resolving the claim.

Equal in importance to the process of negotiation is an understanding of the substance of the claim. The negotiator must understand the facts, the standard of care, and the applicable legal principles.

In brief, the process of negotiation involves the following:

1. *Analyzing the needs of both parties to the negotiation:* In addition to deciding what he or she wants to accomplish and prioritizing those needs, the negotiator should assess the needs of the other party. This will facilitate successful collaboration, which requires that both parties fulfill their needs rather than each competing to gain the greater advantage over the other.

2. *Determining whether expectations are reasonable:* The focus should be on concluding the negotiations satisfactorily to both parties. This result is far more likely when the parties' expectations are reasonable.

3. *Setting realistic goals:* Goals are based on needs and expectations; however, they must be tempered by reality. For example, a claims manager's goal may be to settle a claim involving a scar on the face of a five-year-old girl for $1,000 in order to keep average per-claim payments under $5,000. Although that goal may meet certain needs, it will be viewed as unrealistic if recent reported settlements or court awards for similar injuries have been in the $20,000 to $30,000 range.

4. *Obtaining appropriate authorization for settlement:* The negotiator must have limits to his or her settlement authority in order to enhance flexibility in negotiation. In other words, the negotiator should not be able to commit the institution at the negotiation table. Having final agreements subject to ratification allows the negotiator to use the ratification as an excuse to delay the negotiations, seek further concessions, avoid making additional concessions, or finalize the agreement.

When professionals are sued, they believe their competence is at issue. The successful negotiator approaches the task of negotiation objectively, setting aside the ego needs of the people involved. A position based on logic rather than personal issues is far more likely to succeed. In addition, the successful negotiator will have prepared well and enhanced his or her bargaining power by learning all the facts, using documentation to support the position, and being patient.

Negotiators may employ a variety of techniques, including:

Figure 26-2. Reserve Rationale Form

1. Liability Issues:

   For each issue, indicate
   + = favorable or
   − = unfavorable.

   _____
   _____
   _____

Prepared by: _____

2. Damages:

   Hospitalization: _____

   Physicians: _____

   Rehabilitation:
   _____

   Future medicals:
   _____

3. Worst case
   estimate: _____

   Probable adverse
   verdict: _____

   Probability (%) of
   losing: _____

   Insured's liability
   exposure (%): _____

   Permanent injury:
   _____

   Lost wages: _____

   Lost earning power:
   _____

   Pain and suffering:
   _____

   Total: _____

4. Legal Basis for
   Allocation among
   Defendants:

   _____
   _____
   _____
   _____

5. Indemnity Reserve: _____
   _____

   Expense Reserve: _____
   _____

   Total: _____

6. Reserve by Coverage:

   Primary: _____

   Excess: _____

   Excess: _____

   Claim no.: _____

   Date: _____

7. Allocation (%) of
   Indemnity and Expense
   Reserve:

   Hospital: _____

   Physician(s): _____

   Other(s): _____

Source: Neumann Insurance Co., Englewood, CO.

- Emphasizing mutual interests
- Using questions
- Using delays
- Creating "straw" issues
- Using humor and other diversions
- Presenting "good guys" and "bad guys"
- Walking out in the middle of a negotiation
- Using deadlines
- Using threats
- Being silent
- Using alternative positions
- Using concessions
- Making the other party appear unreasonable
- Calling for a caucus or recess
- Moving to close the arrangement
- In complex negotiations, carefully documenting what has been agreed to and getting consensus on what has been documented

Before structured settlements were introduced, medical malpractice claims were resolved by cash payments. However, with the introduction of a method whereby payments are paid out, or structured, over a period of years, settlements may be easier to negotiate because the total settlement value can be greatly increased without increasing the cost to the payer. When initially introduced, structured settlements were recommended for cases where the values were in the million-dollar range; however, it is now quite common to structure cases with values of several thousand dollars.

The final step in the settlement process is executing an appropriate release. The purpose of the release is to document the payment of damages for a particular injury by a named party and to foreclose future claims against that party for injuries arising out of the same occurrence. Thus, all parties having an interest in the subject matter of the claim should be named in the release. The risk manager should consult legal counsel for advice in the drafting and execution of the release, because claims involving minors, incompetents, and the deceased may have special requirements. Although there may be small claims in which obtaining a release may not seem necessary, it is always preferable to obtain an appropriate release.

☐ Defense Counsel

Underlying successful claims management is the careful selection and effective use of defense counsel. There should be appropriate criteria for assigning defense counsel and procedures for ensuring effective communication between defense counsel and the risk manager. Equally important are instructions designed to ensure that defense counsel and the risk manager work together to provide the highest quality of legal representation available.

The health care entity may be self-insured, in which case the risk manager is responsible for selecting defense counsel, or it may be commercially insured, in which case the risk manager merely needs to recommend defense counsel. The following criteria should be considered in either situation.

General Requirements for Defense Counsel

A law firm selected to serve as defense counsel should have the following:

1. Significant experience litigating medical malpractice cases. Factors to consider in evaluating the level of experience of a law firm include the number of health care

clients represented by the firm and the types of legal representation provided; the number of insurance carriers (commercial or captive) or self-insurance trusts represented by the firm, and the nature of the representation provided; the number of medical malpractice actions defended by the firm, including the actual number of trials conducted; and the firm's record in medical malpractice litigation.

2. More than one attorney capable of litigating medical malpractice cases, and adequate support staff, including paralegals or trained investigators.
3. Representation that has been limited to defense, with no clients preferred over other clients.
4. Billing rates that are competitive with other firms of similar experience.
5. Reasonable geographical proximity to the insured defendants.

In assigning or recommending counsel for a case, the risk manager should also take the following additional factors into consideration:

1. The attorney's current caseload and ability to handle the litigation effectively and efficiently
2. Prior experience with the subject matter and with the allegations raised in the case
3. Prior experience with counsel chosen to represent the plaintiff

Conflicts of interest in representing clients are common. To ensure that the best possible legal services are provided in all circumstances and that there is no conflict of interest, the risk manager should select at least two law firms to which assignments for representation in litigation may be made.

How to Communicate with Defense Counsel

The risk manager's responsibility is to coordinate the defense of lawsuits filed against the health care entity and to communicate effectively with defense counsel. Therefore, it is helpful to develop guidelines to assist defense counsel. A defense firm's compliance with those guidelines should be part of the risk manager's periodic review and evaluation of the effectiveness of defense counsel. The following are useful instructions:

1. The attorney assigned to the defense of a case shall acknowledge receipt of the assignment, in writing. Where the health care entity is commercially insured, this acknowledgment generally is addressed to the insurance company, and a copy is sent to the risk manager.
2. The attorney shall conduct a comprehensive investigation into the facts surrounding the allegations, making use of independent adjusters, hospital risk management personnel, and any investigation of the claim previously conducted.
3. The attorney shall file an answer in a timely fashion and provide copies of all pleadings.
4. The attorney shall file appropriate interrogatories and schedule appropriate depositions as soon as practical. Copies of interrogatories and responses to them, as well as summaries of depositions, are to be provided in a timely fashion.
5. The attorney shall not file counterclaims, cross-claims, or third-party actions without the risk manager's authorization.
6. The attorney shall provide copies of all correspondence relating to the claim.
7. The attorney shall notify appropriate parties of any hearing dates or trial dates and provide written summaries of all proceedings. In the case of a trial or proceeding before a health claims arbitration panel, the attorney is expected to maintain daily telephone contact throughout the proceedings.
8. The attorney shall provide an initial report, a pretrial report, and status reports. The attorney's initial report (figure 26-3) should be filed within 30 days of the receipt

Figure 26-3.   Attorney's Initial Report

Case caption: _____

_____

_____

1.   Law firm: _____

2.   Law firm file no.: Claim no.: _____

3.   Date of assignment: _____

4.   Service: Is service proper? Yes _____ No _____
     If service is not proper, state reason and recommendations: _____
     _____
     _____

5.   Venue: Is venue proper? Yes _____ No _____
     If venue is not proper, state reason and recommendations: _____
     _____
     _____

6.   Statute of limitations: Is statute of limitations an issue? Yes _____ No _____
     If statute of limitations is an issue, state reason and recommendations:
     _____

7.   Analysis of facts, issues, and legal defenses (include case citations, if applicable):
     _____

8.   Case value (based on facts currently known; include case citations where applicable):

     (a)   Estimated judgment value: _____

     (b)   Prejudgment interest rate: _____ and effective date: _____

     (c)   Probability of successfully defending case (%): _____

     (d)   Estimated cost of defense (not including trial): _____

9.   Recommended reserve: _____

     Reasons: _____

10. Settlement: Is settlement recommended at this time?

     Yes _____ No _____

     Reasons: _____

     Recommendations: _____

11. Trial: _____

     Estimated trial date: _____

     Estimated cost of trial: _____

     Attorney who will try case: _____

(continued on next page)

Figure 26-3. (Continued)

12. Plaintiff counsel: _____

Experience and expertise:

_____

Prior experience with plaintiff counsel:

_____

13. Recommendations for future handling:

Investigation: _____

_____

Discovery: _____

_____

Expert reviews: _____

14. Other comments: _____

_____

Attorney preparing report _____ Date _____

Source: Neumann Insurance Co., Englewood, CO.

of the case assignment by the law firm. The attorney's pretrial report (figure 26-4) should be filed no later than 90 days prior to the scheduled trial or arbitration hearing date. Status reports should be filed as necessary.

9. The firm shall process all billing in a timely fashion. All bills should be itemized and should list the attorney or paralegal providing the services, their billable rate, hours worked, and a description of the work performed. General bills submitted without this type of information are not acceptable. Bills may be submitted by the law firm on a monthly basis; however, bills should be submitted at least quarterly. Where the health care entity is commercially insured, the law firm may send bills directly to the insurance company; however, risk managers should have the opportunity to review them.

The attorney assigned to the defense of a case must maintain a close working relationship with the risk manager. The attorney should rely on the risk manager to assist in investigating the facts and developing the defense. The risk manager should assist the defense attorney in arranging interviews of hospital staff, gathering information for answering interrogatories, and locating pertinent hospital records, policies, and procedures. Having the risk manager serve as the conduit for communications between the defense attorney and health care professional staff minimizes the risk of communication by members of the staff to unauthorized individuals. All staff involved in the claim should be cautioned to treat the case as confidential and advised not to discuss it with anyone, especially attorneys or adjusters, unless authorized to do so by the risk manager.

Figure 26-4.   Attorney's Pretrial Report

Case caption: _____
_____
_____

1.   Law firm: _____

2.   Law firm file no.: Claim no.: _____

3.   Trial location: city/state: _____

4.   Court and docket no.: _____

5.   Trial date: _____

6.   Jury trial Nonjury trial Arbitration: _____

7.   Plaintiff trial attorney (name/firm): _____
     _____

8.   Experience of plaintiff counsel: _____

9.   Defense trial attorney: _____

10. Discovery: Complete Incomplete: _____

     If discovery is not complete, list further discovery needed: _____

11. Special damages: _____

12. Should this case be settled? Tried? _____

     Reasons: _____

13. Settlement value: _____

14. Plaintiff's demand: _____

     Do you recommend: Acceptance Rejection _____

     Reasons: _____

15. Possibilities for contribution/indemnity: _____
     _____

     Recommendations: _____

16. Possibility of successful defense (%): _____

17. Probable verdict range: _____

18. Probable cost of defending case through trial: _____
     _____

19. Recommended reserve: _____

     Reasons: _____

20. Recommended course of action: _____

21. Other comments: _____
     _____
     _____

Attorney completing report Date _____

Source: Neumann Insurance Co., Englewood, CO.

Defense Counsel Review

The risk manager should review the performance of each law firm at least once a year. That review should consider the following factors:

1. The firm's compliance with the procedural requirements as set forth in the instructions to defense counsel
2. The degree of responsiveness to and cooperation with the hospital risk manager
3. The firm's track record in litigation over the previous year
4. The firm's billings over the previous year
5. The firm's ability to understand the underlying medical issues and manage the claim

See figure 26-5 for a sample defense counsel evaluation form.

☐ How to Work with Insurance Companies and Brokers

The risk manager may interact with commercial insurance companies in several ways. If the institution is commercially insured and has no deductible or a very small deductible, the insurance company may take a very active role in claims and litigation management. If the institution is commercially insured and has a self-insured retention, the insurance company's role will depend on the amount of the retention. The greater the retention, the less active the insurance company's role. Finally, if the institution is self-insured but has purchased excess commercial coverage, the excess insurance company will most likely assume a passive role.

However, regardless of the level of insurer involvement, the risk manager should clarify the following issues with the commercial carrier:

- Requirements for reporting potentially compensable events (PCEs), claims, and lawsuits
- Responsibilities for investigation
- Responsibilities for negotiation
- Authority to appoint defense counsel
- Responsibility for providing periodic status reports
- Settlement authority

The risk manager also needs to understand the role of the insurance broker. Insurance brokers can be a valuable resource for the risk manager in the following ways:

- Assisting in evaluating coverage
- Explaining terms and conditions of coverage
- Serving as the agent for purposes of reporting PCEs, claims, and lawsuits
- Maintaining loss runs
- Acting as an advocate for the insured

Regardless of the risk-financing arrangement, the risk manager plays a major role in claims and litigation management. It is incumbent upon the risk manager to clarify his or her role with insurance brokers and commercial carriers in order to more effectively execute his or her responsibilities. This clarification should be in writing in order to avoid disputes. Similarly, it should be emphasized that insurance brokers and commercial carriers can provide a service to the health care entity, and the risk manager should take appropriate advantage of that service.

Figure 26-5. Defense Counsel Evaluation Form

File no.: _____

Date: _____

Firm: _____

1. **Responsiveness**

   How accessible was defense counsel throughout the duration of this claim file?

   (1) Unaccessible
   (2) Usually unavailable
   (3) Generally available
   (4) Most accessible; prompt response to all inquiries
   (5) Always accessible; frequently initiated communication

2. **Communication**

   How well did defense counsel keep the file updated regarding significant claim activity throughout the duration of this claim file?

   (1) Infrequently updated; had to request most information
   (2) Erratic information flow
   (3) Moderate information flow
   (4) Prompt information flow
   (5) Superior information flow; updates regardless of activity

3. **Competency**

   How well did defense counsel identify, enunciate, and apply the underlying medical or liability issues involved in this claim?

   (1) Poor understanding; seemed to learn as he or she went
   (2) Fair understanding
   (3) Average understanding; subject matter unfamiliar but researched
   (4) Good understanding; file benefited from attorney's experience
   (5) Excellent understanding; attorney is expert in this field

4. **Management**

   How well did defense counsel govern the progress of this claim?

   (1) Poor control; seemed to *react* to the movement of others
   (2) Fair control
   (3) Average control; not much else he or she could do to speed process
   (4) Good control; aggressive representation
   (5) Excellent control; attorney in command as much as possible

5. **Billing**

   Overall, how well did defense counsel comply with billing guidelines and how expensive, comparatively, were defense costs?

   (1) Did not follow guidelines; fees excessive
   (2) Occasionally followed guidelines; fees higher than average
   (3) Erratic billing system; fees average
   (4) Usually followed guidelines; fees average or below norm
   (5) Always complied with guidelines; fees always in order and reflected only time spent on file

(continued on next page)

Figure 26-5. (Continued)

---

6. **Performance**

   What category would best describe the overall performance of defense counsel in the aforementioned claim file?

   (1) Poor
   (2) Fair
   (3) Average
   (4) Good
   (5) Excellent

   Total score: _____

   Average score: _____

Source: Neumann Insurance Co., Englewood, CO.

☐ The Process of a Lawsuit

A *lawsuit* is the mechanism used by one party (for example, patients or clients) to attempt to establish a legal basis for a claim against another party (for example, a health care professional). In the pursuit of such claims, the U.S. legal system uses the *adversarial process*, that is, a process in which opposing parties produce evidence to support their respective positions. This process demands a neutral forum—a court.

For the process to be effective, certain rules have been developed to govern the conduct of the proceeding. Those rules are referred to as *procedural law.* They provide the structure for the presentation of evidence and arguments of the parties, and they include rules to determine the court where the lawsuit is to be filed, time limits for filing various legal documents, and limits of the discovery process. Those various rules aid the courts in performing two major functions: resolving disputes between parties in a manner consistent with the applicable law and principles of justice, and accomplishing this within a time frame that makes the relief granted meaningful.[1] *Substantive law,* on the other hand, creates, defines, and regulates the rights and duties that are to be enforced. The trial process can be divided into broad categories: pretrial procedure, trial procedure, and posttrial procedure.

Pretrial Procedure

The patient's, or *plaintiff's,* attorney will evaluate the merits of the patient's claim, and if it has merit, will file a *complaint,* or statement of material facts on which the plaintiff is relying to support the claim. When the complaint is filed, either the court or the attorney issues a *summons,* a notice to the parties named in the complaint that an action has been filed against them and that they are required to answer it at a time and place indicated in the summons.

The *defendant* must in turn seek legal counsel. In response to the complaint, the defendant's attorney may choose to file one or more *motions,* asking to have the case dismissed because of lack of jurisdiction, asking for a more definite statement in the complaint, or asking for summary judgment in a case where the facts are not in dispute and the applicable legal principles dictate a decision in favor of the defendant.

The purpose of a motion is not only to obtain the requested relief but also to preserve the record for appeal. Preserving the record is important because the appellate court generally will refuse to consider any legal theories not first presented to the trial court.

The defendant is then required to file an *answer*, in which the defendant admits or denies the *allegations* in the complaint and sets forth any additional information regarding the facts of the case. The defendant may also assert various *affirmative defenses* in the answer, such as the plaintiff's contributory negligence, or the *statute of limitations*, indicating that the time limit for the plaintiff to sue has expired.

In some jurisdictions, the plaintiff is then permitted to file a *reply* in response to the defendant's answer. After those documents have been filed with the court, the issues of the case are said to be drawn, or joined. The basis of the claim is established, and the plaintiff may not later attempt to establish the claim on grounds not presented in those initial pleadings.

The statute of limitations prescribes the time period during which plaintiffs can file a complaint. Generally, if a complaint is not filed within this period, the patient loses the right to proceed with a claim. Once the plaintiff has filed the complaint, other time limits apply to the filing of the remaining *pleadings*, and because extensions of such time limits are routinely granted, months pass between filing the complaint, the answer, and the reply, adding to the overall length of time required for the processing of a lawsuit from filing to final judgment.

Both parties to the suit use the *discovery* process to gather facts, documents, or other materials that are in the knowledge or possession of the other party and are necessary to that party to develop the case.

The mechanisms used to elicit that information include requests for admissions of facts as well as:

- *Interrogatories:* A list of questions to be answered in writing and under oath
- *Depositions:* Oral or written testimony of a witness taken in response to questions, not in open court, but in the presence of an official empowered to administer an oath—usually a notary public—and often intended to be used during the actual trial of a case
- *Subpoenas or subpoenas duces tecum:* A process requiring a witness to appear and give testimony or produce documents or property for inspection

In addition, defendants in medical malpractice cases have the right to request that the plaintiff undergo an examination by an independent medical expert either designated by the defendant or appointed by the court. That examination may provide vital information substantiating or refuting the plaintiff's claim of injuries.

The complex nature of a medical malpractice action usually requires the testimony of *expert witnesses*. That requirement, however, adds to the time involved in the discovery process as well as the trial itself.

After each party to the lawsuit has had an opportunity to fully delineate the issues to be addressed and to obtain all necessary information, the judge assigned to the case generally will call a pretrial conference. The purpose of this conference is to attempt to settle the case without resorting to trial. Because all discovery should have been completed by that time, each side should be fully aware of the facts and better able to assess the likelihood of prevailing at trial.

If the attempt at settlement fails, then the pretrial conference serves to clarify issues still in dispute. It is also an opportunity for each side to set forth the facts of the case from its point of view, the issues, and the applicable law, and to identify the witnesses who will testify and the exhibits that will be submitted for the court's consideration. At the pretrial conference, the parties might also enter into *stipulations* agreeing upon particular facts or other matters not in dispute in the proceedings. The parties to the lawsuit generally do not attend those conferences, but they may attend if they choose.

Trial Procedure

The case generally has been set for trial prior to the pretrial conference. By the time the case comes to trial, often a year or more has passed since the filing of the complaint, and at least two or three years have passed since the actual incident occurred.

The plaintiff may, and usually does, ask to have a jury trial. In such cases, the court then proceeds to *impanel a jury.* Each prospective juror is questioned by the attorneys representing the plaintiff and the defendant to determine possible bias or partiality. This process, known as *voir dire,* allows each party to attempt to select a jury that will be most favorable or at least impartial to the issue at hand. If a juror appears biased, either party may challenge the juror "for cause," and that person will be dismissed.

In addition, all jurisdictions permit a specific number of "peremptory" challenges that allow a prospective juror to be removed without giving any reason.

In a jury trial, the jury's role is to determine the facts of the case from the evidence presented and any conflicting testimony. It is the province of the judge to rule on questions of law, such as the scope of pretrial discovery, the competency of a witness to testify, or the admissibility of evidence. If a plaintiff waives the right to a jury trial, the trial proceeds with the judge deciding questions of fact as well as questions of law.

After the jury has been selected, jurors are sworn in and attorneys for both sides present their *opening statements,* setting forth the basis upon which the claim or defense is made and what evidence the parties intend to present to prove their respective cases. It is important to note that opening statements, however persuasive and well reasoned, are *not* evidence.

At the conclusion of the opening statements, the plaintiff has the first opportunity to plead the case through the testimony of witnesses and other documentary evidence, such as expert medical reports. Each witness is subject to *direct examination* by the plaintiff's attorney, and then *cross-examination* by the defendant's attorney, to clarify or challenge statements made during direct testimony.

Rules of evidence govern the questioning of witnesses and the presentation of documentary evidence and exhibits. Attorneys for either the plaintiff or the defendant may *object* to questions asked or exhibits *submitted* for the court's consideration, and the judge will rule on the objection. To be considered admissible, evidence must be relevant and material to the facts at issue in the trial.

After the plaintiff has presented all evidence believed necessary to prove the case, both parties have an opportunity to make motions for a *directed verdict.* If the plaintiff makes a motion for a directed verdict, the judge is asked to rule that the evidence or law is so clearly in the plaintiff's favor that it is pointless for the trial to proceed. If the defendant makes a motion for a directed verdict, the judge, assuming all evidence presented by the plaintiff as factually true, is asked to rule that the plaintiff has no case. If the judge grants the motion on behalf of the plaintiff, the judgment is rendered in favor of the plaintiff. If the judge grants the motion on behalf of the defendant, the case is dismissed with *prejudice* and the defendant has prevailed.

If no motion for a directed verdict is made or if the motion is denied, then the defendant presents the evidence to support the case by calling witnesses and presenting exhibits in the same way that the plaintiff did. The defendant's witnesses are subject to direct examination by the defendant's attorney and cross-examination by the plaintiff's attorney. After the defendant has concluded, the plaintiff has a right to rebut the evidence presented by the defendant by either recalling witnesses or calling new witnesses.

Again, the defendant and the plaintiff have the opportunity to move for a directed verdict at the close of all the evidence in the case. If no motion is made or if such a motion is denied, then *closing arguments* are presented to the judge or jury. Just as opening statements are summaries of what the respective parties believe the evidence *will show,* closing arguments are summaries of what the respective parties believe the evidence *has shown.* Like opening statements, they are not considered evidence.

The judge then instructs the jury, if there is one, concerning the applicable law. This is referred to as the *charge to the jury.* The judge may also instruct the jury on how to arrive at an amount of damages to be awarded if it finds in favor of the plaintiff. The purpose of those instructions is to provide a framework for the jury to weigh the evidence.

In a jury trial, the jury then retires to consider the evidence and reach a verdict. In a nonjury trial, the judge will retire to review the evidence and reach a decision. Under some circumstances the judge may decide to take the case away from the jury by *directing a verdict* in favor of one party, by *declaring a mistrial* because of the lack of some requisite, or by *declaring a nonsuit*, terminating the action if the plaintiff failed to present a sufficient case.

The jury (or judge) returns a *verdict*, which may be a general or a special verdict. A *general verdict* is one in which the jury makes a complete finding and a single conclusion on all issues presented to it. In a *special verdict*, the jury makes only findings of fact. It then becomes the duty of the judge to apply the law to the facts as found by the jury. Most states require unanimous verdicts in civil cases, but a few do not. In cases where the requisite number of votes cannot be obtained after thorough deliberation, a *hung jury* may be declared and a new trial will be ordered.

Posttrial Procedure

Depending on the verdict, either the plaintiff or the defendant may allege errors at the trial that constitute grounds for an appeal to a higher court. The person who files the appeal is the *appellant,* usually the loser in the lower court; the other party is the *appellee.* Again, there are time limits applicable to the filing of the appeal. The appellant will first prepare a written document, referred to as a *brief,* setting forth the *assignments of error* (made by the trial court) and file it with the appellate court. The appellee then will respond to the appellant's brief. These briefs will include statements and arguments regarding points of law.

The appellate court will rely on the transcript of the trial court proceedings and the briefs and arguments made by counsel in reaching its decision. Usually, there will be oral arguments as well. The parties rarely attend the appellate hearing. The appellate court will issue a written opinion setting forth the decision, applicable law, and the rationale for the court's decision. The appellate court may affirm or reverse, in whole or in part, the lower court's decision, or it may remand (send the case back to the lower court for a new trial).

An appellate court is a court of review. Its purpose is not to retry the case, but to scrutinize the record of the trial court to determine whether reversible error has been committed. Most appellate courts do not review factual issues because the determination of such issues is the sole province of the trial judge or jury. In general, a party has a right to a first appeal, but a second appeal to a higher court often requires the consent of the court.

If the final judgment is for the defendant, the case is concluded except for the payment of court costs, usually by the plaintiff. If the plaintiff prevails, the defendant must comply with the judgment—in the case of a medical malpractice action, usually the payment of monetary damages. Failure to do so could result in being cited for *contempt of court* with a *writ of execution,* a written order to put in force the judgment of a court levied against the defendant's property to satisfy the judgment.

How to Answer Interrogatories

Answering interrogatories might well be viewed by risk managers with the same disdain with which a billing clerk views the filing of insurance forms. Both, however, are necessary evils. Just as the cash flow of the health care entity depends in large part on third-party reimbursement, so, too, does the success of the litigation depend on the information provided in the answers to interrogatories.

Interrogatories can be useful or bothersome. Obtaining information by interrogatories may disclose facts that appreciably improve the health care institution's case. On the other hand, having to answer lengthy and detailed interrogatories can be annoying and expensive.

The following are guidelines for responding to interrogatories:

1. The risk manager should generally be the one to respond to interrogatories on behalf of the institution. Although some information may not be in the risk manager's immediate possession, letting a member of the senior administrative staff who may have all the information answer interrogatories may subject him or her to a deposition and allow the plaintiff to go on a "fishing" expedition.
2. The risk manager should not be intimidated into answering burdensome questions. It is perfectly appropriate to object to such questions.
3. The risk manager should *never* allow the defense attorney to file answers to interrogatories without reviewing and approving the final answers.

When interrogatories exceed the bounds of reasonableness, the answering party may be excused from compliance by requesting a protective order from the court. Short of a protective order, the answering party has the right to object to answering interrogatories by stating specifically the grounds for the objection. The following are standard objections that can be raised:

1. The answers sought are readily known to the inquiring party and the request amounts to an undue burden upon the answering party.
2. The information sought is in the possession of the party requesting the information.
3. The information sought is a matter of public record and equally available to both parties.
4. The interrogatories are burdensome and time-consuming. This objection must be supported by detailed reasons.
5. The interrogatories require a legal opinion. Such matters are beyond the scope of "factual" interrogatories.
6. The scope of the interrogatories is too broad.
7. The interrogatories are inapplicable to the instant case. The plaintiff's attorney may have used "stock" interrogatories without tailoring them to the specific claim.

Although the risk manager may be annoyed by having to answer interrogatories, propounding them on the other party can be a useful tool. Some reasons for submitting interrogatories include the following:

1. When first notice of a claim is the lawsuit, interrogatories may aid in securing preliminary information.
2. Interrogatories are an excellent means of reducing the issues and avoiding extensive and time-consuming depositions.
3. Answers to interrogatories will provide some essential facts needed to obtain such additional information as employment records or, if there was subsequent treatment at another facility, hospital records.
4. Information contained in the answers to interrogatories may disclose that all of the essential parties have not been joined in the lawsuit.

Following are some reasons for *not* using interrogatories:

1. The complexity of a factual issue may be too involved to provide a clear understanding in a written answer.
2. Unlike oral depositions, the plaintiff's attorney will read and approve the language used in answering interrogatories by the plaintiff. Crucial questions of fact might be better asked in an oral deposition.[2]

The Process of Testifying

A *deposition* is the testimony of a witness who is examined out of court by a party who has given notice to all other parties so that they can be present to cross-examine the *deponent*. The examination takes place before an official, usually a court reporter, who is empowered to administer an oath. Testimony of a witness being deposed takes the same question-and-answer format as testimony in open court.

Objections to questions may be made but cannot be ruled upon at the time because the person before whom the deposition is being taken is not a judge. Such objections will be noted in the stenographic record of the deposition and can then later be ruled upon by the court. The taking of testimony by depositions was originally the means of taking testimony of witnesses who would be unable to appear at the trial. However, depositions may also be taken (and today, more commonly are taken) for discovery purposes—that is, as a means for the parties to learn all relevant facts pertaining to their case prior to trial.

The mechanics for taking a deposition are relatively simple. The party desiring to take the deposition is merely required to give written notice to all other parties to the lawsuit of the time and place for taking the deposition and the names of the witnesses to be examined. A subpoena may be used to compel the attendance of a witness if necessary; such a subpoena may also require the witness to bring specifically designated documents—the medical record and hospital policies, for example.

Depositions taken on oral examination are more effective than a written examination because an answer to a question may disclose information or suggest a clue to a new line of inquiry, which, in turn, may open up other areas.

The only limitation in the scope of questioning during a deposition is that the inquiry be confined to any matter relevant to the subject matter of the suit, including not only what may be evidence at the trial but also what may lead to evidence.

The Deposition Process

It is helpful, in preparing a witness, to explain in some detail the process of a deposition, including, for example, who will be present, how the room will be arranged, how those in attendance will be seated, and what the order of questioning will be. That information allows the deponent to become oriented immediately to the surroundings and then concentrate on the substance of the deposition.

Most depositions are held in the offices of the attorney for the party requesting the deposition. However, in medical malpractice cases involving the depositions of several health care professionals, it is not uncommon to hold the depositions in the hospital, thereby accommodating the schedules of the deponents and avoiding disruption of the delivery of health care services. Because depositions are used for discovery by all parties to a lawsuit, the risk manager may be coordinating depositions for both the plaintiff and defendant.

The room chosen should be large enough to accommodate the deponent and his or her attorney, the attorney who requested the deposition, the attorneys for other parties involved in the lawsuit, the court reporter, and the plaintiff(s) or defendant(s), if they choose to attend. The seating for a deposition is dictated by a number of factors. First, the court reporter needs to be in a position to hear clearly the testimony of the deponent. The attorney who has requested the deposition needs to be in a position to be heard by the deponent and to hear the deponent's responses. The deponent is usually seated directly across from the attorney who will be asking the questions, and the court reporter is seated off to the side but facing the deponent. The deponent's attorney will be seated immediately beside the deponent. The parties to the lawsuit and any other attorneys will then seat themselves accordingly.

The deposition will commence as soon as all parties are present. At that point, the court reporter will be asked to swear or affirm the witness; from that point on, every word spoken during the course of the deposition is under oath and recorded.

Suggestions for Witnesses

The risk manager will help prepare the hospital's employees for deposition or trial. The following is a list of suggestions for witnesses:

- *Remember that appearance is important:* The witness should present a good appearance. The opposing attorney will appraise the witness and evaluate the witness's probable impression on the jury. Therefore, it is important that he or she dress neatly and conventionally. A business suit or similar attire is appropriate, as is a uniform if the deposition takes place at the hospital.
- *Maintain a courteous demeanor:* In answering questions, the witness should be polite and cooperative and avoid showing displeasure at the inconvenience of having to go through the deposition. The witness should rely on the hospital's attorney for protection against harassment or improper questioning.
- *Enunciate clearly:* The witness must speak loudly and enunciate clearly so that the court reporter can correctly record what is said. Witnesses who nod their heads or use other body language will be asked to respond audibly. Witnesses should avoid body movements, such as nodding in agreement with the attorney posing questions, as those movements might be misinterpreted by the attorney and lead to a different line of questioning that may either obscure or distort the main issues.
- *Be prepared to give personal/professional information:* The witness should be prepared to answer questions about place of residence, age, and marital status, including the dates of marriages or divorces. Although such information often seems irrelevant to the issues of a particular lawsuit, it may be relevant to the witness's credibility. Of even greater importance are questions having to do with educational background, including schools attended, the dates attended, the degrees awarded, and additional academic work that may not have led to a degree.

  In addition to this general information, attorneys often ask specific questions concerning certain courses taken—mathematics, for instance, and what grade the witness received. This kind of questioning may be intended to show the witness in a bad light.

  The witness will be questioned concerning employment background. The witness who reviews this information prior to the deposition will answer questions with confidence and self-assurance.
- *Know the facts:* It is always appropriate for the witness to review the facts of the occurrence. This includes reviewing the medical record and the documentation made by the witness, as well as any notes made at the time of the incident. No purpose is served by an attempt to "play dumb" in a deposition. In fact, professional credibility often is damaged when such tactics are used.

  The witness who is asked a question beyond the scope of that person's professional competence should say so in response to the question. Often a plaintiff's attorney will ask a witness who is a nurse to render an opinion on the care provided by a physician. This question is inappropriate and should be objected to by the hospital's attorney.
- *Prepare diagrams and sketches, if appropriate:* If the particular incident that is the subject of the lawsuit involves placement of persons or objects, and those placements are particularly relevant, it may be helpful to make a sketch or diagram of the scene either before or during the deposition, if requested to do so.
- *Be prepared to answer questions regarding matters of time, amount, and distance:* Often in medical malpractice cases, the time of an event—an order, a transfer to the operating room, a page to the attending physician—is important. Also, the amount of certain items—fluids administered intravenously, blood, medication—is a crucial issue. The witness might be asked to estimate a time or an amount. If the witness cannot make a reliable estimate, the appropriate response is, "I'm only guessing," or even, "I don't know."

- *Identify exhibits:* The basis of almost every medical malpractice action is the documentation contained in the medical record. Thus, it is quite likely that during a deposition the witness will be handed the medical record of the patient involved in the case. If this happens, the witness should take time to review it carefully before either identifying it or saying, "I don't know." In responding to questions concerning the exhibit, the witness should make clear reference to the title of the document and its various parts and make sure the answers given are related to the documentation provided in the exhibit. Witnesses are not required to interpret notations made by other members of the health care team.

  In addition to the medical record, hospital policies and procedures may be introduced as evidence to prove the standard of care in a particular situation. Again, time should be taken to identify the document, checking carefully for the effective date of the policy's application.
- *Understand the question:* The witness must be sure that the question is clearly stated before answering. Often deponents, in an effort not to antagonize the attorney asking questions, will hesitate to ask the attorney to repeat a question. An inaccurate answer in response to a misunderstood question can materially affect the results of the case. In addition, if the clarification does not come until the transcribed deposition is reviewed or even later, as at trial, the witness's motives in changing a response may be questioned.
- *Pause before answering:* After being asked a question, a witness should pause long enough to reflect and be certain he or she understands the question being asked and to allow time for the deponent's attorney to raise any objections. When the hospital's attorney objects to a question, the witness should refrain from answering further until the matter has been resolved. The attorney will direct the witness if an answer is required.
- *Answer briefly:* Answers to questions should be stated as briefly as possible. If yes or no will suffice, then no further information should be given in response to the question. Lengthy responses give the questioner much more information than asked for; furthermore, it may be information the questioner would not have thought to have extracted. The witness should be coached to answer only the questions asked. Witnesses are not required to guess or speculate as to what the answer might be. "I don't know" or "I don't remember" is a perfectly acceptable response, as long as it is truthful.
- *Do not qualify favorable facts:* Witnesses should avoid qualifying favorable facts, avoiding such expressions as "I think" or "I guess" in the response. The response should convey a sense of authority and definiteness that serves to increase credibility. Vague responses draw into question not only the timing of certain crucial events, but professional integrity.
- *Tell the truth:* When a witness receives a subpoena notifying him or her to appear for a deposition, he or she typically inquires, "What shall I say?" The response is simple: "Tell the truth." It is unnecessary and often harmful to try to "improve" upon the facts of the case. The opposing party invariably recognizes such conduct and can later exploit any inaccuracy to its advantage. Furthermore, if at a subsequent time the judge or jury believes that a witness has exaggerated on one point, they may well surmise that other points have been exaggerated.
- *Review the transcript:* The witness will be asked to review the transcription of the deposition and to correct any errors. Often the risk manager will perform a preliminary review and then meet with witnesses to review matters needing clarification. The witness will then sign the transcript, authenticating its accuracy.

How to Testify at Trial

All the previous suggestions also apply to testifying at trial. The major difference, of course, is that the witness will be in a courtroom and, in addition to the attorneys and parties, a judge and perhaps a jury will be present. Also, members of the general public, the press, and other interested parties may be present. However, the nature of the questioning is the same. Whoever calls a witness will have the first opportunity to ask questions. Afterward, the opposing party's attorney will have the opportunity to question the witness.

By offering to prepare a witness either alone or in conjunction with the defense counsel and sharing with him or her the previous guidelines, the risk manager can assist the witness in presenting a professional and credible image.

References

1. Hemelt, M. D., and Mackert, M. D. *Dynamics of Law in Nursing and Health Care.* Reston, VA: Reston Publishing Co., 1978, p. 5.

2. Morrill, A. E. *Trial Diplomacy.* 2nd ed. Chicago: Court Practice Institute, 1972, pp. 188–91.

☐ Bibliography

Cohen, E. S. How to be a good witness. *The Coordinator* 3(7):11, Aug. 1984.

Donaldson, J. H. *Casualty Claim Practice.* 3rd ed. Homewood, IL: Richard D. Irwin, 1976.

Hemelt, M. D., and Mackert, M. D. *Dynamics of Law in Nursing and Health Care.* Reston, VA: Reston Publishing Co., 1978.

Holder, A. R. *Medical Malpractice Law.* 2nd ed. New York City: John Wiley & Sons, 1978.

King, J. H. *The Law of Medical Malpractice.* St. Paul: West Publishing Co., 1977.

Klimon, E. L. The legal process and medical malpractice. *Nursing Economic$* 3(1):44–48, Jan.–Feb. 1985.

Klimon, E. L. Do you swear to tell the truth? *Nursing Economic$* 3(2):98–102, Mar.–Apr. 1985.

Kraus, G. P. *Health Care Risk Management: Organization and Claims Administration.* Owings Mills, MD: National Health Publishers, 1986.

Laubach, P. B., Rand, R. L., and others. *The Process and Technique of Negotiating.* Chicago: Foundation of the American College of Hospital Administrators, 1984.

Miller, C. E. *How Insurance Companies Settle Cases.* Santa Ana, CA: James Publishing Group, 1989.

Morrill, A. E. *Trial Diplomacy.* 2nd ed. Chicago: Court Practice Institute, 1972.

The Neumann Insurance Company Claims Management Policy and Procedure Manual. Englewood, CO: The Neumann Insurance Company, 1988.

Troyer, G. T., and Salman, S. L. *Handbook of Health Care Risk Management.* Rockville, MD: Aspen Publishers, 1986.

Wade, R. D. *Risk Management HPL: Hospital Professional Liability Primer.* Columbus, OH: Ohio Hospital Insurance Company, 1983.

Chapter 27

Insurance

Sanford M. Bragman

The most common method of risk transfer/risk financing is to purchase insurance. However, most health care risk managers come to the discipline with very little knowledge about the workings of insurance.

The risk manager's primary insurance responsibility is to determine whether insurance is an appropriate, cost-effective method for treating risks in health care operations. To make that judgment, the risk manager will need a basic understanding of the nature of insurance and will need to know how to read an insurance policy and understand what it covers. The risk manager must know what is going on in the institution to determine when insurance issues need to be explored.

Insurance principles can be understood easily and applied effectively by risk managers who use common sense and know when to ask questions, what questions to ask, and where to look for additional reference material. This chapter introduces the basic principles common to all types of insurance and provides a brief analysis of specific types of coverages that are important to health care risk management.

☐ What Is Insurance?

Barry Smith defines insurance as "a system by which a risk is transferred by a person, business, or organization to an insurance company, which reimburses the insured for covered losses and provides for sharing of costs of losses among all insureds. Risk, transfer, and sharing are vital elements of insurance."[1] The insurance company provides that service for a fee, known as the *premium*. Risk is transferred through the issuance of a written policy, which is a *contract*; contract laws apply in interpreting the policy's terms.

Once a risk has been identified through the risk management process, insurance may be the best method to finance that risk. To determine whether insurance is the appropriate choice, a risk manager should recognize the following realities:

- Part of the premium cost of purchasing commercial insurance is the commercial insurance company's profit.
- A prudent risk manager should look at factors in addition to cost when selecting a given company.

Important elements to consider in selecting an insurance carrier are (1) the solvency of the carrier, (2) the rating given the carrier by *Best's Review* (a publication of the A. M. Best Company, which provides comprehensive reports on the financial position, history, and transactions of insurance companies), (3) the licensing and filing status of the carrier under various state laws, and (4) the services the carrier offers. These may include fast and efficient claims service, loss-prevention consulting, inspection of the facility, willingness to meet the insured to understand the unique nature of a particular risk, and the opportunity to establish a long-term relationship that will provide continuity and stability to the risk management program.

Risk managers should understand that state insurance regulators monitor the financial condition and operations of insurance companies and that rules and regulations differ from state to state. Nearly all states give their insurance commissioners the power to regulate rates, license insurers and insurance company representatives, approve policy forms, and respond to consumer complaints.

☐ How to Purchase Insurance

The health care risk manager will most likely gain access to the commercial insurance market through the use of an insurance broker or an independent agent.

Brokers

Brokers traditionally are independent insurance professionals who represent the insurance purchaser rather than the company. The broker represents an insured in seeking, negotiating, or purchasing coverage and renders assistance in preparing appropriate applications to a variety of prospective insurance carriers. In some cases, the broker may also be an agent of the insurer.

Agents

Traditionally, agents legally and contractually represent the interests of an insurer, not the insured. An independent agent may represent a number of insurance carriers.

In practice, despite the technical distinction between brokers and independent agents, the actual differences are slight. Both the broker and the agent act as go-betweens for the insurance company and the insurance buyer. Both are in the business of helping the risk manager to identify particular insurance needs and providing insurance for those needs. Both usually are compensated by the insurers in the form of commissions. To educate themselves regarding the unique nature of the specific types of coverage being provided, risk managers should ask their brokers or agents to provide policy interpretation and analysis.

Coverage

Risk managers have a primary responsibility to understand and be able to explain what their institutions' various insurance policies cover. Insurance contracts should be kept by the risk management department. The question asked most frequently of all risk managers is, "Is it covered?" The risk manager must know not only what is covered, but also who is covered and when the coverage is in effect. To determine what the insurance policy covers, the risk manager must read the policy, including the "exclusions," or the list of exposures excluded from coverage.

☐ The Insurance Contract/Policy

Every provision of property and liability policies logically falls into one of the following five divisions:

- Declarations
- Insuring agreements
- Exclusions
- Conditions/miscellaneous provisions
- Definitions

These divisions may not be labeled specifically in the policy, but they accurately categorize the general provisions found in most property and liability policies.

Declarations

The declarations of an insurance policy identify the named insured and describe each property or activity to be insured. The declarations usually specify the following:

- Name and address of insured
- Policy number
- Number of forms and endorsements attached
- Policy limits
- Policy term
- Premium and method of payment
- Deductibles
- Additional interests (mortgagee)
- Perils covered

Insuring Agreements

The insuring agreements provide the language wherein the insurer states its obligations under the terms of the contract—in other words, the promises of the insurer. They define the coverage afforded by the policy in broad terms. An example of an insuring agreement of a liability policy is, "The insurer agrees to pay on behalf of the named insured all sums which the named insured becomes legally obligated to pay as damages because of bodily injury or property damages arising out of an occurrence covered by this policy."

Exclusions

Exclusions refer to policy provisions that eliminate coverage that the insurer does not intend to provide. Exclusions eliminate unintended coverages whether or not the provision is labeled an exclusion. Such an unlabeled exclusion can be in the form of a limiting endorsement. What the insuring agreements appear to give, the exclusions may take away. Many insurers will negotiate additional premium to delete exclusions. A typical exclusion found in many general liability insurance policies states, "This insurance will not apply to damage to property in the care, custody and control of the insured." That exclusion has been a source of friction between insurers and hospitals because property such as dentures and other patients' belongings typically are excluded. Risk managers should work with their brokers to attempt to have such exclusions deleted.

It is as important for the risk manager to know what is specifically covered by the policy as it is to know what is specifically excluded. *The insuring agreements and exclusions must be read together to understand the coverage of a given policy.*

Conditions/Miscellaneous Provisions

The *conditions* are a series of clauses that spell out the obligations of the insured, as well as the insured's rights and privileges. Examples of important conditions are the insured's obligation to provide prompt notice of loss to the insurer, the insured's obligation to cooperate with the insurer in investigating and settling loss, the insured's obligation to pay premium in a timely manner, and the conditions under which the policy may be canceled.

Failure of an insured to adhere to the policy's conditions could result in the insurer refusing to honor a claim.

Definitions

Insurance policies often contain technical terms or words that are used in a very specific way. Many policies contain a separate section labeled "Definitions." Without these specific definitions, words are assumed to refer to their dictionary definition. The risk manager should review each insurance policy to determine any special meanings contained therein.

☐ Specific Types of Insurance

Two of the most common types of coverage found in property and casualty insurance contracts are first-party and third-party coverage.

First-Party Insurance

First-party insurance provides coverage for the insured's own property or person so that the insured will be restored to the same financial position that he or she had prior to the loss. The contract is between the insured and the insurer for the benefit of the insured. First-party insurance for the insured's own person usually is in the form of disability or health insurance.

Most health care risk managers will deal with the risks associated with the ownership and occupancy of property by purchasing traditional insurance. Property insurance is usually readily available and affordably priced. The health care entity frequently is a desirable risk for the insurer. In fact, most hospitals are classified as a *highly protected risk* (HPR) because of the fire-resistant construction and sprinkler and alarm systems found in most facilities. Also, hospitals are occupied and staffed 24 hours a day, increasing the facility's ability to respond to a loss before significant damage occurs. The insurer provides loss-prevention services that the risk manager should use. However, the benefits of complying with the insurers' recommendations should be balanced against the cost of compliance. An example of a property insurer's loss-prevention recommendation is that sprinkler protection be added.

Health care risk managers should consider purchasing property insurance in the form of a comprehensive package. Direct damage to buildings and contents represents one of the largest exposures the health care facility faces. Those policies are designed to combine various elements of coverage for similar types of risk. The following types of risk, which are explained in more detail below, are commonly covered by sections of a single property insurance policy:

- Fire and extended coverage, or all-risk, on buildings and contents
- Business interruption
- Boiler and machinery
- Builders' risk
- Electronic data processing
- Flood and earthquake
- Crime/dishonesty

Property insurance policies specify the exact property and contents to be covered, the property's stated value, and the types of loss the property is covered for. Property insurance may protect any covered person or organization that has an "insurable interest" (see glossary) in the property.

Property insurance policies may contain a coinsurance provision, which requires the insured to carry an amount of insurance that at least equals a specified percentage of the total value of the property (usually 80 or 90 percent). If a limit of insurance is purchased that represents less than the specified percentage of the total value of the property at the time of loss, the insured will be penalized in the settlement of a claim.

Risk managers should work with their finance department, the engineering department, and an appraisal service to determine the risks and values to be insured. Departments involved in property acquisition should coordinate with the risk management department to make sure that adequate insurance protection is afforded.

Fire and Extended Coverage/All-Risk

Almost all property insurance policies are written to cover the insured for losses arising from fire and lightning. The reference to extended coverage acts to extend the policy to cover the insured for other specifically named perils—usually windstorm, hail, riot, explosion, vehicle damage, aircraft, smoke, and so on. Those are only some of the perils usually named in a property insurance policy. Each policy should be carefully read to determine the perils insured.

An all-risk policy covers the insured property against all risk of direct physical loss to which the policy applies. Exclusions must be carefully read to determine what losses or property may not be covered. The risk manager should also know whether the property is covered for actual cash value or replacement cost. *Actual cash value* refers to the valuation of the damaged property based on replacement cost less depreciation for age and use. *Replacement cost* refers to the valuation based on the cost of replacement at the time of loss. A risk manager must recognize that the broader the protection, the more costly the insurance.

Business Interruption

Business interruption losses result from an occurrence involving a named peril or all risk that interrupts the revenue stream to the insured facility. A health care facility that suffers a fire loss and can no longer care for patients may suffer a significant business interruption loss. Damage to computers and media may also cause a significant loss of revenue. Business interruption insurance pays for the loss of earnings and continuing expenses resulting from a covered loss. It also will pay for extra expense incurred to keep the facility in operation while repairs are being made. This coverage provides a *contribution clause,* which operates much like a coinsurance clause. In order to ensure that the facility's limit meets the policy requirements, limits should be reviewed annually with the insurance carrier. The deductible for this insurance is usually stated in the number of hours following the casualty that coverage begins. Typically, the deductible applies for 24 to 48 hours.

Boiler and Machinery

Boiler and machinery insurance usually provides for named peril coverage as well as protection against accidental damage or mechanical breakdown of boilers and pressure vessels essential for premises operation. In addition to damage to the boilers and pressure vessels, coverage is provided for resulting damage to other owned property if it is not covered by the facility's property policy. Coverage would also extend to damage to the property of others for which the facility is held responsible.

Builders' Risk

This covers exposure associated with new construction, usually on the premises of the insured property. Hospitals are always in various phases of new construction or remodeling. Builders' Risk covers the potential for loss to the property under construction, which may include the interest of the owner as well as the contractor.

Electronic Data Processing

This coverage protects owned or leased data-processing equipment, data, media, and computer programs. The coverage provided is beyond the scope of most other property policies. Standard property insurance policies pay only for the loss of media and not the loss of information; this coverage will pay for the replacement of information displayed on cards, disks, drums, or tapes.

Flood and Earthquake

This coverage can be included in the facility's property insurance policy or in a separate policy referred to as a *difference in conditions* policy.

Crime/Dishonesty

Burglary and theft losses can be covered under the basic property insurance policy. However, employee dishonesty and some forms of robbery are not usually covered by the basic property policy. A comprehensive crime policy supplementing property insurance will almost always provide a menu of coverage options, including employee dishonesty, theft of money and securities, disappearance of property for no known cause, burglary of the facility's safe, robbery, destruction of property, and computer fraud. Those policies may have a deductible.

Automobile Physical Damage

Prudent health care risk managers will want to cover vehicles owned by the health care institution for loss resulting from damage to those vehicles. Automobile physical damage usually is purchased as part of a broad form automobile policy that will include liability coverage. Coverage is afforded for collision and comprehensive, usually subject to a deductible. The premium is determined by a rate applied to the number of vehicles. Rates are a product of the number, age, use, value, and garaging location of vehicles, as well as historical loss experience.

A risk manager responsible for a large fleet of vehicles may be able to negotiate a rate significantly below general market conditions. Coverage can be negotiated to cover leased, nonowned, rental, and temporary substitute vehicles. Most vehicles that are financed will be required to carry collision and comprehensive coverage that protects the lender.

If the facility has decided not to provide coverage for nonowned vehicles, the risk manager must decide whether to assume or to transfer that risk. Because health care facilities provide services to the community, its employees may be using their own vehicles on company business.

Third-Party Insurance

Third-party insurance is a synonym for liability insurance. Liability insurance always involves three parties—the one who is harmed, the insurer, and the insured who caused the harm or damage. Liability insurance protects the insured from loss arising out of its liability to others for their injury caused by the insured's negligence. The most common forms of third-party coverage that the health care risk manager will encounter are the following:

- Professional liability
- General liability
- Excess/umbrella liability
- Automobile liability
- Garage liability
- Garage keepers' legal liability

- Directors' and officers' liability
- Fiduciary liability
- Heliport/nonowned aircraft liability
- Educational institution/child care center liability

One other area of important coverage considered third-party but not based on negligence is Workers' Compensation. Workers' Compensation is considered social insurance predicated on an employer's obligation created by statutory law. An employer does not have to be negligent for an employee to be eligible for compensation.

Professional Liability

Professional liability, or malpractice coverage, is designed to protect the assets of the facility from the negligent acts or omissions of the hospital's employees that result in patient injury. Patients who believe that they have been injured in the hospital setting often will sue, alleging separate acts of negligence against the treating physicians, the hospital, and its employees.

The facility's employees usually are additional insureds under the institution's policy of professional and general liability insurance. If a hospital employee is named individually in a lawsuit filed against the hospital, the employee's coverage for judgments, settlements, and all costs associated with defending the claim usually will be paid by the hospital's policy. Personal coverage for the clinical activity of employed physicians and surgeons is usually not covered under the standard "employees as additional insureds" endorsement. If individual coverage for them is required in the facility's coverage, a separate endorsement or rider is required. The policy can be written so that its liability insurance is primary over malpractice policies that employees purchase. If a hospital employee is separately insured, the risk manager should find out from the employee who the insurer is so that the defense of the claim can be coordinated with all parties in interest.

Hospital employees, particularly nurses, frequently ask the risk manager whether they should carry their own insurance. In responding to the question, the risk manager should tell the employees what and who the hospital's policy covers. Many health professionals provide their services outside the hospital and may need additional personal insurance coverage. The hospital's policy usually will cover them only for negligent acts and omissions within the scope of their employment. The risk manager should also remind employees that, although the hospital's policy protects them from costs of lawsuits, hospital employees will have no decision-making authority over how their defense is conducted—something they may have with their own policy.

Most physicians on the medical staff carry their own professional liability insurance policies. If the physician and the hospital are both found to be negligent, the hospital may be held financially accountable when the physician has inadequate insurance limits. To keep from being the "deep pocket," many facilities require physicians on the medical staff to carry malpractice insurance with specified limits. Where physicians have challenged the hospital's ability to impose that requirement as a condition of staff membership, the courts have said that the hospital may do so as long as the requirement is not arbitrarily or capriciously applied.

The policy forms used for this professional liability coverage generally contain insuring agreements similar to the following:

The Company (Insurer) agrees to pay on behalf of the Insured (Hospital) all sums the insured shall become legally obligated to pay as damages because of injury to any person or entity arising out of the rendering of or failure to render the following professional services. . . .

The agreement usually is worded to cover the specific nature of services provided by the insured. Each insurer uses different policy forms, and the language of each may contain important basic differences. The risk manager must examine the wording of the facility's professional liability policy and ensure that all services offered to patients are covered. One important distinction made in professional liability policies is between occurrence coverage and claims made coverage.

Occurrence coverage provides protection from claims that arise from events that occur during the policy term, regardless of when the claim is made against the insured. A claim conceivably could be filed today that alleges negligence on the part of the insured 20 years ago, and the insurer who provided the coverage 20 years ago would be obligated to respond on behalf of the insured.

Claims made coverage provides protection only from claims reported or filed during the year that the policy is in force for any incidents that occur either during that year or during any previous period for which the policy holder was continuously insured by the same insurer. There are various options available to insurers using claims made forms that will provide extended coverage. Those options may be referred to as *tail or prior acts coverage.* The majority of insurers writing professional liability coverage will write only claims made coverage in the current environment. Because of the length of time between an incident of malpractice and the actual judgment or settlement of the claim, insurers find it easier to adjust their premium in response to claims activity utilizing claims made.

General Liability

General liability coverage is usually provided by the same insurer that provides professional liability coverage to the health care facility. Those two types of protection frequently are combined in a single policy and differentiated by various coverage parts and endorsements. *General liability,* also known as "premises" liability, provides protection from claims that assert negligence against the insured for events arising out of their nonpatient-care activities. The most common claim is injury suffered by visitors who trip or fall because of some alleged failure of the facility to keep the premises safe.

In addition to bodily injury and property damage, general liability policies may provide coverage for *personal injury,* frequently defined as false arrest; malicious prosecution; wrongful eviction; and libel, slander, or defamation of character. They also cover libel and slander that may arise out of advertising activities, as well as infringement of copyright, title, or slogan.

The risk manager must keep informed about the health care facility's activities so that he or she can ensure that the policy is broad enough to cover new ventures. Some common areas of concern are advertising liability exposure, exposures from child care provided for employees and the community, environmental impairment/pollution exposures, and exposures through management contracts and consulting. The risk manager should review all contracts to determine the insured's requirements for insurance as well as other risk management concerns.

The possibility of a single catastrophic loss covered by general liability insurance presents a greater dollar exposure than the possibility of loss covered by professional liability insurance. For example, injuries to many people as a result of a fire or elevator accident are covered by general liability insurance. Coverage will be provided with a maximum limit per claim as well as an aggregate limit for all claims during a policy term. The insurer will not be responsible for paying claims in excess of the stated limit. For example, a hospital may be covered for up to $1 million per claim but not more than $3 million in the aggregate for all claims arising during the policy term.

Excess or umbrella liability insurance can be purchased to provide additional coverage after the first or primary liability policy has exhausted its limits. Excess coverage usually is purchased at the same time and covers the same policy term as the primary policy. The risk manager should avoid gaps in coverage by ascertaining that all liability policies that are covered by the excess have the same policy-effective dates.

A key element of liability coverage is that the primary insurer has an obligation to pay on behalf of the insured for the insured's legal liability, and retains the right to investigate, defend, and make settlement on behalf of the insured. This means that the insurer has the right to settle a claim even if the insured does not agree. Fortunately, most insureds and insurers resolve claims cooperatively.

Automobile Liability

Health care entities are exposed to liability through the use of motor vehicles. A typical automobile liability policy will provide protection for losses arising out of the ownership, maintenance, and use of owned, hired, and nonowned automobiles. Coverage should be broad enough to provide protection for newly acquired vehicles and leased vehicles.

Most commercial automobile liability policies can be modified to provide additional coverage for garage and parking operations. Garage liability covers the insured for liability caused while hospital employees are driving cars to be parked that are involved in accidents resulting in bodily injury or property damage to others. This coverage does not provide reimbursement for damages to the car the hospital employee is driving.

Garage keepers' Legal Liability Coverage can be purchased to provide Physical Damage Coverage for damages to vehicles in the care, custody, and control of the insured if the insured is held legally liable for the damage.

Insurers determine rates for automobile liability based on loss experience, territory of operation, and the type and use of vehicles. As in physical damage coverage, the risk manager should be able to negotiate a better rate by demonstrating loss-prevention activities and a sizable fleet of vehicles. Other auto coverages that may be needed are uninsured motorists' coverage and personal injury protection that meet state statutes.

Workers' Compensation

All states create a statutory obligation on the part of employers to provide compensation to employees for injuries arising out of and in the course of their employment. Employers may choose to transfer that risk to an insurer, who then acts on behalf of the employer in fulfilling the employer's obligation under the law. *Workers' compensation* is a no-fault insurance system created by state law so that workers may be compensated for any work-related injury regardless of whether they or their employer was at fault. Because workers' compensation is an exclusive remedy for injured employees in most states, employers are protected from the threat of suit brought by employees and the possibility of unlimited damage awards. Some employers may be authorized by a state regulatory board to self-insure their exposure.

Traditionally, insurers providing this coverage include loss prevention and claims service as a means of controlling losses. The cost associated with work-related injuries to health care workers exceeds malpractice costs in some jurisdictions. The premium usually is determined by varied rates set state by state and applied to gross payroll by employment classification as a measure of exposure. Claim history is an important factor in determining ultimate cost. Risk managers should work closely with their human resources and employee health departments in dealing with this risk.

Directors' and Officers' Liability

Directors' and officers' (D & O) liability insurance is designed to protect individuals serving in a governance role from liability claims arising out of errors in judgment, breaches of duty, and other wrongful acts. Individuals serving on hospital boards may delegate authority for day-to-day operations of the institution, but the responsibility for governance cannot be delegated. Coverage is provided on a claims made basis. The policy usually is written to reimburse the named directors and officers for claims brought against them. Claims against directors and officers of hospitals used to be infrequent; however, suits filed by physicians for credentialing decisions and issues of wrongful termination are becoming common. The risk manager should be aware of the exclusions of the hospital's D & O policy and ensure that risk management techniques other than insurance will protect directors and officers for claims of antitrust violations, discrimination claims, and other intentional acts that probably are excluded from insurance coverage. The risk manager also should make sure that the D & O policy covers volunteer members of the board and medical staff committees involved in the quality assurance process and credentialing decisions.

Fiduciary Liability

Fiduciary liability insurance can be obtained to provide protection for those who manage the financial affairs of others. It usually is needed to cover financial officers and pension and health trust administrators, and it can include risk managers who manage self-insured trusts and captives. Coverage provides protection for those named in the various pension plan documents for negligent administration of pension and other similar funds.

Heliport/Nonowned Aircraft Liability

Health care entities that have a dedicated heliport or occasionally have a helicopter land on their premises should carry heliport liability coverage. The coverage is usually reasonably priced and can provide protection not found under traditional liability policies.

Nonowned aircraft liability coverage, also usually priced reasonably, provides coverage for claims asserted against the insured arising out of use of a nonowned aircraft. Frequent air travel by employees or board members should be evaluated to determine the need for this type of coverage. Claims have been made against corporate entities arising out of their sponsorship of meetings wherein employees were victims in commercial air disasters as well as chartered aircraft crashes. Risk managers also should evaluate the adequacy of insurance provided by charter companies and helicopter services.

Educational Institution/Child Care Center Liability

As health care facilities broaden their activities to provide child care services to employees and visitors, additional insurance may be required to cover areas that general and professional liability policies may exclude. Additionally, many health care facilities are affiliated with schools and universities that require special protection for claims that may arise out of the educational environment. Examples of types of claims that may arise under these coverages are failure to educate, wrongful suspension from a program, inadequate supervision, corporal punishment, and failure to maintain sanitary conditions in a child care center, resulting in the spread of contagious illness.

☐ Conclusion

Insurance remains only one tool in the risk management process. The risk manager's primary insurance responsibility is to determine what the institution's exposures are and whether insurance is an appropriate method for treatment of risk. Using insurance will require the risk manager to develop a good working relationship with brokers and insurers. To use insurance effectively, the risk manager must become skilled at developing specifications, directing the broker in selecting markets, evaluating loss experience, and understanding how to interpret coverage.

Reference

1. Smith, B. D. *How Insurance Works: An Introduction to Property and Liability Insurance.* 1st ed. Malvern, PA: Insurance Institute of America, 1984, p. 4.

☐ Bibliography

Best's Insurance Reports. Oldwick, NJ: A. M. Best Co. Updated annually.

MacDonald, M. G., Meyer, K. C., and Essig, B. *Health Care Law: A Practical Guide.* New York City: Matthew Bender & Co., 1987.

Smith, B. D. *How Insurance Works: An Introduction to Property and Liability Insurance.* 1st ed. Malvern, PA: Insurance Institute of America, 1984.

Smith, B. D., Trieschmann, J. S., and Wienong, E. A. *Property and Liability Insurance Principles.* 1st ed. Malvern, PA: Insurance Institute of America, 1987.

Tiller, M. W., Blinn, J. D., and Kelly, J. J. *Essentials of Risk Financing: Volume I.* 1st ed. Malvern, PA: Insurance Institute of America, 1986.

Troyer, G., and Salman, S. *Handbook of Health Care Risk Management.* Rockville, MD: Aspen Publishers, 1986.

Chapter 28

Risk Financing and Funding

Brad R. Norrick

The previous chapter provided an overview of the types of insurance of greatest concern to the health care risk manager. This chapter will explain risk financing, the risk manager's role in risk financing, and why the risk manager should be aware of alternative risk financing approaches.

As insurance becomes more expensive, understanding the strengths and weaknesses of various risk financing alternatives to insurance allows the risk manager to choose a long-term strategy that best serves the institution.

☐ Overview

Before discussing alternatives to conventional insurance, a brief review of insurance pricing and other relevant concepts may be helpful.

Insurance Pricing

An insurance company requests information from the hospital that it uses to determine what the hospital's exposures to loss are so that coverage can be "rated." Typical measurements of exposures requested include number of beds, number of outpatient procedures, number of employed physicians by specialty, total square footage of the institution, number of owned automobiles, and other standard items. For professional liability coverage, the insurance company, using an item of information such as the number of beds, multiplies that number by an industry standard "rate." This rate is calculated by an insurance industry service organization and is based on claims experience in a particular area or industry. As the cost to insurance companies of paying professional liability claims increases, the service organization develops an increased rate. These rates are compiled into a rate manual available to insurance companies. This concept is called *spreading the risk*. As the cost of claims for all hospitals rises, rates for all hospitals increase, regardless of each individual hospital's claims experience.

For example, the annual rate per bed for $1,000,000 in coverage may be $2,000. If the hospital reports an exposure of 200 beds, the rate is multiplied by that number of beds to arrive at a *manual premium* of $400,000. (The insurance company has used rates from the manual to calculate this premium, hence, manual premium.) In addition to this $400,000 figure, outpatient visits might also be multiplied by a rate of $10, for example. Thus, 5,000 outpatient visits would represent $50,000 of premium for the same $1,000,000 of coverage.

If this process were all there was to pricing insurance coverage, premiums would tend to remain fairly stable from year to year. However, two additional elements need to be taken into consideration: the hospital's past claims experience and the competition among insurance companies. Industrywide claims statistics that are compiled to produce manual rates represent the cost for an average hospital. This average cost usually is adjusted to recognize the differences between state laws and other factors. For example, rural hospitals may experience different claims from those of urban hospitals. Insurance companies also use the past losses of an individual hospital to predict future losses for that hospital in much the same manner that the industry service organization predicts average future losses for all hospitals. Thus, the hospital's experience becomes a factor in the premium calculation.

Competition among insurance companies also has an impact on a hospital's premium. The competitiveness of the insurance marketplace is cyclical. For a few years, prices decrease; then, for a few years, they increase. Sometimes the variations in cost are dramatic. In the mid-1970s and mid-1980s, insurance buyers experienced a "hard" market characterized by little competition among insurers, little capacity for high limits of coverage, and high premiums. Between those hard markets was a "soft" market, which brought steady premium reductions and greater availability of coverage.

It is difficult to explain why such cycles occur. The insurance industry is subject to a variety of outside pressures in addition to the cost of claims. Changes in tax law, the rates of return from various investment opportunities, and the complicated process of predicting future losses based on past claims makes it very difficult for an insurance company to project the ultimate cost of its product. An insurer may not know its final cost for many years, so correcting an inappropriate price takes time.

In addition to the *cost* of insurance varying significantly as a result of the insurance cycles, *availability* of coverage at *any* price can be affected. During 1985 and 1986, insurers felt they had lost money on previous years' coverage, so it was not uncommon to see insurers simultaneously reduce limits of insurance, raise deductibles, demand new exclusions, and increase premiums. In some cases, increases were so dramatic that hospitals "went bare" and did without professional liability coverage.

The health care risk manager needs to be aware of these cycles and do everything possible to anticipate and prepare for high insurance premiums and restrictive insurance policies. Searching out alternatives to conventional insurance will allow the health care risk manager to level the peaks and valleys of the insurance market cycles and maintain appropriate coverage at appropriate costs.

Concepts of Conventional Insurance

Most hospitals' professional liability and other liability programs are "layered" to develop the appropriate limits of coverage. Typically, a primary insurer provides the first layer of coverage and excess insurers provide higher layers above this limit. Figure 28-1 displays a liability program that might be purchased from a single insurer or from several insurers. The figure shows four layers of coverage—a primary $100,000 layer (costing $1,000,000 in premium), a layer of $400,000 in excess of $100,000 (costing $750,000), and so on. The total program features a $2,000,000-per-claim limit and costs $3,025,000. Additional limits of coverage in excess of the $2,000,000 displayed might also be purchased. Note the cost of insurance as the layers stack upon one another. The first layer, which has the first $100,000 of coverage for each claim, costs $1,000,000, whereas the layer that has $1,000,000 excess of $1,000,000 costs $600,000. The first layer costs more because the

Figure 28-1. Layers of Coverage: Simplified Version

Total Limits	Layers/Premium	Total Premium
$2,000,000 (Layer 4)	$1,000,000 in excess of $1,000,000/$600,000	$3,025,000
$1,000,000 (Layer 3)	$500,000 in excess of $500,000/$675,000	$2,425,000
$500,000 (Layer 2)	$400,000 in excess of $100,000/$750,000	$1,750,000
$100,000 (Layer 1)	Primary/$1,000,000	$1,000,000

first $100,000 of coverage is almost certain to have several claims brought against it. The upper layer will respond to claims far less often. That is, it would be far more common to have several $25,000 claims than to have several $1,025,000 claims. The insurer providing the first layer needs to collect enough premium to pay those several expected $25,000 claims, meet its expenses, and make a profit.

Insurance companies normally provide two limits of protection on liability policies—a limit for each occurrence and another limit for the annual aggregate. The *each occurrence limit* (also known on some policies as each claim, each injury, each incident, each person, or each disease) is the maximum the insurance company will pay for any one incident. This limit should be set at a level high enough to protect the hospital from an unexpected disaster. For example, the professional liability policy limit should pay claims alleging professional incompetence if failure of an emergency generator affects incubators in the neonatal intensive care unit. Several wrongful death or blindness claims from this single occurrence could cost millions of dollars.

How much coverage is enough? There is no good answer to this question. The risk manager should evaluate a number of important factors in deciding, including the jurisdiction of the hospital, the hospital's past claims experience, and the types and numbers of procedures performed. Damages for claims of medical malpractice have been awarded in excess of $10,000,000; therefore, high limits of coverage should be seriously considered.

The *annual aggregate limit* (also known on some policies as *stop loss* or *loss fund*) is the maximum the insurance company will pay for all occurrences within the insurance policy's annual period. Annual aggregate limits usually are not of concern in policies such as automobile liability, because the possibility of dozens and dozens of unrelated accidents occurring under that coverage is fairly remote. Medical professional liability insurers are very concerned about annual aggregate coverage because a number of unrelated incidents may cause damages to several different individuals in the same policy period.

Figure 28-1 was simplified to give the idea of a layered insurance program. Figure 28-2 displays more completely a typical layered program of medical professional liability insurance. It shows limits for each occurrence and annual aggregate. The primary layer is now expressed as "$100,000 each occurrence, $300,000 annual aggregate." Note that the annual aggregate limit is three times the each occurrence limit. Many insurers will provide this kind of multiple aggregate limit; others will limit their coverage to an annual aggregate limit equal to the each occurrence limit. The important concept in both figure 28-1 and figure 28-2 is that a specific premium is associated with each layer of coverage.

Figure 28-2. Layers of Coverage: Descriptive Version

Each Occurrence Limit	Layer Description	Annual Aggregate Limit
$2,000,000 (Layer 4)	$1,000,000 each occurrence and $3,000,000 annual aggregate in excess of the limits of layer 3.	$6,000,000
$1,000,000 (Layer 3)	$500,000 each occurrence and $1,500,000 annual aggregate in excess of the limits of layer 2.	$3,000,000
$500,000 (Layer 2)	$400,000 each occurrence and $1,200,000 annual aggregate in excess of the limits of layer 1.	$1,500,000
$100,000 (Layer 1)	Primary	$300,000

Access to Capital

Purchasing insurance to protect the institution from claims can be thought of as the cost of access to capital. The money that institutions pay in premium goes into a pool so that, if necessary, an institution can withdraw a large amount of money from the pool to pay a claim. It does not make sense to pay for this access to capital if some other financial arrangement is more cost-effective. It also does not make sense to pay a premium to an insurance company for capital that definitely will be withdrawn, because the insurers will collect not only the cost of the required capital but also an amount to pay taxes, profit, and overhead. An institution that has averaged 10 claims of $10,000 each year for the past decade will pay an excessive premium if it buys insurance coverage for the first $100,000 in claims. Purchasing insurance for expected claims is called *dollar trading* and is cost-prohibitive.

Options other than buying and paying for insurance include using revenues generated by business to pay claims as they are incurred, using available reserve funds to pay claims, or borrowing money or issuing stocks or bonds to access capital.

Depending on the size of claims and how quickly they must be paid, the hospital without insurance coverage may be forced to sell assets. If risk management is defined as finding cost-effective ways to protect the institution's assets, a more formal, premeditated approach to paying claims is preferred.

☐ Alternatives to Conventional Insurance

The risk manager can employ several alternatives to conventional insurance to protect the institution against claims. The most widely used methods are discussed here.

Deductibles

Agreeing to a large deductible amount is an effective method of reducing the cost of insurance. As the amount of deductible increases, the cost of insurance provided by the policy should decrease. The risk manager should carefully consider the cost-benefit ratio when determining what a deductible should be. Accepting a $5,000 deductible on a homeowner's policy may save premium, but it makes sense only if there is a means of paying the $5,000 in the event of a claim. There is a risk management maxim that states "don't risk a lot to gain a little." Saving $100 to move a deductible from $50 to $100 probably makes sense. To save $100 by moving the deductible from $50 to $5,000 does not.

The medical professional liability insurance marketplace routinely provides deductible programs. Normally, when a deductible is employed, the insurance company will continue to provide claims adjusting and other services. Depending on the size of the deductible, an insurance company may require the hospital to have collateral for claims the insurance company will pay that fall within the deductible. The hospital will then be asked to reimburse the company for the amount of the deductible. This collateral may take the form of an escrow deposit, a letter of indemnification, a letter of credit, a promissory note, or some other commitment to repay.

The key to determining the viability of using deductibles is an analysis of past claims experience. If losses within the deductible typically are less costly than the premium for insuring that layer, a deductible makes sense. Insurance consultants, brokers, and actuaries can assist in analyzing past loss information to help make these decisions. Because all insurance premiums inevitably are based on the cost of claims, an assessment of how the hospital's experience compares with the average is essential. Some institutions have poorer loss histories than average; purchasing conventional insurance may be in their short-term best interests. (In the long term, they may find insurance unavailable.) On the other hand, only 60 to 70 cents of each insurance premium dollar is earmarked for the payment of claims; therefore, accepting a deductible or other "loss responsive" program may save money in the long run.

Retrospective Rating

Another alternative to conventional insurance, which is offered by insurance companies, is retrospective rating. *Retro* plans are less common in medical professional liability coverage than they are in other lines, such as workers' compensation. Instead of providing an immediate cost reduction, as in a deductible plan, a retro adjusts the premium based on actual loss experience. Typically, six months after policy expiration, a calculation is made to determine how much money the insurer actually needed to pay claims and cover taxes, profits, and overhead. After this calculation, annual readjustments are performed. If loss experience is good, premium dollars may be returned. If loss experience is poor, additional dollars may be due. Retros are loss-responsive and can reward or penalize an institution for its own claims experience. Unfortunately, because retros are administered by insurance companies, such items as the company's tax and overhead expenses will still be paid by the hospital.

Because a professional medical liability claim usually is not paid until long after the incident occurs (the "long tail"), retros have not been popular for this coverage. The claims adjusting that occurs after the claim is made and, if the claim is in litigation, the trial, can take several years. The administrative burden of calculating and adjusting premiums for several years as claims develop and are reported tends to offset some of the retro's advantages. However, because tax laws in most cases recognize retro premiums as deductible, some for-profit institutions are pursuing retro programs. Some group plans featuring retros are available to both for-profit and not-for-profit institutions. In some cases, retros have been provided in excess liability programs.

Excess Coverage

Deductibles and retro programs are alternatives to complete coverage or conventional insurance. They do not, however, replace insurance entirely. Excess coverage should be purchased above the deductible or above the retro plan. This excess coverage provides the high limits of protection that an institution needs. Because of the infrequency of loss in upper layers, excess insurance normally is not purchased on a loss-responsive basis. However, some excess programs do feature *maintenance deductibles*. After a primary program's aggregate limits are exhausted, the excess policy's maintenance deductible applies to each claim. For example, assume an excess policy includes a $100,000 maintenance deductible. If the underlying policy's limits are used up, the insured becomes responsible for the first $100,000 of each additional claim brought.

Other Alternatives

No matter how much insurance is purchased, risk still exists. Some claims will not be covered by insurance policies; others may be so catastrophic that they exceed the total amount of insurance available. Alternatives to conventional insurance are loss-responsive—that is, the cost of the insurance will increase as claims increase and decrease as claims decrease. Each alternative demands that a hospital accept some risk. Therefore, these alternatives are harder to budget than conventional insurance and demand strong commitment to loss control and quality assurance.

Table 28-1 provides a framework for evaluating some of a hospital's alternatives. Various institutional objectives are matrixed against insurance programs and several alternative risk funding programs. Ns and Ys ("no" and "yes") show whether or not the particular program meets an objective. For example, a deductible, prefunded approach (explained below) does not improve cash flow, but does keep overhead low. The alternative programs and the objectives listed are far from all-inclusive. The risk manager should also consider what the marketplace is like for purchasing coverage in excess of these programs. For example, a program featuring a $100,000 deductible may meet the risk manager's objectives, but if insurers will offer coverage only in excess of a $500,000 deductible, another option may become more attractive. Each of these alternative programs can be considered on both an individual institution basis and a group basis. Before a group alternative can be evaluated, the group itself needs to be evaluated. The more popular group approaches will be discussed later in this chapter.

Prefunding

Loss-responsive programs must be funded, whether through a fund established and administered by the hospital (prefunded) for that purpose or out of operations at the time claims are paid (postfunded). If the hospital has a large deductible or other loss-responsive program, *prefunding*—that is, setting aside funds to pay "expected" future claims—is strongly recommended. Prefunding establishes the credibility of the hospital in the minds of excess insurers. It also ties current costs to current revenues, which makes auditors and regulators happy. As funds accrue in excess of actual loss payments, greater retentions or assumptions of risk are possible in the future. In some cases, excess insurance will not be available without prefunding.

Self-Insured Retention

A self-insured retention (SIR) program looks much like a deductible, except that under an SIR the hospital (or a company that sells this service) rather than an insurer adjusts the claims, including investigating the incident, getting witnesses' statements, determining the value of the claim, and assessing the hospital's culpability for the incident. The hospital also chooses defense counsel and negotiates the amount of the final settlement for damages.

An SIR should be prefunded. Forecasting future claims is a complicated task that requires reviewing past losses and projecting these losses into the future. Actuaries, consultants, and brokers can assist the risk manager in forecasting costs of losses so that the risk manager can be certain that the money is there when claims need to be paid.

Table 28-1. Risk Funding Programs

Objectives	Full Insurance	Retrospective Rating	Prefunded			Postfunded			
			Deductible	SIR	Captive	Deductible	SIR	Spread Loss	Noninsurance
Low overhead	N	N	Y	Y	N	Y	Y	Y	Y
Claims control	N	N	N	Y	Y	N	Y	Y	Y
Ease in budgeting	Y	Y	Y	Y	Y	Y	N	N	N
Good cash flow	N	N	N	N	N	Y	Y	Y	Y
Security required	N	N	N	N	Y	Y	Y	Y	N
Broad coverage	?	?	?	Y	Y	?	Y	Y	Y
Tax deductibility	Y	Y	N	N	N	N	N	N	N
Assurance of continued operations	Y	Y	Y	Y	Y	N	N	N	N
Formal program to access in-excess insurance	Y	Y	Y	Y	Y	?	N	Y	N
In-house administration costs	N	N	Y	Y	Y	Y	Y	Y	Y

Note: Y = yes; N = no; SIR = self-insured retention.

A dedicated self-insurance trust fund is the vehicle of choice for funding SIRs for not-for-profit hospitals. Funds are placed in trust with a financial institution where they can earn investment income until claims require payment. Because excess insurers recognize SIRs as an appropriate method for structuring a program, they will sell excess insurance over the per-occurrence limit for the trust. The use of a properly set-up trust also meets Medicare reimbursement requirements. A trust is relatively inexpensive and easy to administer. For-profit hospitals will find setting aside funds to be an expensive proposition when compared with paying premiums because prefunding an SIR is not tax deductible. However, as claims are paid, the amounts paid are deductible, and the for-profit institution has the use of the funds in the meantime.

Having an SIR trust fund with the hospital's bank may help the hospital's overall financial health. The hospital's financial institution may be willing to extend credit to the hospital only if it has "compensating balances" in deposits. In some cases, self-insurance funds can be recognized as fulfilling an institution's compensating balance requirements, thereby providing some compensation for the loss of tax deductibility.

Possible restrictions on the use of SIRs exist. Operating or management agreements, leases, mortgages, loan agreements, or bond indentures may prohibit anything other than full insurance. In many cases, the use of SIRs can be negotiated with creditors and lessors as long as the program is rational and adequately funded.

Administering an SIR program is less costly, especially for a not-for-profit hospital, than most other alternatives. However, because the institution must either self-administer claims and claims information or contract with providers of those services, some associated costs must be taken into consideration when comparing an SIR program with a fully insured plan. In addition, various costs of litigating claims, trustee fees, and actuarial expenses must be considered. Figure 28-3 returns to the layered insurance program and displays a $500,000 SIR replacing the first two layers shown in figure 28-1. Note that the self-insured retention funding amount is only $250,000 less than the conventional insurance was for this layer. Why aren't there greater savings? Trust fund contributions remain the hospital's money-earning investment income. If losses are controlled through aggressive quality assurance and claims administration programs, surpluses will result, and the hospital can use those surpluses to meet other needs. However, no alternative to insurance will ever cost less than the actual cost of claims. Alternatives to conventional insurance are designed to smooth the market cycles so that costs remain stable and coverage remains more available. Costs can be reduced only as far as claims are reduced.

Figure 28-3. Self-Insured Retention Program

Total Limits	Total Layer/Premium (Funding)	Cost
$2,000,000 (Layer 3)	$1,000,000 in excess of layer 2 limits/$600,000 premium	$2,775,000
$1,000,000 (Layer 2)	$500,000 in excess of layer 1 limits/$675,000 premium	$2,175,000
$500,000 (Layer 1)	Self-insured retention funding $1,500,000 premium	$1,500,000

An SIR program supported by a trust offers several advantages to a hospital, but does not solve all problems. Unless carefully designed and funded and properly presented to insurers and reinsurers, excess coverage may not be obtainable. Medicare reimbursement requirements eliminate flexibility in the use of investment income. The income earned by the trust must become part of the fund. If the hospital plans to combine its insurance with contract physicians' insurance or with coverage for a joint venture, an SIR trust probably would not work, because for-profit and not-for-profit dollars cannot be mixed.

Spread Loss Programs

A *spread loss program,* also known as a banking excess plan or chronological stabilization program, funds claims when they are ready for payment but on a prearranged basis. The spread loss program is a financing plan to get the money it needs to handle claims when they are ready to be paid, without actually purchasing insurance. Risk is not transferred but is retained by the hospital. The benefit of this approach is that it spreads the effect of poor loss experience over several years. When claims must be paid, the hospital borrows capital and repays the borrowed money over time. A spread loss program can include participation by both an insurance company and a lender (bank or savings and loan). This approach can be broken into five steps:

1. Before it experiences losses, the hospital determines its maximum ability to repay funds loaned to pay losses (for example, $1,000,000 per year).
2. The hospital negotiates a line of credit with prearranged interest and repayment schedules (for example, $5,000,000 to be paid over five years at prime interest).
3. If the hospital decides that an insurance policy is necessary to satisfy management agreements or other requirements, it contracts with a "fronting" insurance company. The fronting insurance company does not provide actual insurance; instead, it provides a document that looks exactly like an insurance policy. To state agencies, suppliers, and physicians, it appears to be insurance. The hospital can provide certificates of insurance or even a complete policy if requested, but no insurance exists. If claims occur, the hospital and its financial institution, not the fronting insurer, pay them.
4. The hospital and the fronting insurer negotiate a fee for the use of the insurer's policy and other services. The hospital and the fronting insurer also negotiate any required security (for example, a letter of indemnification and letter of credit), to assure the insurance company that it will not actually have to pay any claims.
5. If significant losses occur, the hospital borrows sufficient funds from the lender, as it has prearranged, to pay the losses and begins the repayment schedule.

In some cases an insurance company will both front the spread loss program and act as the lender. If a policy, certificates, or other services are not needed, the program can be set up without an insurance company.

Positive aspects of a spread loss program include (1) the ability to combine not-for-profit entities with for-profit entities, (2) little up-front cost, and (3) the security of having a loan agreement in place before funds actually are needed. Unfortunately, two or three years of poor experience can produce an overwhelming repayment burden to a hospital. Medicare reimbursement also is complicated because of the postfunding mechanism instead of prepayment. Excess insurance may be difficult to purchase because insurers may not consider a spread loss program to be prudent.

Captive Insurance Companies

A *captive insurance company* is a limited-purpose insurance company, set up in a jurisdiction that is favorable to such companies (that is, "procaptive") to provide insurance to entities that are usually also the company's owners.

"Limited purpose" means that the captive insurance company has been incorporated, capitalized, and organized with the intent of providing insurance coverage for a single entity or a single association. Unlike a standard insurance company, a captive insurance company will not provide multiple lines of insurance to unrelated entities.

Procaptive jurisdictions include Bermuda, Vermont, and several others. Whether or not a jurisdiction is considered procaptive depends on how it regulates insurance companies. Anticaptive states require several million dollars in capital to create a new insurance company and may also require lengthy annual reports, regular state audits, and other paperwork. On the other hand, Bermuda, which is procaptive, requires only $120,000 in initial capital to set up a captive insurance company and very little paperwork; it allows captives tremendous flexibility in investment policy and premiums paid. A jurisdiction's regulations regarding such issues as how reinsurance may be purchased and involvement in insurance insolvency or guaranty funds also determine whether it is considered procaptive.

The hospital may set up a captive insurance company in Bermuda so that it can write insurance for the hospital. The risk manager may decide that rather than establishing a $500,000 SIR, the captive insurance company will issue a $500,000 insurance policy. Money that would be put aside in a trust fund under an SIR plan is instead paid as premium to the Bermuda captive. As claims develop and need to be paid, money is transferred from the Bermuda captive to pay those claims. Claims administration, selection of defense counsel, and all other day-to-day handling of the captive program parallel the SIR plan. The captive insurance company simply has taken the place of the trust as the depository of funds for future claims payments.

Captive insurance companies can be direct insurers (also known as policy-issuing captives) or reinsurers for the conventional insurance market (fronted captives). In the former instance, no insurance company involvement is required, and the captive insurance company itself provides the insurance policy and any appropriate insurance certificates or other required services. In the latter case, the fronted captive "reinsures" an insurance company. The insurance company issues a policy and provides required services but reinsures or passes off a portion of its risk (for example, the first $500,000 of any one loss) to the captive carrier. When claims need to be paid, the fronting company bills the captive. If certificates of insurance and other company services are needed, this fronted approach may make sense. Unfortunately, insurance companies providing these services usually charge substantial percentages of premium for their involvement.

Why set up a subsidiary insurance company and incur incorporation, management, legal, and accounting costs? Why capitalize an insurance company and be required to attend board meetings and pay fronting costs? Why not simply set up an SIR/trust and avoid the effort and inconvenience? For a large not-for-profit hospital with no interest in combining physician or for-profit ventures, there is probably no good reason. However, if the hospital wants to combine various entities or pool resources with other institutions, or if it has other needs an SIR approach cannot address, a captive may make sense.

Within the past several years, many states have approved legislation that makes them attractive captive jurisdictions. In addition to Bermuda and Vermont, Hawaii, Colorado, and Georgia (and many others) have procaptive legislation. However, more than half the world's captives are in Bermuda.

Bond-Financed Self-Insurance

Bond-financed self-insurance combines the best elements of an SIR program with the better aspects of spread loss approaches. Using this concept, the hospital assumes an SIR and immediately prefunds potential liabilities by issuing tax-exempt bonds. Usually, tax-exempt financing produces the lowest interest cost for an institution and ensures that there will be sufficient funds to meet any immediate claim obligations. In Texas, bond issues may be undertaken to finance self-insurance for a single hospital, a hospital chain, or a group of unaffiliated hospitals. The laws of the state in which the hospital is located and the hospital's financial condition and tax status will determine whether bond financing makes sense for the institution.

Combination Programs

Few health care providers have the financial resources or the mettle for total self-insurance. As the various risk-financing alternatives are considered, the risk manager must be concerned with whether excess insurance can be placed over the program. Capping loss potential above the limits of an SIR, captive, or spread loss program does not necessarily require a return to conventional coverage, however. An SIR can be topped by a retrospectively rated layer. Many policies placed through a captive company have small deductibles so that small claims will not require that funds be moved out of an offshore jurisdiction on a regular basis. An example of a combination program follows:

- *First layer:* $10,000 deductible to handle small claims
- *Second layer:* $500,000 reinsured through a standard insurance company to the institution's captive insurance company
- *Layer $1,500,000 in excess of $500,000:* Written with an insurance company providing a retrospective rating plan that allows a reward or penalty of up to 25 percent of premium based on loss experience
- *Coverage in excess of $2,000,000:* Written on a conventional basis with several standard insurance companies in the United States and overseas

Combinations for coverage become even more complicated when group purchasing arrangements are used.

Group Approaches

Several of the approaches already covered can be used successfully for groups or associations of health care providers. For example, several insurance companies owned by groups of hospitals currently exist. Bond financing for groups is also possible. Two newer alternatives involving group coverages are getting attention: risk retention groups and purchasing groups.

Risk Retention Groups

In 1986, Congress enacted amendments to the Product Liability Risk Retention Act of 1981 that expanded the act to apply to all liability risks, not just product liability. Those amendments created the *risk retention group* (RRG). An RRG is an insurance company that provides liability coverage to its members/owners. Members must be "similar or related entities" with respect to liabilities to which they are exposed. This language is interpreted to allow hospitals and physicians to be members of the same RRG.

An RRG must be licensed as an insurance company in at least one of the 50 states. The states that have chosen to attract captive insurance companies are logical choices for licensing RRGs because their regulatory climate and capitalization requirements are attractive to small insurance companies. In fact, many domestically domiciled captives automatically qualify as RRGs. Unlike a captive, which must be licensed or fronted in every state in which its insureds do business, an RRG need be licensed in only one state. This difference significantly lessens the regulatory requirements an RRG must meet. RRGs are exempt from non-licensing states' laws governing insurance companies except in the following areas:

- An RRG may be required to demonstrate its financial responsibility if required to do so as a condition for obtaining a license or permit.
- State antitrust, consumer protection, and criminal laws are not preempted.
- State requirements regarding unfair claim practices, premium taxes, and participation in residual market programs, such as assigned risk pools, still apply.
- Members must be notified that state insolvency guaranty funds will not be available in the event of an RRG failure.
- Requirements may be imposed that are different from state to state.

317

Several questions regarding states' authority over RRGs are still being sorted out. Despite federal legislation, several states are claiming jurisdiction over out-of-state RRGs and are attempting to regulate them. However, by the end of 1987, at least 37 RRGs were functioning. Of those, 11 were health care related.

An RRG is attractive to a group if the members want to combine a number of different entities or address risks regionally or nationally. Premiums paid into an RRG will be tax-deductible, assuming the RRG has sufficient membership and "pools" the risks of its members. To meet Internal Revenue Service requirements for deductibility as an insurance premium, the RRG must "spread" the risk among several members and "transfer" risks by sharing the financial burden of claims. Advantages of RRGs are still being sorted out. If states continue to assert their rights to regulate RRGs, much of the RRG's benefit will disappear. A more intrinsic disadvantage of an RRG is that it is a group plan. Unless an entity can find an attractive and homogeneous group to join, it may not want to pool risks and stand the chance of paying for other entities' pooled claims experience. In 1989, we saw the financial failure of two RRGs. States may use these failures to justify greater regulation to protect consumers. These failures also serve as a warning to the prudent risk manager to fully and carefully research any RRG proposal.

Purchasing Groups

The purchasing group, a hybrid of standard insurance and RRGs, also was created by the Risk Retention Act. *Purchasing groups* allow members to purchase insurance from standard insurance companies on a group basis without state regulation. Purchasing groups must be made up of "similar or related" entities. There are no specific requirements about the structure of a purchasing group except that one of its purposes must be to buy insurance. Existing groups, such as trade associations, may, by board resolution, become purchasing groups. Per the act, a purchasing group is not subject to state insurance regulators' examination, but the insurance company providing coverage to the group is subject to all standard state controls.

Purchasing groups provide an opportunity for individual entities to pool their buying power so that they get more competitive pricing than they can individually. Purchasing groups also sidestep difficult issues such as capitalization, organization, and risk sharing. As a result, purchasing groups can be put together with very short lead time. Unfortunately, purchasing groups are still subject to the cycles of the conventional insurance marketplace. Also, by teaming with others, a purchasing group member may find that it is forced to accept a standard set of coverages that is not tailored to its individual needs.

Like RRGs, purchasing groups are under scrutiny by state regulators. In 1987, several states had legislation pending that would interpret the federal act in their jurisdictions. For example, in 1987, Arkansas charged a $400 annual filing fee and required annual information about purchasing groups on specified state forms. Until some of those regulatory questions are fully answered, RRGs and purchasing groups will not reach their full potential.

Combining Coverages Using Group Purchasing

A hospital may explore several alternatives to insurance on a group basis using a combination of approaches. For example, an individual institution may accept a deductible and pool the next layer of protection with a group. Conventional insurance may then be purchased above the group layer.

Because many large medical professional liability insurance companies will become involved with a hospital only if it has a large "retention," small institutions may be unable to get such coverage. In such cases, using an approach with a group of similarly situated hospitals may be attractive to small institutions.

☐ Conclusion

In addition to those discussed here, new risk financing alternatives are certain to become available in the future. For example, because of its tax-deferred interest accumulation, life insurance currently is being used to fund some liability exposures. As tax laws change and interest rates vary, new financial mechanisms will evolve. The risk manager who is knowledgeable about techniques for risk financing can help the institution to accurately predict its cost for payment of claims and thus save money. In this area more than almost any other, the risk manager can demonstrate the value to the institution of a risk management program. Fully considering all the alternatives to funding risks and providing protection for the institution's assets are at the heart of risk management. As the insurance marketplace, laws, and the health care industry change, it behooves the risk manager to keep abreast of the various alternatives to meet the challenge of risk financing.

☐ Bibliography

American Agent & Broker. St. Louis: Commerce Publishing Co. Published monthly.

Best's Review: Property/Casualty Insurance Edition. Oldwick, NJ: A. M. Best Co. Published monthly.

CPCU Journal. Malvern, PA: Society of Chartered Property and Casualty Underwriters. Published quarterly.

Insurance Review. New York City: Insurance Information Institute. Published monthly.

National Underwriter Property & Casualty/Risk & Benefits Management. Chicago: National Underwriter Co. Published weekly.

Risk Management. New York City: Risk Management Society Publishing. Published monthly.

Part Six

Other Risk Management Issues

Although there are tasks common to all risk managers, each risk manager's job description is different. Some risk managers are lawyers and combine risk management with corporate legal work. Some are radiology technicians and take radiology calls once each week in addition to their risk management duties. Some were previously employed as nurses and have responsibility for quality assurance as well as risk management. This last section includes information on issues in which risk managers may or may not be involved. However, even risk managers who do not have contract review programs, who do not advise on employment issues, or who are not directly involved in managing records can assist those who do have these responsibilities by learning the principles discussed in these chapters.

Chapter 29

Contract Review

Linda Marie Harpster

Although hospitals have developed an increased awareness of the value of good business practices, many have not yet developed contract review programs. Outside counsel shudder at suggestions that risk managers who are not lawyers can assume responsibility for reviewing contracts. Lawyers who have never worked in hospitals probably are unaware, however, of the proliferation and the variety of contracts to be found there.

In many hospitals, contracts are not reviewed by an officer of the corporation, much less by outside counsel. Many are negotiated and signed by the manager of the department whose business is affected by the contract, and if they are read at all, they are read by that manager. Hospitals that are aware that a contract review program is an important element of loss control may have the hospital's risk manager set up such a program or may have in-house counsel in addition to a risk management program.

Contracts are called by a variety of names, including "contract," "agreement," "letter of agreement," "memorandum," or "memorandum of understanding." Some contracts are not called any of those names but are reached through correspondence between the parties. Some are not in writing but may nevertheless be enforceable as contracts. Because the risk manager understands the hospital's operation and is, by training and experience, the person best equipped to anticipate problems, risk management review of contracts will prevent costly contract disputes.

☐ Review by Outside Counsel

If the hospital does not have in-house counsel, the risk manager can make decisions about which contracts need to be reviewed by outside counsel. The more experienced the risk manager is in reviewing contracts, the fewer the number of contracts that will need outside review.

However, certain contracts will always be sent for outside review because the law is constantly changing, the exposure is great, or an independent party needs to have the responsibility. Contracts with physicians fall in this category, even if the risk manager is a lawyer. Also, outside counsel should review any joint venture agreements in which the hospital will be sharing profit and risk with an outside party, whether the outside party is a for-profit or not-for-profit entity. Ventures with outside entities may involve the hospital in prohibited antitrust activity or activity that violates Medicare fraud and abuse laws or, in the case of not-for-profit hospitals, jeopardizes the hospital's tax-exempt status. Institutions that contract with pharmaceutical companies for the development of new drugs or with other companies developing products and equipment using new technology will want to protect themselves from product liability claims. Joint ventures between organizations can have the effect of aggregating the employees of both organizations for the purpose of imposing IRS tests for nondiscrimination in employee benefits.

For any of those exposures, the penalties are severe enough to require outside legal review. A good rule for the new risk manager to follow is to get outside review of any agreement that is not within the experience of hospital personnel or where there may be considerable exposure that risk management review may not protect against.

However, risk managers, whether or not they are lawyers, can and should set up contract review and central contract maintenance programs in their hospitals. Figure 29-1 shows a sample policy describing a contract review program. Many contracts for equipment purchase or service agreements for equipment, educational affiliation agreements, and contracts with allied health professionals may need minimal legal review if the risk

Figure 29-1.   Sample Corporate Policy: Contract Review

Policy: All lease, purchase, affiliation, professional, consulting, and consignment agreements with third parties should be reduced to writing, reviewed by the risk manager (or in-house counsel), and signed by a corporate officer, or, when appropriate, by the department manager of purchasing.

Responsibility: Management committee; department managers; risk manager.

Implementation:

1. The following is a list of types of agreements within the hospital:

    a. Major hospital services
    b. Physician services
    c. Professional services
    d. Educational affiliation agreements
    e. Transfer agreements
    f. Deeds, leases, easements, permits
    g. Consignments
    h. Equipment contracts
    i. Maintenance and service agreements
    j. Agreements with consultants
    k. Shared service agreements
    l. Provision for any other service or equipment not otherwise listed

2. Drafting of contracts:

    a. The party contracting with the hospital may provide the contract.
    b. If a contract is not provided, the risk manager will assist in developing an agreement or will review a manager's draft.
    c. All contracts will be reviewed by the risk manager prior to signature by the appropriate vice-president or by the president.
    d. At least two signed originals of all agreements will be secured—one for the hospital and one for the contracted party(ies).
    e. The department manager/management committee member responsible for the execution of the contract may request a copy for reference to the terms of the agreement.
    f. File maintenance for contracts and leases is provided for in corporate policy #_____.
    g. Requests for outside legal services should be made to the risk manager.

management review is done knowledgeably and carefully. A nonlawyer risk manager can save the hospital time and money by knowing what lawyers look for in contracts and sending to outside counsel only contracts that need to be reviewed by someone who has expertise in an area outside the risk manager's knowledge.

☐ The Nature of Contracts

A contract is the final, written product of a planning process. During that process, each party involved in the relationship has anticipated what it needs from the relationship and what problems may arise. The parties have negotiated contract terms that will resolve those problems if they arise. A thorough contracting procedure makes the hospital's future more certain and its financial position more stable.

A risk manager who becomes involved in the contracting process may encounter resistance from some hospital department managers. For example, a manager who is negotiating for the purchase of a piece of equipment may fear that suggesting changes to terms of the vendor's standard contract is an expression of mistrust of the vendor and that questioning standard contract terms will disturb a well-functioning relationship. The risk manager, however, is a more objective third party not directly involved in negotiation who can assist by posing "what if" questions about problems that could arise during the contract term. By offering that service, the risk manager helps operational managers understand what the risks are in certain contract provisions and helps them devise a negotiating strategy to use with the vendor. Regardless of the manager's trust and confidence in the vendor's sales representative during negotiation, the terms of the contract probably will be carried out by other people in the company who may not be as competent or as honest and trustworthy.

The company may not necessarily fulfill verbal promises made by salespeople and relied on by the buyer but not incorporated into the final written agreement. Most contracts have a clause toward the end of the document stating that no other promises, negotiations, or understandings have become part of the final agreement. As the buyer of the products or services, the hospital must make sure that all the key terms upon which it relied in making the purchase are included in the document. If they are not, it will be difficult to prove that they were part of the agreement. Even without a specific contract clause, a general rule of contract law is that the final written agreement incorporates the entire understanding of the parties. It is in the best interests of all the parties to a contract to avoid the expense and time involved in having to sort out fault or liability after a difference arises as to what the terms of a contract really are.

☐ Common Misconceptions about Contracts

There are several common misconceptions about contracts that can affect risk management in health care organizations.

Changes in Company-Supplied Contracts

One misconception is that company-supplied contracts cannot be changed. Lawyers, with their love of small print, arcane language, and 8½" × 14" paper, have made contracts seem unnecessarily formidable. Contracts appear to be nonnegotiable because when they are presented to the hospital, they have been typeset and single-spaced. However, changes can and should be made in those contracts even if the hospital has been told "This is our standard contract," and "No one has ever before objected to it." Despite the manager's reluctance, there are a variety of acceptable methods by which amendments can be made to preprinted documents. Changes can be made by striking through the written text, by writing in margins, by adding additional terms in an addendum that the parties will sign, by adding a cover letter incorporated into the contract that makes it clear that there are new or different terms to be included in the contract, or by requiring the vendor to make changes in its document. Each new term, additional term, or any of the text that is struck out should be signed or initialed by both parties. The hospital's risk manager must encourage operational managers to be a little braver in dealing with vendors if changes or additions to a vendor-provided contract will help protect the hospital.

Lengthy Contracts and Comprehension

Another myth about contracts is that lengthy contracts are difficult to comprehend. If all the terms that have been negotiated by the parties are included in a contract, and if the parties have done a good job of anticipating and resolving problems that could arise in the future and have incorporated the solutions into the contract, it will probably be a lengthy document. Although a one-page letter of understanding may be far easier to work with in the short run, such a letter cannot address the problems that will arise during the course of the parties' relationship. The more the parties put into writing, the less is left to an uncertain future.

Oral versus Written Contracts

Some people mistakenly believe that contracts must be in writing to be valid. Many oral contracts are, in fact, enforceable. Hospital managers or nonmanagement employees may be entering into a number of oral agreements over the telephone or in other ways that they may not realize that they will be bound to. Whenever possible, such agreements should be put into writing. Contracts can also come about if the parties demonstrate by their conduct that they intended to have a contract. The greatest problem with oral contracts or contracts implied by the parties' conduct is that it is difficult to prove what the terms of the contract are if a dispute arises.

If the parties take a dispute over unwritten contract terms to court, the court will look at the evidence presented to determine what the intent of the parties was at the time they entered into the contract. The same test is used when written contract terms are ambiguous or the written contract has not addressed the issue in dispute. During the dispute, each party will present evidence of what the parties actually intended *at the time* the contract was made. The party that prevails in such a dispute will be the one who has the most persuasive evidence of actual intent.

Penalties for Breaches of Contract

Another misconception is that a party who breaches a contract will be penalized. Generally, the law does not penalize a party who breaks a contract. A court will award contract damages sufficient to compensate the nonbreaching party for actual damages, but the intent is not to punish the breaching party. The court is interested only in either restoring the nonbreaching party to where it would have been without the breach or giving it the advantage it would have received had the contract been fully executed. Punitive damage awards belong in the law of tort, not in contract law.

☐ Specific Contract Clauses of Interest to Risk Managers

Risk managers who know specific contract terms to look for will save the hospital money in outside counsel fees by doing some of the work in-house. The following are some of the things to look for when reviewing contracts.

Effective Date and Termination Date

Generally, contracts will have three dates. There will be the effective date of the contract, which is the date the contract takes effect. There will be a termination date, which is the date at which the contract is fully executed. The date of signature of the contract also may be indicated, probably at the end with the signature lines. The contract may be signed before, after, or concurrent with its effective date. Ideally, the contract is signed on or before the effective date. If the written contract is not signed by the time parties have begun executing it and a dispute arises over what the terms are, it may be more difficult to resolve the dispute amicably.

Many contracts have clauses describing responsibilities that one or both parties assumed under the contract and which continue beyond the termination date. Such responsibilities may include maintaining certain records, being responsible for liability that may arise from negligent performance of the contract, warranties that may survive the contract termination, promises not to compete for a designated length of time after the termination date, promises not to hire personnel for a certain length of time, and the like. If the hospital agrees to terms that give it continuing responsibilities beyond the termination date, it will at least want to include a reasonable time limit on them so that the contract does not remain open-ended after it is fully executed. There also must be a mechanism to ensure that someone is aware of those contract terms and is prepared to carry out the responsibilities and to protect the hospital against any adverse outcome from them.

Many times, the termination clause provides that the contract will automatically renew if it is not specifically terminated by the parties. Those provisions can benefit the hospital if they lock in favorable pricing terms. However, automatic renewals without a system for periodic review may mean that the contract is not reviewed on a timely basis. Automatic renewal provisions should be thought through carefully, and unless they are favorable to the hospital, should be eliminated in favor of definite termination dates. A "diary" or "tickler" system, such as the one described in the section entitled "Elements of a Contract Review Program," reminds the risk manager to review contracts at appropriate intervals.

It is also possible to include a clause in a long-term contract that provides for periodic renegotiation of only certain of its terms. Frequently those will be price terms. If any portion of a contract is renegotiated, the entire contract should be reviewed in light of the effect that the renegotiated term may have. If the contract is reviewed and none of the provisions needs to change, a letter signed by the parties agreeing to continue the terms of the contract is, as a general rule, sufficient to extend the contract for the designated length of time.

Signatures

The importance of signing a contract correctly frequently is overlooked. The name of the hospital or of the appropriate corporation or partnership that is the party to the contract will precede the signature of the person who is signing. The capacity in which the person is signing will follow the signature. If signed that way, it is clear that the person who signed is signing as the agent of the corporation and not as an individual. The following example illustrates the signature line of a contract entered into by St. Elsewhere Hospital, with Ms. Mary Jones signing as agent for St. Elsewhere in her capacity as president:

Entered into this _____ day of _____, 1990

St. Elsewhere Hospital (the entity)

by Mary Jones (its agent)

President (the agent's capacity)

Contracts may have a signature line for someone to witness the signature. The theory of having a signature witnessed is that, should a dispute ever arise about whether the person whose signature appears is actually the person who signed, the person who witnessed the signature will testify as to whose signature it is. The witness does not need to know the contents of the document, only that he or she actually witnessed the signing of the document.

Sometimes contracts are notarized, particularly those that will be recorded in the clerk's office or that are required to be notarized by the law of the jurisdiction. Otherwise, a notary's signature generally is not required on contracts.

Insurance

If risk managers review nothing else in hospital contracts, they should review the insurance provisions to make sure that all the exposures created by the hospital's business relationship with the contracting party are appropriately covered. Depending on the exposure being insured, the hospital can provide the insurance, the other party or parties can provide the insurance, or coverages can be split between the parties and the named insureds specified in the policy. In some business situations, which party carries what coverage and in what amounts is open for negotiation. For example, if the hospital owns medical office space and leases it to physicians, it may carry casualty insurance on the building and require tenants to carry insurance for protecting themselves against loss of their property and equipment. The contract will specify which party or parties will carry general liability insurance and who will be covered by the policy.

Deciding who will be responsible for a particular insurance coverage depends on several factors, among them the amount of control the hospital wishes to exert over cost and over who the company, agent, or broker will be. The hospital can maintain control of those factors if it agrees to carry the insurance. If cost and control are not issues to the hospital, the other party may agree to carry insurance to cover a particular exposure. Limits of the coverage, regardless of whose responsibility it is to secure it, can be spelled out in the contract. The contract price may vary, depending on who buys insurance, because the party buying insurance may wish to build in insurance as a cost.

A more thorough analysis of insurance issues can be found in chapter 27. This discussion will illustrate some insurance issues raised in the context of reviewing hospital contracts. The following examples discuss specific kinds of hospital contracts and the insurance provisions to be included.

Example 1: Affiliation with a School

In a clinical affiliation with a school of nursing, the primary exposure to be covered by contract is the potential injury to the hospital's patients as a result of the students' negligence. Because the students are not parties to the contract, the school should either provide malpractice liability insurance covering students' errors or omissions or show written evidence that each student entering into the clinical affiliation has professional liability insurance.

Covering the possibility of injury to a student or a faculty member as a result of accident or illness while in the hospital may be more difficult. The school's workers' compensation policy will cover faculty, but students may not be covered under either the school's or the hospital's policy. If students are not covered, the hospital may want to require them to carry health insurance, so that in the event of illness or injury the hospital is assured of payment for treatment it may agree to provide. If students or faculty are required to use their automobiles in the course of the clinical experience, there should be insurance provisions for personal injury, liability, and perhaps loss or damage to property.

Example 2: Purchase of Equipment

If the contract is for the purchase of a piece of equipment, the risk manager must know when title to the equipment will pass to the hospital so that the hospital's insurance coverage can begin when title passes. For example, if the equipment is lost or damaged in transit, a dispute may arise if the party who owns the equipment has not insured it. Because the insurance required to be provided by common carriers frequently is insufficient to pay the replacement cost of expensive pieces of equipment, either the vendor or the hospital should provide additional coverage.

Once the risk manager has determined the kinds of insurance that are necessary and has negotiated which party is to provide the insurance, the next issue is in what amounts insurance should be carried. The hospital's insurance agent or broker, as part of the service provided, generally is willing to review contracts to determine the kinds and amounts of insurance needed. If it is important to the hospital to make sure that the other party to the contract is carrying the appropriate insurance in the appropriate amounts, that party can be required by contract to provide certificates of insurance, to have its insurance agent or company notify the hospital of any changes in that party's coverage, or even to name the hospital as an additional insured on the policy in the appropriate situations.

Performance Standards

Risk managers may be less involved with the provisions of contracts that specify the parties' performance than they are with contract formalities or with the insurance provisions. However, the person responsible for the execution of the contract must be familiar with the standards built into the contract by which performance is to be measured. For example, if the hospital buys an expensive piece of equipment to perform mammograms, a good revenue stream from the service depends on the equipment experiencing little or no downtime. A performance standard for such equipment that can be measured and included in the contract provisions makes it easier for the hospital to demonstrate that the equipment does not perform as promised. The contract may specify, for example, that the equipment will perform satisfactorily 95 percent of the time in use over a certain period of time. Expectations of performance, including the date the equipment will be received and installed, should be discussed with the company representative before the contract is signed. When agreement is reached, those performance expectations will be included as written terms to the contract.

Written performance expectations are enforced more effectively if they are followed by specific remedies if the equipment fails to meet the agreed-upon standard. It is not enough to state what the expectation is if the parties do not anticipate and put into the written terms what the remedy is. In the preceding example, the hospital may want the company to pay the hospital an amount equal to the revenue lost because the equipment did not work. However, "lost revenue" clauses are extremely difficult to negotiate. The company may be open to other suggestions, such as extending the warranty period for a mutually agreeable length of time, providing loaner equipment during repair, paying any costs the hospital incurs as the result of having to transfer patients to another facility, or, if attempted repairs are not successful after a designated length of time, replacing the equipment.

Many times contracts will have liquidated damages clauses as remedies for less-than-expected performance. *Liquidated damages provisions* state that a specified amount of money will be paid to the nonbreaching party as total and "final" compensation for the breach. Liquidated damages are a good idea for the hospital, but may not be enforceable unless carefully drafted. The amount stated as liquidated damages must be rationally related to the actual damages that the hospital can be expected to suffer. If it is not made clear on the face of the contract that the amount is rationally related, the entire clause may be found to be unenforceable as a penalty for the breach of contract.

The way to protect the validity of such a clause is to expressly state the formula or method by which the amount was arrived at so that it is clear that the amount is a reasonable estimate of actual damages. In the previous example, the hospital's estimate of lost revenue from downtime of the mammography equipment should be based on past experience or on a realistic assessment of demand for the test, rather than on a projection of the most income it would be possible to make.

Amendments

Contracts may be amended, but amendments should be in writing and signed by the parties in the same manner as the original contract. The amendment first should state clearly which portions of the original contract are no longer valid. Then the new terms should be clearly stated. Unless otherwise written, the amendment or amendments will run concurrently with the existing contract and will terminate when the contract terminates.

Hold Harmless Provisions

A hold harmless or indemnification provision in a contract is a method by which Party A to the contract requires Party B to assume costs of claims when both are sued and Party B is found to be the negligent party. For example, a hospital that contracts with a physician group to staff its emergency department may include a hold harmless provision in the contract. If enforceable, the clause will require that the physician group reimburse the hospital for the costs the hospital incurred as a result of the claim if a physician was the negligent party. The physician group will not be responsible for costs of claims if the hospital is the negligent party. The hold harmless provision may be general and include "all costs" associated with the claim, or it may specify costs of "judgments, settlements, court costs, legal fees, witness costs, investigative fees," or other specified costs.

If the party contracting with the hospital provides its standard contract with a hold harmless provision in it, the risk management responsibility is to make sure that the clause is worded narrowly and describes specifically what problems or claims are anticipated to be covered. If the clause is too broadly stated, it should be narrowed to protect only against those exposures the parties anticipate that it is appropriate for the hospital to cover. In a contract calling for maintenance of a piece of equipment, a hold harmless clause should not include holding the vendor harmless for "all claims," because "all claims" will include claims for personal injury resulting from negligence in servicing the equipment. It is not appropriate for the vendor—or the hospital, for that matter—to hold itself harmless for its own errors or omissions, because such a clause probably is not enforceable. But it may be appropriate for the hospital to hold the vendor harmless for claims resulting from repairs or modifications that the hospital made to the equipment or from negligent operation of the equipment by hospital employees.

For example, in a software licensing agreement, a narrowly worded hold harmless clause could be drafted in which the hospital will specify that it will be indemnified by the software supplier against any costs or other liabilities that the hospital incurs as a result of any claim for trademark or service-mark infringement. When the hospital uses service-marked software through a license agreement, it has no way of controlling or protecting itself against such claims; only the vendor has that ability. In that instance, it is appropriate for the hospital to be indemnified against for a claim over which it had no control.

The hospital's first approach when presented with a vendor-prepared agreement that includes a broadly drafted, one-sided hold harmless provision is to negotiate the provision out of the contract. If a company insists on keeping the hold harmless provision in, the hospital should insist that the provision be reciprocal. To make it so, the risk manager should add a second hold harmless paragraph that tracks the language of the first hold harmless paragraph exactly, but reverses the names of the parties, using the company's name as the party providing the indemnification and the hospital's name as the party being indemnified.

The risk manager may also ask the hospital's insurer to review the contract to make sure that including a hold harmless clause does not adversely affect the hospital's insurance coverage.

Access to Books and Records

Federal law requires that contracts with parties who will provide a service to the hospital that could cost more than $10,000 per year give the controller general of the hospital or his or her designate access to the books and records of that contractor and any subcontractors. The clause should specify that access will be given to the books and records for up to four years after the expiration of the contract. Figure 29-2 provides sample language for the access-to-books-and-records clause.

Situs

Toward the end of every contract, there generally is a clause specifying under what state laws the contract will be construed. Usually, vendors specify the state that is most convenient to them—the state in which their home office is located and their corporate attorneys are headquartered. Unless the law of the vendor's state is more favorable for the hospital, the hospital can insist that the contract be construed under the laws of the state in which the hospital is located. Generally, the hospital does business only in its home state, whereas the vendor may do business in several states. The vendor has come to the hospital's state specifically to provide the product or service that is the subject of the contract. It is not unreasonable for the hospital to expect that because the vendor is doing business in the hospital's home state, the vendor is knowledgeable about state laws and can litigate any contract disputes in that state.

□ Elements of a Contract Review Program

If an organized system of contract review does not exist in the hospital, the risk manager who expends the energy to set one up will find that managing the system can fit easily into the risk management routine. A comprehensive system to manage the institution's contracting process should be outlined in hospital policies. There should be a written policy delineating who has the authority to commit the institution by signing contracts, a policy requiring risk management review of all contracts, and a policy designating who has the authority to seek outside legal review.

Important risk management practices for safekeeping of hospital contracts also should be included in a policy. Those elements include a central file in the administrative office, under the jurisdiction of either the risk manager or an officer of the corporation, in which the originals of all contracts are kept; a backup system that contains copies of all contracts,

Figure 29-2. Sample Language for Access-to-Books-and-Records Clause

If _____ is determined to be a "subcontractor" under the provisions of subparagraph (i) of Section 1861(v)(1) of the Social Security Act, and if this Agreement is determined to be a "contract for services" with a value or cost of $10,000 or more over a twelve (12)-month period, also as defined by the foregoing Act,_____ shall, until the expiration of four (4) years of the furnishing of services under this Agreement, make available upon the request of the Secretary of Health and Human Services, the Comptroller General, or their representatives, this Agreement and the books, documents, and records as may be necessary to certify the nature and extent of the costs incurred hereunder by the Hospital, and _____ shall make a similar requirement of any "related organization" performing services pursuant to this Agreement if such "services" have a value or cost of $10,000 or more over a twelve (12)-month period, all as defined by the foregoing Act.

in case the file of originals is destroyed; and a tickler system that pulls up contracts within a specified number of days before their anniversary date or expiration date so that they can be reviewed at least annually.

Determination of Signatory Authority

If no policy exists to provide guidance to managers on who can sign contracts, the risk manager and the chief financial officer can develop one. Generally, the policy will use the contract amount to determine at what level of the organization the contract can be signed, but sometimes the length of the contract or the kind of contract is determinative. For example, a capital lease for equipment differs significantly from a three-month lease for temporary, replacement equipment, and may require signing at a higher level. Alternatively, the hospital's malpractice exposure may be greater under a service agreement for patient care equipment than for a more expensive or longer-term service agreement for office equipment in the administrative suite, thus requiring a high-level signature.

In determining the organizational level at which a contract should be signed, the risk manager will look for total exposure under the contract, not just the contract amount. An educational affiliation agreement, for example, may not call for payment at all, but it does expose the hospital to significant liability for negligence of students that results in harm to patients. The greater the exposure under the contract, including payment amount and liability exposure, the higher should be the rank of the person signing. Contracts for which the hospital's exposure exceeds a designated amount or whose term exceeds a designated length, usually one year, should require the signature of an officer of the corporation.

Central File Maintenance

An effective contract review system depends on maintaining all contracts in the same location. Wherever a written contract exists, the hospital should have a document that has on it *original* signatures of all the parties. Ideally, those contracts will be kept in a centrally located, locked, fireproof cabinet. Once a contract has expired or has been terminated, it should be removed from the active file to a file of executed contracts. Only those who are authorized by policy should have access to the file of active contracts, not only to ensure confidentiality where appropriate, but also to ensure that originals are never removed from the file except by the person whose responsibility it is to maintain the file. Managers who are responsible for administering contracts will need working copies of the contracts in their offices, but they should not have the originals. Figure 29-3 is a sample policy describing a system of centrally maintaining contracts and leases.

Good risk management practice is to have a second, backup file for all contracts in case anything happens to the file of originals. As a safeguard, a comprehensive list of all contracts in the file may be maintained and updated monthly, and a second copy kept in a place different from the original.

Periodic Contract Review

Because contracts may never be looked at again after they are signed, instituting a system *requiring* review of all contracts at least annually may prevent costly contract disputes. If the business practices of the parties are different than was contemplated when the contract was entered into, it will be difficult during a contract dispute to determine what the terms of the contract are—whether they are what the written document says or what the actual practices of the parties are. Another risk is that if one party permits the other to vary from the written terms, it may be construed in court as a waiver by the party permitting the variation.

Figure 29-3.   Corporate Policy File Maintenance for Contracts and Leases

---

Policy: A file of all contracts and leases for hospital services, physician services, professional services, transfer agreements, educational affiliations, real estate agreements, and consignments will be maintained in an up-to-date and easily accessible manner in the administrative offices.

Responsibility: Risk manager (or in-house counsel); management committee; department managers; director, internal audit.

Implementation:

1. The purchasing office maintains originals of all purchase orders.
2. As soon as signatures have been obtained, all original contracts, leases, and agreements will be sent to the risk manager to be filed, except those assigned a purchase order number. Those will be maintained in the purchasing department.
3. Upon receipt of the properly executed contract, lease, or agreement, the risk manager will follow these procedures:

   a. All contracts, leases, and agreements will be filed in a locked filing cabinet.
   b. An alphabetically sequenced master list and a categorically sequenced master list will be maintained for cross-referencepurposes. Those lists will include name of the party the hospital is entering into the contract with, effective date, expiration date, term, and category.
   c. All requests for copies of a contract, lease, or agreement must be approved by the risk manager.
   d. Operational managers will be notified of contract expiration at least 90 days prior to actual expiration.

4. The contracts, leases, agreements, alphabetically sequenced master list, and categorically sequenced master list maintained in the administrative offices may be removed temporarily by the director of internal audit once a year in support of the annual financial audit conducted by the hospital's certified public accounting firm.
5. The corporate policy on record retention indicates length of retention of outdated contracts and the form in which they are retained.

Because health care is heavily regulated, changing federal and state laws require frequent reexamination of the hospital's business relationships. Contract review not only encourages hospitals to include contract provisions mandated by legislation, such as the access-to-books-and-records clause, but also allows hospitals to rethink business relationships as the laws change and to negotiate terms that accommodate the changing regulations.

A tickler system for periodic review of all contracts helps avoid problems and is easy to administer once it is in place. Using a comprehensive list of all hospital contracts, the risk manager assigns annual review dates to each. The annual review date of every contract, regardless of its terms, should be at least 90 days prior to its anniversary or termination date. Added to the minimum period for review will be the amount of time that the contract specifies that notice must be given of termination or renegotiation. At the beginning of each month, the contracts to be reviewed that month are pulled from the file and sent to operational managers for review of business practices, performance specifications, and contract price.

At the same time, the risk manager will review that month's contracts to determine whether all exposures are either eliminated or minimized, or whether new legislation or regulations require contract changes. When all reviews are completed, operational managers will renegotiate contracts as necessary and remand contracts that have reached the end of their terms to the file of fully executed contracts. If a given contract is to continue on the same terms, a letter so stating may be sent to the other party to the contract.

☐ Hospital-Based Physician Contracts

Contracts with hospital-based physicians, such as for emergency services, radiology, anesthesiology, or pathology, provide the hospital with an advantage that it does not have with other physicians on its medical staff. The hospital can build provisions into such contracts that it may be reluctant to impose on or unable to demand of staff physicians who are not bound by a contract or employed by the hospital. Contracts with hospital-based physicians always should be reviewed by an attorney because they have implications for Medicare and Medicaid reimbursement and may have an impact on the hospital's tax-exempt status and bond financing. However, the risk manager can also review those contracts, including elements that outside attorneys may not be asked to look at.

The risk manager may be particularly interested, for example, in what the contract says about credentialing the contracted physicians through the medical staff procedure, including credentialing physicians whose only role is to provide coverage, physicians who may be moonlighting with the group, and allied health professionals who may be employed by the group and provide service at the hospital. Effective physician participation in risk management and quality assurance programs should be detailed in the contract with the hospital.

Particularly with the emergency services contract, the risk manager may want to negotiate the physicians' participation in community relations programs, such as community education or medical screenings open to the public. Such programs provide visibility for the physicians in the community. Having the physicians interact with neighborhood residents before they provide service may make the filing of malpractice suits less likely.

Other areas in physician contracts for risk management input include the allocation of control between the hospital's administration and the physician group. Although the hospital needs advice from physicians when deciding to purchase expensive pieces of equipment, for example, it must maintain control of the cost of the equipment. It also must ensure that consideration has been given to the equipment's safety features, training of personnel to use the equipment, cost and quality of maintenance, ease of securing replacement parts, and other administrative issues. The contract should specify that the physician group may not bind the hospital as its agent in the purchase of equipment and supplies.

Another administrative control issue involves the hiring, firing, and disciplining of staff. Hospital staff in radiology, emergency services, and pathology get medical direction from the physicians in the department and administrative supervision from hospital management. For the hospital to maintain its Medicare reimbursement and to maintain high-quality medical care, there must be medical direction of hospital staff. However, the hospital is responsible for overall supervision of its staff, and it must decide administrative issues of productivity and compliance with policies and procedures. On the issues of hiring, firing, and disciplining of hospital staff, the contract must state unequivocally that the hospital maintains administrative control and that medical direction is provided by the physicians.

The risk manager should be particularly interested in the insurance provisions of physician contracts. The kinds and amounts of coverage, who is covered, and whose responsibility it is to provide insurance should be specified in the contract. The hospital should require that it be notified by the physician's carrier 30 days in advance of cancellation, expiration, or other termination of coverage.

The risk manager should anticipate such issues as how physicians will be covered for acts and omissions incurred during the contract but not reported until after the physician has left the group or after the contract with the group terminates. The risk manager should look closely at the individual and aggregate limits of the policy and at whether the physicians are insured individually. It is important to know whether the group uses moonlighting physicians and, if so, how these physicians are covered through the insurance provisions.

☐ Student Affiliation Agreements

The hospital faces risk of loss when nursing students, physical therapy students, biomedical technician students, and the like work with patients or patient care equipment in the hospital. If there are no written agreements with educational or training organizations to cover those exposures, the risk manager must persuade hospital administration that, even though the students are not paid employees, there should be a contract describing the clinical affiliation arrangement with the educational or training organization. Clinical affiliations with persons who are not students of a school should be avoided because there is no successful way to protect the hospital from the risk that those people may present in a clinical setting. They should be encouraged to affiliate through a school.

When reading clinical affiliation agreements, risk managers should check to see that the following items appear:

1. The hospital should reserve the right to refuse access to anyone who it believes does not comply with its policies and procedures; who does not meet hospital expectations with regard to appropriate dress, behavior, and health practices; or to anyone who poses an immediate hazard to or disruption of patient care. The decision not to admit certain students to the program or to deny a student access to the facility should be made by the hospital, at its sole discretion.
2. Provisions regarding confidentiality of patient information should be clearly stated and a remedy for breach of this provision should be included.
3. The school should be required to cooperate in claims investigation procedures and in securing the cooperation of witnesses if there is a claim involving a student.
4. The hospital should not accept responsibility for loss or damage to property of students or faculty, including autos parked in the hospital's lot.
5. The school should be required to carry malpractice insurance covering its faculty, if faculty are going to be in the hospital, as well as its students, or should warrant that students carry their own professional liability insurance in an amount acceptable to the hospital. In addition, the hospital should make sure that the school has workers' compensation coverage for any of its faculty who may be injured on hospital property. Students should be covered by workers' compensation if such coverage is possible under the laws of the state and if it is available.
6. The hospital, if it decides to provide emergency health care service to students, may wish to require that the students show evidence of coverage under a policy of health insurance so that the hospital is assured of a third-party payer for follow-up care. If the hospital does provide emergency care, all follow-up care should be the responsibility of the student unless the hospital makes an exception in order to avoid a claim. If the hospital's emergency department or employee health service offers health care services to students, there may be some additional exposure for the hospital if the student alleges negligent treatment. If health care is provided by emergency department physicians, the exposure will belong to the physicians or perhaps be shared between the physician and the hospital.
7. The hospital should require that students have a health examination of the same kind and quality as is required of other hospital employees.
8. Regardless of whether the hospital or the school has supervisory responsibility for the students, the contract should state specifically that the hospital maintains administrative control of its patient care areas.

☐ Contracts for the Purchase of Equipment

Most contracts for the routine purchase of equipment and supplies are handled through the hospital's purchasing department. The risk manager should be familiar with the hospital's standard purchase order and influence the development of terms advantageous to the hospital.

Many times, major pieces of equipment are covered by contracts other than the hospital's purchase order. Even if not provided for in a separate contract, there will be risk management issues to be analyzed in equipment purchases. A good risk management tool is a capital equipment form for internal use that includes questions regarding safety features of the equipment. Prior to the selection of a vendor, the form should be circulated to all departments that will be involved with the equipment. Using the form to evaluate equipment will bring out issues that should be incorporated in the contract terms. The American Hospital Association, and probably other professional and trade organizations, can provide samples of such forms that a risk manager can use as a starting point for developing a hospital-specific form.

Following are some risk management/contract considerations that should be included in this form:

1. Whether and how often the equipment will be inserviced and who will provide the training. The company should be required to leave training materials with the hospital.
2. The warranties that the vendor provides and what activities of the hospital invalidate the warranties.
3. How maintenance will be done, whether by contract service or in-house. If done in-house or by a vendor other than the vendor who sold the equipment, how the warranties will be affected.
4. If the equipment is technically innovative, how upgrading of the equipment will be handled. Much diagnostic equipment has a computer component. The hospital may want to get both hardware and software upgrades as they become available.
5. Provisions for confidentiality of information, where applicable.
6. If the hospital leases rather than owns the equipment, who insures it, who calibrates it, and who maintains it.
7. The shelf life, composition, handling, precautions to be taken with, and safe disposal of, any hazardous chemical used with the equipment.
8. Accessibility of replacement parts for repairs of the equipment.
9. The right to terminate without penalty for delivery of goods that do not conform to the quality or quantity specified or for failure to maintain the delivery schedule, and provisions for liquidated damages.
10. A mechanism for dealing with recalls of, significant incidents with, claims against, suits against, or governmental investigations of the equipment or product.
11. Adequacy of insurance during transit and during installation.

☐ Service Agreements for Equipment

Service contracts for hospital equipment seldom are reviewed by the hospital's attorneys unless the hospital has in-house counsel. Because most such agreements follow a standard format, the risk manager who undertakes a contract review program will soon become familiar with the standard terms of service contracts and will be able to review most of them quickly. The risk manager's focus will be on service contracts for equipment that affects patient care. When reviewing service contracts, the risk manager, working with the purchasing department (if service contracts go through that department) and the operational manager, should be aware of the following concerns:

1. *Termination provisions:* The hospital needs to know under what conditions the vendor is able to terminate the contract. If there is only one suitable vendor of the service, the hospital will want to negotiate specific termination conditions so that the vendor cannot terminate without cause, which would leave

the hospital without a service vendor. The conditions under which the hospital can terminate also should be spelled out.

2. *Access to books and records:* Because service on major pieces of equipment will exceed $10,000 annually, the hospital must have on record that the vendor agrees to open the books relating to its service to the U.S. Department of Health and Human Services. This clause probably will not appear in most service contracts. An alternative to negotiating it into the contract is to have the vendor sign a separate statement agreeing to access that the hospital can keep on file.

3. *Hours of service:* Contracts for patient care equipment should include provisions for emergency and after-hours service and should specify the time limit within which the company must provide service once notified.

4. *Storing equipment and parts:* If the hospital agrees to store on its premises equipment, parts, and tools belonging to the company, the contract should specify who is responsible for damage or loss.

5. *Warranties:* The hospital should be aware of what, if any, warranty is provided by the vendor. If the equipment is serviced by the same vendor that sold the equipment, the contract should include a paragraph similar to the following:
   - Any provisions of the agreement for purchase of the equipment or the warranty statement that are more favorable to the hospital than the provisions of this agreement remain in effect.

6. *Exclusions from service:* The operational manager must be aware of and agree to any service that is excluded from the contract and the conditions under which any warranty for the service may not apply. Typically, the service warranty will not apply if the hospital has added nonapproved parts or made other engineering changes, has not controlled the environment according to the equipment specifications, or has had other maintenance or repair service done by nonauthorized personnel.

7. *Assignment:* The contract terms should specify whether the vendor is able to assign the contract to another vendor without the hospital's consent or to have the service performed by someone with whom the hospital has not contracted.

8. *Workers' compensation:* The hospital must be assured that the workers' compensation insurance is provided for the company's service representatives.

9. *Limitations of liability:* The risk manager should read carefully the section of the contract describing the vendor's liability and advise the person signing the contract of its impact. Vendors almost always specify that they will not be liable for lost profits or for incidental or consequential damages. Many provide that the hospital's sole remedy for damages resulting from repair is limited to actual damages or the contract amount, whichever is less. Any clause limiting the vendor's liability for damages must, at the least, include a statement such as the following:
   - This limitation of liability will not apply to claims by the hospital or a third party for personal injury or damage to property attributable to the negligent acts or omissions of the company, its agents, or employees arising out of services provided under this agreement.

An indemnification clause such as the following, if the vendor agrees to include it, better serves the hospital:
   - The company agrees to indemnify and hold the hospital harmless from and against any and all claims, demands, suits, and expenses by reason of injury or death of any person(s) or damage to any property attributable to the negligent acts or omissions of the company, its agents, or employees arising out of services provided under this agreement.

☐ Independent Contractors

Many hospitals use nonphysician independent contractors to provide health-related services, including speech pathologists, occupational therapists, or exercise teachers for hospital-sponsored exercise classes. When the hospital contracts with an individual rather than with a company, there are a variety of liability issues to be anticipated and provided for through a contract with the individual. An independent contractor will not be covered by the hospital's workers' compensation policy and may not be eligible to buy workers' compensation insurance. When contracting with an individual rather than a company, the hospital must determine in advance how to protect itself from suit should the individual be injured while on the hospital's property.

Determination of Independent Contractors versus Employees

A major issue for risk management is that unless carefully drafted, contracts with independent contractors may be construed to be employment contracts. If an independent contractor is determined to be an employee rather than an independent contractor, the hospital may be found to be liable for contributions of federal and state taxes not paid by the individual. It may be required to provide other benefits to the contractor that it did not initially intend to provide, or it may face a wrongful termination suit or defend against malpractice liability for the contractor's actions and for which it was intended that the contractor be held liable. To avoid problems with those contracts, risk managers should make sure that they contain a clause that states specifically that the individual is not receiving health insurance benefits, life insurance, paid vacation time, or any other benefits that employees receive. Additional protection is added by a clause that says that the individual is an independent contractor and not an employee. But this clause by itself is not enough if the other provisions of the contract give the impression that the individual is functioning as an employee and receives the benefits of employees.

Assurance of Confidentiality

The hospital should anticipate and provide for the protection of confidential patient information, and, just as critical, the protection of hospital proprietary information. An independent contractor who works in a hospital's marketing department, for example, can easily move from that hospital to another and share the hospital's proprietary information with other hospitals unless specifically prohibited from doing so by contract.

Other Considerations

The hospital must assure itself that individuals with whom it contracts have the appropriate current professional licensure and also any required occupational licenses that the local jurisdiction may require. The hospital may require the individual to sign a contract with noncompete provisions in appropriate circumstances. If the clauses include the appropriate time and geographic limitations, they will be enforceable. The hospital should insist that the individual carry the appropriate professional liability insurance coverage if it is available. Although the contract should describe performance specifications, they should not be drafted to look like a job description or be in the hospital's job description format, to protect against the contract being mistaken for an employment contract.

☐ Conclusion

As the hospital's risk manager gains experience in contract review, the variety of contracts that he or she can review competently will grow. License agreements for computer software seem to be fairly standard from company to company. A risk manager who has worked with the hospital's in-house counsel or an outside attorney on one such agreement may develop the expertise to make standard license agreements part of the contract review process and refer only nonstandard clauses to attorneys. Most maintenance and service agreements for hospital equipment are reviewable in-house if the reviewer, either the hospital's risk manager or in-house counsel, has developed expertise in the area.

There are many instances when a hospital has an advantage in a contracting situation if the hospital provides the initial draft of the contract to the outside party. The hospital-drafted contract will likely contain provisions that are more favorable to the hospital than will a vendor-provided contract and give the hospital a better bargaining position than the vendor. A risk manager who is knowledgeable about hospital operations can work with other hospital personnel to oversee the drafting of such contracts and then send the draft to in-house counsel or the outside attorney for comment, where appropriate.

The more work that can be done in-house, either by in-house counsel or the risk manager, even if the risk manager is not a lawyer, the more the hospital can save in legal fees. *But a word of caution is in order.* Any savings can easily be wiped out if the risk manager does not make appropriate decisions about getting legal advice. Where doubt exists about the legal impact of any hospital contract, the cost-effective approach is to get expert advice. Paying outside counsel to step in after a problem is discovered usually is a lot more expensive than seeking counsel's advice to avoid problems.

Chapter 30

Employment Issues

James H. Kizziar, Jr., and Gregory E. Alvarez

Although the functions of a health care institution could not be performed without employees, the hospital's relationship with its employees has become an increasing source of claims and potential liability. Federal, state, and even local governments continue to regulate the employment relationship ever more closely, and courts increasingly constrain employers from taking arbitrary and subjective actions toward members of their work force. This chapter will provide an overview of statutory and regulatory requirements imposed by governmental authorities, as well as actions that can be taken to minimize risks in these areas.

☐ Selection of Applicants

Hospitals seek to employ highly motivated and knowledgeable employees who are dedicated to providing high-quality patient care. In order to secure such a work force, hospitals must recruit and select qualified individuals while complying with a myriad of governmental requirements and restrictions.

Recruitment and Advertising

A hospital should ensure that the means used to announce vacancies and recruit applicants are not suspect under equal employment laws. A hospital's reliance principally on word-of-mouth recruiting could be viewed as discriminatory if the makeup of the hospital's work force does not substantially reflect the racial, ethnic, or sex composition of the appropriate labor market.[1] Word-of-mouth recruiting may tend to perpetuate the current makeup of the work force and exclude qualified minorities from the hiring process. Hospitals should utilize a wide variety of recruitment sources for both general and licensed employees. For example, vacancy notices could be provided to state and local government employment agencies, nursing and technical schools, minority and women's placement services, and other sources that provide racial and ethnic minorities, as well as both males and females, with information on employment opportunities. Contact with such diverse recruiting sources may also be required to ensure that hospitals with federal government contracts meet their affirmative action obligations under Executive Order 11246.[2]

Hospitals should carefully scrutinize print advertisements for language or inferences that may be interpreted as discriminatory. Hospitals should avoid sex-designated job titles or descriptions and use, for example, the term "repair person" rather than "repairman." Hospitals also should ensure that advertisements are not listed under a sex-designated column such as "Help Wanted—Female." They also should avoid references to age unless a minimum age is required by statute or regulation. Finally, each advertisement should state that the hospital is an equal opportunity employer (EOE) to reaffirm its non-discriminatory recruitment and hiring practices.

Employment Application

Generally, questions asked of potential employees that do not have a bona fide business justification may be suspect under federal, state, or local equal employment statutes, regulations, and ordinances. Moreover, some preemployment inquiries that do not appear improper on their face may still present legal problems if information the hospital obtains through them is used for an improper purpose, such as to limit, segregate, or restrict the employment of individuals within protected categories.

Hospitals should seek only information that is relevant to the determination of whether applicants have the requisite qualifications for the jobs for which they are applying. Seeking information on an employment application that identifies a person's minority status, sex, age, marital status, religion, or potential handicap conditions is ill-advised and may create a perception that the hospital is considering those factors in selecting employees. In developing employment applications, hospitals should also consider a job applicant's right of privacy. Employers do not need to know certain personal, nonjob-related facts, such as current personal relationships and sexual history. Asking questions about such facts could be construed as a potential invasion of privacy.

One approach to obtaining information is to have two forms: an employment application and a postemployment data sheet; the latter is completed following the applicant's selection by the hospital. This procedure allows the hospital to seek information on the application form that is pertinent to making a hiring decision while avoiding potential liability for invasion of privacy or violation of equal employment laws. The follow-up form would allow the hospital, after hiring, to obtain such data as marital status, number and age of children, race, sex, and other facts necessary for insurance, security, Equal Employment Opportunity Commission (EEOC) reporting, or other legitimate business purposes. Such information should be maintained in a separate record apart from the employee's personnel file.

Preemployment Physicals

Inquiring about an applicant's disabilities or illnesses may raise questions under federal and state law. Such inquiries could be construed as seeking to identify applicants' handicaps and using that information to disqualify them.

The Vocational Rehabilitation Act of 1973 provides that no otherwise qualified individual shall be excluded from participation in or be subjected to discrimination under "any program or activity receiving Federal financial assistance."[3] Therefore, any hospital participating in the Medicare program is subject to the Rehabilitation Act. Under the federal regulations promulgated in connection with the act, any hospital requiring a determination of an applicant's or employee's handicap may require the applicant or employee to provide medical documentation or, as an alternative, may require the applicant to undergo a medical examination.[4] The results of the physical examination must remain confidential and be used solely for the purposes of affirmative action and proper job placement.[5] The information may not be used to exclude or otherwise limit the employment opportunities of qualified handicapped individuals.

When considering the employment of an applicant, a hospital may make an offer of employment conditional upon a physical examination. A hospital's policies should state that the physical is only to determine the extent of an applicant's handicap and the possibility of reasonable accommodation and not to exclude qualified handicapped persons from employment. The hospital should explain that policy to every applicant who receives a conditional employment offer.

With regard to preemployment medical examination questionnaire forms, there are some questions a hospital should not ask—for example, the applicant's date of birth. That question could conceivably be used as evidence of age discrimination.

Also, a hospital should not ask the individual's height and weight. The EEOC and the courts have ruled that minimum height and weight requirements are illegal if they screen out a disproportionate number of minority group individuals or women, and if the employer cannot show that those standards are essential to the safe performance of the job in question.[6] A safer practice would be to have the physician who conducts the physical examination ask the applicant those questions directly if the physician feels that the questions are necessary to assess the individual's overall physical condition as it relates to the individual's ability to perform work for the hospital.

Negligent Hiring Claims

Under the legal doctrine of *respondeat superior*, employers are responsible for the work-related actions of their employees because they have the responsibility to direct and supervise the way that employees do their jobs. Employers also have been faced with claims by injured third parties asserting that the employer has an affirmative duty to hire only competent employees who do not pose a threat to patients, coworkers, or the general public.[7] At least 26 states now permit recovery under this "negligent hiring" theory.[8]

Although the elements of a negligent hiring claim may vary, in general a claimant must prove:

1. The existence of an employment relationship between the hospital and the person who caused the claimant's injury
2. That the employee was incompetent or unfit for the job, which resulted in an unreasonable risk to the public (for example, patients, coworkers, or hospital visitors) coming into contact with the employee
3. That the hospital knew, or could have known with reasonable effort, of such incompetence or danger
4. That the employee's act or omission actually caused the claimant's injury
5. That the hospital's negligence in hiring or retaining the employee directly caused the claimant's injuries

To reduce the risk of negligent hiring claims, hospitals should carefully review an applicant's background before extending an offer of employment. This review may vary, based on the position and the prospective employee's anticipated contact with patients, visitors, and the general public. Precautions may include:

1. Examining the employment application to determine whether it seeks sufficient information on an applicant's background, qualifications, licensure, prior work record, and criminal conviction history
2. Ensuring that the applicant properly completes the employment application and does not omit any information requested therein
3. If applicable, confirming an applicant's license or certification and, where applicable law permits, inquiring with the appropriate regulatory agency in each state where

the licensed applicant has worked about complaints or sanctions that may have been issued against him or her

4. Verifying prior employment references, especially where the applicant worked in the same position for which he or she is presently seeking employment

5. Documenting in writing and retaining all information obtained regarding the applicant, particularly verbal employment references

☐ Claims Arising from the Employment Relationship

The following sections discuss the most common potential areas for claims arising from employment relationships.

Employment Discrimination

There are four general theories on which claimants may bring charges of employment discrimination:

1. Treatment of certain individuals that is less favorable than treatment of others in similar circumstances (that is, disparate, or different, treatment) because of race, color, religion, sex, or national origin

2. Policies or practices that perpetuate the effects of past discrimination

3. Policies or practices that are neutral on their face but nevertheless have an adverse impact on a specific minority, age group, or sex that is not justified by business necessity

4. Failure to reasonably accommodate an employee's handicap condition or religious practices

All claims of employment discrimination arise under one or more of those theories.

Title VII of the Civil Rights Act of 1964[9] (Title VII) and the other federal laws and orders prohibiting employment discrimination[10] require that covered employers provide equal employment opportunities in all aspects of employment, including recruitment and selection of employees, compensation, training, promotion, evaluation, discipline, and discharge. Title VII covers hospitals with 15 or more employees and prohibits discrimination in employment because of race, color, religion, sex, or national origin.[11]

Under the Age Discrimination in Employment Act of 1967,[12] applicants and employees aged 40 and over are protected from discrimination based on their age. In 1987, the EEOC issued Guidelines on Age Harassment[13] that require employers to take affirmative action to prevent the occurrence of age harassment in the workplace. Under those guidelines, hospitals may be held liable for harassment by their supervisors and agents on account of age. A hospital also may be responsible for harassment by nonsupervisory employees if it knew or should have known of the employee's conduct and failed to take prompt corrective action.

In 1980, the EEOC issued Guidelines on Sexual Harassment[14] that provide that sexual harassment is a form of discrimination prohibited by Title VII. Sexual harassment is defined as unwelcomed sexual advances, requests for sexual favors, or other verbal or physical conduct of a sexual nature that creates a hostile, intimidating, or offensive work environment.

Hospitals may be liable for the actions of supervisors and agents where an employee's response to a request for sexual favors is an explicit or implicit term or condition of employment or is used as the basis for an employment decision. This liability may result even if the hospital has no knowledge of the conduct and has promulgated policies prohibiting sexual harassment in the workplace. Therefore, careful selection of supervisory personnel and training on sexual harassment are essential to avoid potential liability. Hospitals also may be liable for sexual harassment of employees by coworkers or nonemployees if they create a hostile, intimidating, or offensive work environment where the hospital knew or should have known of the offensive conduct and failed to take prompt corrective action.

In its decision in *Meritor Savings Association v. Vinson,*[15] the United States Supreme Court stated that an employer *may* avoid liability for sexual harassment that creates a hostile, offensive, or intimidating work environment if, upon knowledge of the offensive acts, it takes prompt corrective action.

Therefore, hospitals should not only prevent the occurrence of sexual harassment in the workplace, but also establish a complaint procedure regarding sexual harassment that encourages employees to report questionable conduct. A hospital's sexual harassment policy should set forth a definition of sexual harassment, provide specific examples of conduct that would be considered prohibited or offensive, and declare that sexual harassment by management, supervisors, or employees will not be tolerated or condoned. The policy should also contain a viable complaint procedure for employees and provide that they can report offensive conduct directly to management without going through their supervisors. This is particularly important where the supervisor may be the individual harassing the employee.

If a hospital receives a complaint of sexual harassment, it should undertake a prompt and confidential investigation. The hospital should obtain voluntary statements from the complaining employee, the employee accused of misconduct, and all witnesses. The results of the investigation should be set out in writing to both the complaining and accused employees. If the investigation fails to indicate sexual harassment, the complaining employee should be so advised. Under Title VII, employees are protected from retaliation or harassment for raising complaints of discrimination, including sexual harassment. Therefore, hospitals should not discipline or discharge employees if a claim of sexual harassment fails to be substantiated, nor should they tolerate harassment or retaliation against the complaining employee by the accused or others.

If the complaint of sexual harassment is found to be valid, the hospital must take prompt and appropriate corrective action based on all the circumstances involved. Such corrective action may include, but would not be limited to, separating the harasser and complaining employee through transfer, implementing discipline or discharge against the harasser, and notifying the complaining employee regarding his or her protection against harassment and retaliation. All actions should be taken in confidence so as to avoid claims of defamation against the hospital by the harasser.

In addition to a claim under Title VII, employees suffering from sexual harassment may raise tort claims against the hospital and/or individual employees. Such tort claims could include assault and battery, invasion of privacy, negligent or intentional infliction of emotional distress, and negligent hiring, retention, or supervision. The availability of such claims may vary, depending on the jurisdiction. However, the potential damages against the hospital or supervisors from such claims could include actual damages, such as lost wages and benefits, compensatory or punitive damages, and legal expenses including court costs and attorneys' fees. Further, those tort claims may be raised notwithstanding a hospital's prompt corrective response to an incident of sexual harassment under Title VII. Clearly, a hospital's best defense against claims of sexual harassment is the publication of a strict sexual harassment policy, education of supervisors and employees, and monitoring of workplace conduct to eliminate potential incidents.

The Vocational Rehabilitation Act of 1973 and the Vocational Rehabilitation Act Amendments of 1986[16] prohibit discrimination against individuals with handicaps by federal contractors and those facilities that participate in federal programs. The Department of Labor has defined a handicapped individual as any person who (1) has a physical or mental impairment that substantially limits one or more major life activities, (2) has a record of such an impairment, or (3) is regarded as having such an impairment.[17] Hospitals that participate in the Medicare program will be subject to the handicap discrimination publications of the Rehabilitation Act. However, hospitals also should determine whether state or local handicap requirements exist to ensure overall compliance with applicable requirements. Hospitals are not required to hire an applicant or excuse employee non-performance because that person is handicapped. The Rehabilitation Act requires only reasonable accommodation of "qualified, handicapped individuals," who are defined as persons "capable of performing the essential functions of the job . . . with reasonable accommodation to his or her handicap."[18] A hospital's accommodation obligation is limited to reasonable actions that do not constitute an undue hardship by disruption of operations or excessive expense.

Contagious diseases also may be covered handicaps under the Rehabilitation Act. In its 1987 opinion in *School Board of Nassau v. Arline,*[19] the U.S. Supreme Court ruled that a teacher with tuberculosis, a contagious disease, was protected by the Rehabilitation Act. The 1988 enactment of the Civil Rights Restoration Act[20] codified the decision in *Arline.* The Supreme Court specifically did not expand that decision to include all contagious diseases. The Court stated that in determining whether an individual with a contagious disease is "otherwise qualified" for a job, an employer must analyze whether there is a substantial risk of harm to others in the workplace, either with or without reasonable accommodations. Cautioning against too broad an application of the case, the Court pointed out that it was not ruling on whether an AIDS victim could be considered a handicapped person under the act solely on the basis of contagiousness. However, in an October 6, 1988, opinion, the Justice Department said that Section 504 of the Rehabilitation Act covers persons infected with the human immunodeficiency virus (HIV), including asymptomatic carriers, and that no justification exists to consider contagion as a legitimate basis for discrimination.

Title VII and many state laws protect employees against religious discrimination in the workplace. Most claims of religious discrimination focus on two issues: (1) Did the employer reasonably accommodate the exercise of an employee's religious beliefs where they conflict with work? (2) Is the employer excused from further accommodation efforts on the grounds of undue hardship? The courts have narrowed employers' obligations for reasonable accommodation in recent years, saying that the cost to the employer of making the accommodation and the disruption of the workplace that may result from the proposed accommodation may be taken into account. Factors that hospitals should consider in determining whether an accommodation is reasonable include the nature of the employee's job, the disruption caused by the accommodation, the availability of substitutes to perform the required duties, the cost of the accommodation, the ease of rearranging the employee's schedule to permit the religious observances during non-working time, and the advance notice provided by the employee.

Wage Discrimination

The Equal Pay Act of 1963[21] prohibits discrimination in compensation on account of sex. That federal law prohibits hospitals from providing different compensation to males and females unless based upon (1) dissimilar job duties, (2) a valid seniority system, (3) a valid merit pay system, and (4) any other factor except sex. Hospitals should evaluate their compensation systems to confirm that employees performing similar work, whether under one or more job titles, are receiving equal pay, subject to legitimate differences for seniority, merit, or other considerations not based on sex. Wage and salary studies should be undertaken regularly to ensure that the institution is not inadvertently treating employees dissimilarly in violation of this statute.

Workers' Compensation

All states have enacted laws to protect and compensate employees who are injured in the course and scope of employment. Many workers' compensation statutes are limited to physical injuries and often provide the sole remedy for employees. Some states require a specific accident or personal injury for the disability to be compensable.[22] However, in some instances, injuries such as emotional distress arising in the course and scope of employment may be covered by workers' compensation laws.

Many states also protect employees from discharge or retaliatory treatment because they have pursued a claim for benefits under the relevant workers' compensation act.[23] In other states, the protection of employees from a retaliatory discharge is judicially created.[24] Claims of retaliatory discharge or discrimination may arise from any adverse action by a hospital following a work-related injury. One common source of such claims is a leave-of-absence policy that treats employees who are absent because of job-related injuries less favorably, or under more restrictive procedures, than those employees who are absent because of other medical problems. Similarly, the employee's failure to obtain reinstatement following a work-related injury (in those states that do not require reinstatement) may create a perception of unfair treatment by the hospital, resulting in a claim under the pertinent state statute or judicial precedent.

A hospital can defend against retaliation claims by showing that the termination or other actions are not based on the employee's workers' compensation claim. The hospital must establish that it had a legitimate reason for taking the action against the employee, and that others in similar circumstances have received similar treatment, notwithstanding the absence of a work-related injury. For example, a hospital could show that it discharged an employee for violating policies[25] or making false statements on his or her employment application[26] rather than for filing a claim under the workers' compensation statute.

Workplace Safety

Congress enacted the Occupational Safety and Health Act of 1970 to provide "so far as possible every working man and woman in the Nation safe and healthful working conditions and to preserve our human resources."[27] The act grants the Secretary of Labor as well as the Secretary of Health and Human Services the power to inspect facilities and to enforce employer compliance with safety requirements by administrative and court proceedings. Occupational Safety and Health Administration (OSHA) regulations also require employers to maintain accurate records of, and to make periodic reports on, work-related deaths, injuries, and illnesses other than certain minor injuries requiring only first aid treatment.[28] The act also provides that employers must maintain accurate records of employee exposures to potentially toxic materials or harmful physical agents that are required to be monitored or measured under Section 655 of the act.[29]

Regulation of Wages and Working Hours

The Fair Labor Standards Act[30] and various state laws govern payment of wages for employees. The act establishes minimum wage and overtime pay standards for all covered employees, sets standards for exempting employees from overtime, and regulates other compensation aspects of employment, including but not limited to child labor, deductions from employee paychecks, and independent contractor status. Many states have supplemental or more restrictive wage and overtime requirements. Hospitals should carefully review their compensation program, including employee overtime exemptions, to ensure that they fully comply with both federal and state requirements.

Under the act, an employer's wage data for employees must include: (1) the day of the week and the time of the day when an employee's workweek begins; (2) the total number of hours, including fractional hours, worked each day; and (3) the total number of hours worked in each workweek. With regard to compensation, hospitals must maintain information on: (1) the hours, salary, or basis upon which the employee's wages are paid; (2) the employee's overtime pay rate; (3) the amount and nature of any payments excluded from the employee's regular pay rate; (4) the employee's total regular and over-time earnings for each workweek or pay period; (5) an explanation for each addition to or deduction from the employee's wages; and (6) the date of payment and pay period that it covers.

Willful failure to maintain required wage records or a deliberate falsification of such records is punishable by criminal penalties. Also, the absence of accurate records could raise a significant credibility issue during a wage-and-hour investigation or result in the assessment of back-wages liability by the Department of Labor.

Immigration Reform and Control Act of 1986

Under the Immigration Reform and Control Act of 1986,[31] it is unlawful for an employer to recruit or hire an alien if the employer knows that the alien is not authorized to work in the United States. Employers must verify under penalty of perjury that each newly hired employee is a citizen of the United States, an alien lawfully admitted for permanent residence, or an alien who is seeking amnesty and is authorized under the act to be hired for employment. Also, employers must retain the I-9 verification form and make it available for inspection by the Immigration and Naturalization Service and/or the Department of Labor for three years following the individual's date of hire, or for one year after the individual's employment is terminated, whichever is later.

The act requires employees to attest to their citizenship or lawful alien status and provide verification of identity and eligibility for employment in the United States within 72 hours after commencement of employment. This verification must be substantiated through submission of documents to the employer. Although the documents provided by the employee need only appear genuine on their face, acceptance of documents that are obvious forgeries will not demonstrate good-faith compliance with the act's verification requirements.

Drug and Alcohol Testing

Because of widespread drug abuse in today's society, drug use on the job and the effects of off-the-job drug use are of increasing concern to employers. In an effort to develop a drug-free work environment, Congress enacted the Drug-Free Workplace Act of 1988.[32] This law requires federal contractors and grantees to maintain "drug-free" workplaces. Federal procurement contractors who receive awards of $25,000 or more must establish and communicate policies on drug awareness to employees and report workers convicted of workplace-related drug violations to the procuring government agency. The act also provides that no institution shall receive a grant from any federal agency unless it has certified to the granting agency that it will provide a drug-free workplace.

A federal government contractor also must certify to the contracting agency that it will provide a drug-free workplace. Specific requirements of the act for a drug-free workplace include:

- Publishing a statement notifying employees that the unlawful manufacture, distribution, dispensation, possession, or use of a controlled substance is prohibited in the workplace
- Stating the action that will be taken against employees for violation of this prohibition
- Establishing a drug-free awareness program to inform employees about the dangers of drug abuse, available drug counseling, rehabilitation, and employee assistance programs, and the penalties for drug abuse

Contracts awarded by a federal agency will be subject to suspension of payments or termination of the contract, or both, if:

- The contractor makes a false certification under the act
- The contractor violates its certification by failing to carry out the requirements of the act
- Such a number of the contractor's employees have been convicted of violations of criminal drug statutes as to indicate that the contractor had failed to make a good-faith effort to provide a drug-free workplace

The requirements for recipients of federal grants are similar to those set out above for federal contractors.

Hospitals that are not subject to the Drug-Free Workplace Act may still implement drug and alcohol testing for employees and applicants. The legality of and procedures for drug and alcohol testing have been challenged on many occasions. Although courts have established testing procedures for public employers, it is not clear whether the same restrictions apply to employers in the private sector. Generally, incorporating constitutional due process procedures will protect nongovernmental hospitals' drug and alcohol testing programs. Such protections include:

- Giving prior notice to applicants and employees of the hospital's drug and alcohol testing requirement
- Obtaining written voluntary consent from the applicant or employee prior to administering the test
- Implementing workplace testing for employees on the basis of reasonable suspicion of drug or alcohol usage or other objective criteria
- Providing an appropriate chain of custody and independent laboratory testing of urine, blood, or breathalyzer samples obtained from employees

Other statutory or judicially imposed requirements and restrictions may exist in some jurisdictions, and hospitals should carefully review them before implementing a drug and alcohol testing program. Moreover, hospitals should review testing procedures periodically with legal counsel and update as necessary to ensure continued legal compliance.

Employee Polygraph Tests

The Employee Polygraph Protection Act of 1988[33] restricts most private employers from requiring job applicants or current employees to submit to polygraph tests. It also prohibits most employers from taking adverse employment action against applicants or employees who refuse to take such a test. The Department of Labor may bring injunctive actions to restrain violations of the act and may assess civil penalties up to $10,000 for violations. There is a limited statutory exception permitting employers to administer strictly voluntary polygraphs in connection with the investigation of theft or economic loss. Those tests must be conducted under very specific procedures and employee protections must be outlined in the act. However, the results of such a polygraph without other evidence, or the refusal to take the polygraph, generally may not be used as the basis for an adverse employment decision (for example, discharge, discipline, discrimination, denial of employment or promotion). The act requires employers to post a notice in the workplace summarizing the protections of the act.

Personnel Records and Employee Notices

The EEOC has not adopted any generally applicable requirement that employers maintain personnel records. However, it may require employers to keep records if it determines that such records are necessary to further the purpose of Title VII. Hospitals with 100 or more employees must file an annual Employer Information Report, or Form EEI-1,[34] which sets forth the racial, ethnic, and sex composition of the work force. Hospitals with affirmative action obligations under Executive Order 11246 or state law must assemble more detailed information on the composition of their work force and significant employment actions (for example, hire, transfer, promotion, and termination) with respect to employees. If a hospital elects to maintain personnel records, they must be retained for at least six months following the creation of the entry.[35] Hospitals charged with a violation of federal employment law must maintain all records regarding the employee and the incident giving rise to the alleged violation until the final disposition of the case.[36]

Many federal and state laws require covered employers to post notices in the workplace to provide employees with information on their legal rights. Notices must be posted regarding the minimum wage and overtime pay, equal employment opportunity, the Age Discrimination in Employment Act, and, for private nongovernmental employers, the Employee Polygraph Protection Act of 1988. Those notices are available from the governmental agencies that enforce the applicable statutes. If a hospital has more than one facility, it must post notices in each workplace.

Governmental Investigations

Congress has granted many federal agencies subpoena powers to investigate claims and enforce the obligations of various acts. The EEOC may subpoena documents in the possession or under the control of an employer that is subject to a charge of employment discrimination under Title VII.[37] Before issuing a subpoena, the EEOC generally will submit a written request to an employer for documents relating to the charge. Those documents may include, for example, materials regarding the composition of the work force (such as race, ethnicity, sex, and so on), personnel records regarding the claimant and similarly situated employees, and the hospital's employment policies.

Employers should carefully scrutinize the EEOC's request for information to determine if it is overly broad or unrelated to the allegations of the charge. Hospitals should contact the assigned investigator and attempt to reach agreement on requests for information. This may save the employer considerable time and effort in responding to the charge, while permitting it to undertake a successful defense to the claims.

For example, an investigator may undertake a wide-ranging investigation and request employment records covering too broad a group of employees or time period. By conferring with the investigator, an employer may be able to clarify the issues or underlying factual circumstances involved in a claim and reach agreement to provide less information than originally sought by the investigator.

There are few limitations placed on the EEOC's investigative and subpoena powers. The Supreme Court has held that only minimal information must be included in charges of employment discrimination before the EEOC may obtain judicial enforcement of an administrative subpoena. The Court stated that a charge must meet the requirements of Title VII as a jurisdictional prerequisite to judicial enforcement of an EEOC-issued subpoena.[38] The relevant section of Title VII provides simply that "[c]harges . . . shall contain such information and be in such form as the Commission requires."[39] Thus, a district court does not have to find that a charge is well founded, verifiable, or based on reasonable suspicion before enforcing an EEOC subpoena.

The Wage and Hour Division of the U.S. Department of Labor also has broad powers to enter a covered employer's premises and inspect wage records.[40] That division may obtain and enforce a subpoena if employers refuse to permit inspection of wage records.[41] There are limitations to the division's power to compel the production of general business records. In one instance, a federal appellate court held that in conducting an inspection, the Wage and Hour Division can demand records only of wages paid, hours worked, and tasks performed by the employees.[42]

The Occupational Safety and Health Administration and state agencies with delegated authority for workplace safety also may enter the hospital premises to conduct inspections and investigations.[43] Those inspections may be conducted without prior notice to the hospital. However, the U.S. Supreme Court has held that an employer may require OSHA to obtain an administrative search warrant prior to entering the premises to conduct an inspection.[44] The hospital must request that OSHA obtain a search warrant at the time that the agency representative seeks entry to the premises.

□ Discipline and Discharge

Hospitals can reduce potential employee claims and litigation for wrongful discharge by conducting regular and comprehensive performance appraisals that reflect actual work performance, counseling employees in writing for rule violations or performance deficiencies, and conducting exit interviews. Hospitals should disseminate written policies to employees regarding rules, procedures, and the sanctions for noncompliance. The hospital's management and legal counsel should review the policies and progressive discipline program before they are implemented.

The hospital should state in writing that its personnel policies, and in particular its progressive discipline and discharge program, do not constitute a contract of employment with any employee. Appropriate disclaimers of such a contractual relationship will help hospitals maintain an at-will employment relationship with their employees. By comparison, hospitals subject to collective bargaining agreements may have specific "cause" or "good cause" standards for discipline and discharge of represented employees under the terms of such agreements.

Hospital management must commit to a consistent application of policies and discipline if it desires to avoid claims of employment discrimination. Hospital management should implement training and education programs on hospital policies for supervisors. To minimize claims of wrongful discharge or employment discrimination, hospitals may consider reviewing significant disciplinary actions (such as suspension or probation) and discharge with the personnel department, upper management, or legal counsel before imposing such sanctions on employees.

Wrongful Termination Claims

The employment-at-will doctrine generally has granted employers discretion to terminate employees for any reason or no reason at all. As stated by one court a century ago, employers ". . . may dismiss their employees at-will . . . for good cause, for no cause, or even for cause morally wrong, without being thereby guilty of legal wrong."[45]

During the past century, numerous federal and state statutes have limited an employer's right to terminate employees for reasons unacceptable to society, such as, for example, race or sex. Because of the perceived harshness of the employment-at-will doctrine, courts also have restricted employer rights in this area. Courts in some states have taken the position that employee manuals or handbooks may constitute implied contracts to which an employer is legally bound.[46] Other courts have ruled that there are public policy limits on the at-will doctrine, which may include termination for whistle blowing, refusing to engage in unlawful conduct, and refusing to commit perjury.[47] Other restrictions against at-will termination may be contained in collective-bargaining agreements that require hospitals to discharge only for "cause" or "just cause."

Even where employees of a particular hospital are considered to be employed at-will, claims of wrongful discharge may be raised based upon written materials, the oral representations of management, and the particular circumstances of termination. The potential for wrongful discharge claims can be reduced by effective personnel policies that disclaim contractual relationships with employees, provide that neither cause nor just cause is required for termination, and set out reasonable workplace rules that, if followed, provide rational and lawful grounds for employee discipline and discharge.

Intentional Infliction of Emotional Distress

A claim of intentional infliction of emotional distress may be incorporated in a suit alleging wrongful discharge. Some jurisdictions have recognized intentional infliction of emotional distress as a separate cause of action. The elements of this claim are: (1) outrageous conduct by the employer or its agents, (2) intent to cause emotional distress or reckless disregard for the probability of causing such distress, (3) suffering of the employee from severe or extreme emotional distress, and (4) the employer's actions being the direct cause of the emotional distress. A few courts now permit a claim of intentional infliction of emotional distress without simultaneous physical injury or impact.

Actions by the hospital or its agents may be considered outrageous if the hospital abuses a relationship or position that gives it power to damage an employee's interest, takes actions knowing that the employee is susceptible to injury through mental distress, or acts unreasonably or intentionally outrageously knowing that its acts are likely to result in mental distress. Generally, the fact of an employee's discharge or the mere existence of insulting language will not support a claim for outrageous conduct.

A hospital can reduce the potential for such claims by several actions. First, it should train managers and supervisors to deal with employees in a businesslike manner and avoid arguments and abusive interrogations. Second, it may want to have two supervisors or managers present for employee discipline or discharge conferences to ensure that such meetings are conducted properly and that corroboration exists for their statements and actions. Third, any employee claims of abusive or inappropriate conduct by supervisors should be investigated promptly and, if found to be valid, counseling should be provided to or disciplinary action taken against the supervisor.

Defamation

A claim for defamation is based on: (1) a false written or verbal statement or a statement made with reckless disregard for its truth or falsity, (2) demonstration that the statement related to the plaintiff, (3) evidence of communication or publication of the statement to a third party, and (4) damage to the reputation or standing of the person identified.[48] Defamation claims may arise in various circumstances, but are most likely to occur when an employee is discharged for a reason that he or she believes to be untrue that is communicated to third parties, or where references, comments, or written or verbal statements may have prevented the former employee from obtaining employment.

Generally, an employer has a qualified privilege to make good-faith statements to a prospective employer concerning the services and character of a current or former employee. The privilege is qualified because only relevant, work-related statements are protected. Statements by a hospital or its supervisors containing false, nonwork-related information, such as the employee's sexual preference, would exceed the scope of the hospital's privilege. The qualified privilege also is lost if statements, such as employment references, are made with malice or lack of good faith (that is, if the speaker knows that a statement is false or has reckless disregard for the truth.)[49]

By definition, statements that are defamatory are untrue, and truth is therefore an absolute defense to a charge of defamation.[50] The defense of truth does not require proof that the alleged defamatory statement is literally true in every detail. Rather, substantial truth is sufficient.

The general rule has been that statements to a discharged employee by the employer regarding the reason for the discharge do not constitute "publication" of the alleged defamation (that is, the reason for discharge). Recently, however, some jurisdictions have recognized that if a discharged worker is forced to tell a prospective employer the allegedly defamatory reason that he or she was discharged, then such "compelled self-publication" may constitute defamation by the former employer if the reason for the firing is found to be untrue.[51]

Hospitals can protect themselves from potential defamation suits by adopting a "neutral reference" or "confirmation of employment" policy regarding references and refusing to comment to third parties on the employee's separation from work. Hospitals also can limit their potential exposure to defamation claims by indicating that information provided regarding a former employee is qualified as an opinion and should not be taken as a declaration of fact. Generally, statements of opinion, as opposed to statements of fact, are not considered capable of bearing a defamatory meaning.[52]

Clauses on employment application forms purporting to waive liability for any statements made in the course of checking an applicant's employment record will not always preclude the former employer or its agents from liability.[53] Therefore, hospitals may want to obtain releases from an employee or written agreements on the text of future employment references.

Invasion of Privacy

Generally, an invasion of privacy is an act by one who invades the privacy of another, with resulting liability for any harm caused by such an action. There are three forms of privacy invasion recognized as tortious that could arise in hospital employment: (1) intrusion upon seclusion, (2) publicity given to private facts, and (3) portrayal in a false light.

Intrusion upon seclusion arises when there is an intentional intrusion on one's private affairs. This cause of action generally requires an expectation of privacy and a substantial intrusion on that privacy that would offend, humiliate, or outrage a reasonable person. This cause of action may be brought in connection with a sexual harassment claim or an unauthorized and unwarranted search of an employee's property, person, or locker.

The U.S. Supreme Court has held that public employers have a wide latitude to search the offices, desks, and files of their employees.[54] Although there was no majority opinion in the Court's decision on that issue, five justices concurred that the employer was not required to obtain a warrant or establish probable cause for suspecting misconduct before undertaking a search.

The very element to be considered is the reasonableness of the employer's search. It is only an unwarranted intrusion that is highly offensive to the reasonable person that is actionable. In addressing the employee's reasonable expectation of privacy, the Court suggested that this standard applied to the private sector as well.

> The operational realities of the workplace . . . may make some employees' expectations of privacy unreasonable when an intrusion is by a supervisor rather than a lawful enforcement official . . . [and] like similar expectations of employees in the private sector, may be reduced by virtue of actual office practices and procedures, or by legitimate regulation.[55]

Thus, the communication to employees of a public or private employer's search policy may reduce the employees' expectation of privacy and lessen the likelihood of an action arising from a subsequent search.

The tort of publicity given to private facts generally requires that the facts given publicity by the employer are highly offensive to a reasonable person and that such facts are not of legitimate concern to the public.

Portrayal in a false light is perhaps the most dangerous and frequent claim of invasion of privacy. It arises from a significant misrepresentation of the character, history, activities, or beliefs of the employee that is placed before the public in a false light. The mischaracterization must be highly offensive to a reasonable person and passed on with reckless disregard of its truth or falsity. That claim can arise from employment references or public statements made about employees.

As with defamation, truth is an absolute defense to that claim.

☐ Conclusion

The relationship between hospitals and their employees is subject to increasing regulation at all levels of government and in the courts. To minimize exposure for potential claims and liability, risk managers and human resources officials must be knowledgeable about current statutory, administrative, and court-imposed restrictions. Hospitals should develop lawful and well-founded personnel policies that foster good employee relations and a fair and consistent approach to personnel actions. The failure to comply with applicable laws, or the inconsistent and subjective enforcement of policies, will only lead to claims, litigation, and liability.

References

1. *See* Domingo v. New England Fish Co., 727 F.2d 1429 (9th Cir.), modified 742 F.2d 520 (9th Cir. 1984).

2. Exec. Order No. 11246, 30 *Federal Register* 12319 (1965), reprinted in 42 U.S.C.A. §2000e at 19-24 (1981).

3. 29 U.S. Code §794(a).

4. 41 Code of Federal Regulations (C.F.R.) 60-741.6(b).

5. 41 C.F.R. 60-741.6(c).

6. Dothard v. Rawlinson, 433 U.S. 321 (1977); EEOC guidelines on employee selection procedures 29 C.F.R. 1607 4(c)(2); EEOC guidelines on discrimination because of national origin 29 C.F.R. 1606 6(a)(2).

7. In Hipp v. Hospital Auth., 104 Ga. App. 174, 121 S.E.2d 273, 275 (1961), the parents of a nine-year-old girl claimed that she was sexually molested by a hospital orderly who had previously been convicted of being a "Peeping Tom." The parents alleged that the hospital had been negligent in hiring the employee. Although the trial court dismissed the case in favor of the defendant hospital, an appellate court subsequently reversed this decision, noting that even charitable institutions can be held liable for the torts of employees if they have been negligent in selecting or retaining them.

8. Alabama, Alaska, Arizona, Colorado, Connecticut, Florida, Georgia, Illinois, Indiana, Iowa, Kansas, Maryland, Michigan, Minnesota, Missouri, New Hampshire, New Jersey, New Mexico, New York, Oklahoma, Pennsylvania, Rhode Island, Tennessee, Texas, Utah, and Washington.

9. 42 U.S. Code §2000 *et. seq.*

10. Age Discrimination in Employment Act of 1967, 29 U.S. Code §§621 *et. seq.;* Vocational Rehabilitation Act of 1973, 29 U.S. Code §§701 *et. seq.;* Equal Pay Act, 29 U.S. Code §206; Exec. Order No. 11246.

11. 42 U.S. Code §§2000e(b) and 2000e-2(a).

12. 29 U.S. Code §§621 *et seq.*

13. EEOC Compliance Manual §615.11 (Age Harassment).

14. 29 C.F.R. §1604.11.

15. 477 U.S. 57 (1986).

16. 29 U.S. Code §§701 *et seq.*

17. 29 C.F.R. §32.3.

18. *Id.*

19. 480 U.S. 273 (1987).

20. Pub. L. No. 100-259.

21. 29 U.S. Code §206.

22. Luna v. Denver, 537 F.Supp. 798 (D. Colo. 1982) (claim for intentional infliction of emotional distress is not covered nor barred by the Colorado Worker's Compensation Act, because act

does not include those injuries consisting primarily of mental suffering); Brady v. Royal Mfg. Co., 117 Ga. App. 312, 160 S.E.2d 424 (1968) (neurosis not caused by accident is not compensable).

23. For example, Texas Revised Civil Statutes Annotated, article 8307(c) (Vernon Supp. 1989) provides, in pertinent part:

> Section 1. No person may discharge or in any other manner discriminate against any employee because the employee has in good faith filed a claim, hired a lawyer to represent him in a claim, instituted, or caused to be instituted, in good faith, any proceeding under the Texas Worker's Compensation Act, or has testified or is about to testify in any such proceeding.

24. *E.g.*, Clanton v. Cain-Sloane Co., 677 S.W.2d 441 (Tenn. 1984). (The Tennessee Supreme Court found an exception for retaliatory discharge to the employment-at-will rule. The court reasoned that to deny employees a cause of action for retaliatory discharge under the Worker's Compensation Act would "completely circumvent this legislative scheme.")

25. DeFord Lumber Co. v. Roys, 615 S.W.2d 235 (Tex. Civ. App.—Dallas 1981, no writ).

26. *See* Laclede Gas Co., 86 LA 480 (1986) (failure to disclose previous neck and back injury on employment application was material and purposeful falsification warranting discharge).

27. 29 U.S. Code §§651 *et seq.*

28. 29 U.S. Code §657(c)(2).

29. 29 U.S. Code §657(c)(3).

30. 29 U.S. Code §§201 *et seq.*

31. 29 U.S. Code §§1802 *et seq.*

32. 41 U.S. Code §§701 *et seq.*

33. 29 U.S. Code §§2001 *et seq.*

34. 29 C.F.R. 1602.7.

35. 29 C.F.R. 1602.14(a).

36. *Id.*

37. 29 C.F.R. 1626.16.

38. EEOC v. Shell Oil Co., 466 U.S. 54, 80 L. Ed.2d 41, 104 S. Ct. 1621 (1984).

39. 42 U.S.C. §2000e-5(b).

40. 29 U.S. Code §211(a).

41. Dunlap v. Resource Sciences Corp., 410 F.Supp. 836 (D. Okla. 1976).

42. McComb v. Hunsaker Trucking Contractor, Inc., 171 F.2d 523 (5th Cir. 1948).

43. 29 U.S. Code §657(a).

44. Marshall v. Barlow's, Inc., 436 U.S. 307 (1978).

45. Eastline & R.R.R. Co. v. Scott, 72 Tex. 70, 10 S.W. 99 (1888).

46. Alabama, Alaska, Arizona, Arkansas, California, Colorado, Connecticut, District of Columbia, Georgia, Hawaii, Idaho, Illinois, Kansas, Maine, Maryland, Michigan, Minnesota, Missouri, Montana, New Jersey, New Mexico, New York, Ohio, Oklahoma, Oregon, South Carolina, South Dakota, Texas, Vermont, Washington, West Virginia, Wisconsin, Wyoming.

47. Alabama, Arizona, Arkansas, California, Connecticut, Hawaii, Idaho, Illinois, Indiana, Iowa, Kansas, Kentucky, Maryland, Massachusetts, Michigan, Minnesota, Missouri, Montana, Nebraska, Nevada, New Hampshire, New Jersey, New Mexico, North Carolina, North Dakota, Ohio, Oregon, Pennsylvania, South Carolina, South Dakota, Tennessee, Texas, Virginia, Washington, West Virginia, Wisconsin.

48. Austin v. Torrington Co., 810 F.2d 416 (4th Cir.), *cert. denied*, 484 U.S. 977 (1987).

49. *See* Golden Bear Distrib. Sys. v. Chase Revel Inc., 708 F.2d 944, 948 (5th Cir. 1983).

50. Johnson v. International Minerals and Chem. Corp., 122 LRRM 2652 (BNA) (D.S.D. 1986).

51. Lewis v. Equitable Ins. Society, 389 N.W.2d 876 (Minn. 1986); Churchey v. Adolph Coors Co., 759 P.2d 1336 (Colo. 1988) *(en banc)*.

52. *See* Coleman v. American Broadcasting Co., 119 LRRM 3324 (BNA) (D.D.C. 1985).

53. Kellums v. Freight Sales Center, Inc., 467 S.2d 816 (Fla. Dist. Ct. App. 1985).

54. O'Conner v. Ortega, 480 U.S. 709 (1987).

55. *Id.* 480 U.S. 709 at 717–718.

Bibliography

Bureau of National Affairs. *Fair Employment Practices Manual.* Washington, DC: BNA, 1989.

Bureau of National Affairs. *Wage and Hour Manual.* Washington, DC: BNA, 1989.

Bureau of National Affairs. *Individual Employment Rights Manual.* Washington, DC: BNA, 1989.

Connolly, W. B., Jr., and Crowell, D. R. *Practical Guide to Occupational Safety and Health Act.* 1988.

Diedrich, W. L., Jr., and Gaus, W. *Defense of Equal Employment Claims.* Colorado Springs, CO: Shepard's/McGraw-Hill, 1982.

Eglit, H. C. *Age Discrimination.* Colorado Springs, CO: McGraw-Hill, 1981.

Ginsburg, G. J. *Cases and Materials on Federal Labor Standards.* 2nd ed. Washington, D.C.: George Washington University, 1976.

Larson, A., and Larson, L. K. *Employment Discrimination.* New York City: Matthew Bender & Co., 1990.

Player, M. A. *Employment Discrimination Law: Cases and Materials.* St. Paul: West Publishing Co., 1980.

Rothstein, L. F. *Rights of Physically Handicapped Persons.* Colorado Springs, CO: Shepard's/McGraw-Hill, 1984.

Rothstein, M. A. *Occupational Safety and Health Law.* 2nd ed. St. Paul: West Publishing Co., 1983.

Schlei, B. L., and Grossman, P. *Employment Discrimination Law.* Chicago: American Bar Association, 1983.

U.S. Department of Labor. *29 Code of Federal Regulations.* Washington, DC: U.S. Department of Labor, 1989.

U.S. Department of Labor, Employment Standards Administration, Office of Federal Contracts Compliance Program. *Federal Contract Compliance Manual.* Washington, DC: U.S. Department of Labor, 1979.

Weiner, L. *Federal Age and Hour Law.* Philadelphia: American Law Institute, 1977.

Chapter 31

Medical and Business Record Management

Susan N. Chernoff

The medical record is the basic document underlying all quality assurance and risk management activities. The medical records department and its personnel have the important role of ensuring that records are retrievable, accurate, and up to date and that those people who make entries in a record or examine it for any reason do so in accordance with applicable laws, regulations, accreditation standards, and hospital policy. In addition, the medical records department provides a health care facility's risk manager with the basic data with which to control liability risk in the facility. It is essential to the risk manager's function that medical records be thorough, accurate, and promptly retrievable. Thus, the medical records manager and the risk manager should work in tandem to reduce the institution's risk—the former providing a complete history of patient care in the institution, and the latter using that information to identify potential liability risks and reduce the likelihood that such risks will materialize.

In recent years, the duties of both the medical records manager and the risk manager have become increasingly complex as hospitals have expanded the type of medical care they provide outside the actual facility, such as in outpatient clinics or other hospital-sponsored ambulatory care or home care programs.[1] Those programs expand the duties of both the risk manager and the medical records department to include traditional inpatient treatment provided by hospitals and newer forms of outpatient treatment provided outside the hospital. Certain business records also create critical evidence that could be useful in defending a hospital. This chapter will examine the management of medical records and selected business records and their risk management implications.

☐ Medical Records

The material in this section provides an overview of medical records in general.[2] The medical record consists of four types of data concerning an individual patient: personal, financial, social, and medical. The medical data form the patient's clinical record, a continuously maintained history of the diagnosis and treatment provided to the patient in the hospital. Such data include the results of physical examinations, medical history, treatment administered, progress reports, physician's orders, clinical laboratory reports, X-ray reports, consultation reports, anesthesia records, operative reports, signed consent forms, nurses' notes, and other reports that may be generated during the patient's treatment.[3]

The medical record can be handwritten, typed, or computer-generated. The computerized record can aid the information network on a patient, enhancing completeness and accuracy as well as the immediate availability of the record to authorized personnel.[4] Whether handwritten, typed, or in computer form, the medical record should be a complete, accurate, current record of the patient's history, condition, and treatment as well as the results of the patient's hospitalization or outpatient treatment.

The medical record is used not only to document chronologically the care rendered to a patient, but also to plan and evaluate the patient's treatment and to enhance communication among the patient's physician and other health care professionals treating that patient. The record also provides clinical data for medical, nursing, and scientific research. In addition, individuals who conduct medical and nursing audits and peer review evaluations rely heavily on documentation in medical records.

Medical records also are important documents to the health care provider and to the patient for quality assessment purposes. For example, where hospital bylaws designate standards of care to be established by individual departments, examination of patient records can provide verification that the standards are being maintained. Administrative and clinical assessment programs may be targets of scrutiny by accreditation agencies, and patient records can aid evaluation and justification of the programs.[5]

Medical records are essential to the hospital in the defense of professional negligence actions. Because such actions often are litigated two to five years after the plaintiff received the treatment in question, the hospital record generally is the most detailed record of what actually occurred during the patient's hospitalization. Those who participated in the plaintiff's treatment may not be available to testify on behalf of the defendant(s) or may not remember important details of the case. A good record enables the hospital to reconstruct the patient's course of treatment and to show whether the care provided was acceptable under the circumstances.[6] The contents of the hospital record usually are admissible in evidence for or against the hospital and physicians. It is essential that everyone involved in medical record documentation and management and risk management understand the legal implications of the record so that they will create and maintain a record that will be useful to them in any future litigation.

Content of the Medical Record

The requirement that hospitals maintain medical records is found in state and federal statutes and regulations, municipal codes, and hospital accreditation standards. In a few states, hospital licensing statutes set forth the minimum record requirements.[7] In most states, the regulatory agency for hospitals has the power to promulgate rules and regulations that specify the information that must be kept in medical records of a licensed hospital.[8] State licensing regulations generally fall into three groups: those detailing specific information required; those specifying the broad areas of information required; and those stating simply that the medical record shall be adequate, accurate, or complete.

Federal reimbursement programs also require hospitals to maintain medical records and specify minimum content requirements. Medicare conditions of participation contain such requirements. Finally, some local or municipal codes may require certain information not otherwise required by state law or regulation.

The Joint Commission on Accreditation of Healthcare Organizations requires hospitals to maintain patient care records as a standard of accreditation.[9] The Joint Commission also specifies in considerable detail the information that should appear in the medical record.[10]

In the absence of specific statutory or regulatory direction, a hospital should adopt an institutional policy concerning the content of medical records. The policy may be a detailed list of data required or may reference some other policy, such as the Joint

Commission standards and interpretations. Most accredited hospitals in states that provide no statutory or regulatory direction concerning patient record content rely on the Joint Commission standards.

In all states, however, hospitals should keep abreast of state, federal, and Joint Commission medical records requirements. State and local associations of medical record practitioners often publish changes in the applicable law and accreditation standards. Hospitals also receive notice of those changes from state and national hospital associations and from hospital legal counsel. All health care institutions should develop reliable ways of communicating new laws and regulations to the individuals responsible for making policy recommendations concerning medical record content, particularly medical record practitioners and the medical staff. Risk managers may play an important role in that process.

Record Retention and Destruction

The length of time that a medical record is retained will be determined by federal or state law and regulations or by sound hospital administrative policy and medical practice. It also will be influenced greatly by the nature of the institution and resources available to maintain a long retention period.

A few states have hospital licensing acts and regulations that establish general medical record retention requirements[11] or requirements for specific parts of medical records, such as X rays.[12] Some states have established different retention requirements for different classifications of patients, such as minors, the mentally ill, and the deceased.[13] In states that have adopted the Uniform Preservation of Private Business Records Act, the three-year preservation requirement may apply to the medical records maintained by private hospitals, even though that act does not specifically address medical records.

Medicare conditions of participation for hospitals require hospitals to maintain their medical records, including X rays, for a period of not less than five years.[14] In addition, discharge summaries, clinical summaries, and other medical records relating to Medicare health insurance claims must be retained for a period of five years after the month that the cost report to which the materials apply is filed with the fiscal intermediary, unless state law requires a longer retention period.[15]

Development of a Retention Policy

In developing a record retention policy, hospitals must, at a minimum, comply with all applicable legal requirements. After those requirements are satisfied or in the absence of regulatory requirements, each hospital should, with input from its risk management department, establish its own policy governing medical records retention. It is clear that hospitals should retain medical records for as long as there is a medical or administrative need for them—for example, for subsequent patient care, medical research, review and evaluation of professional and hospital services, and defense of professional or other liability actions.

One factor often considered in developing a retention policy is the statute of limitations for filing contract and tort actions. Except in the case of minors' records, retaining records for this length of time usually is not the determining factor because limitation periods generally are shorter than the period that the record would be maintained for medical reasons. Although most suits by minors are brought before the minor reaches the age of majority, the hospital will be best protected if it retains the records until the minor reaches the age of majority plus the period of the statute of limitations. For example, in states in which the age of majority is 18 and the statute of limitations for torts is two years, the retention period for a newborn's records would be 20 years.

If hospital staffs engage in extensive medical research, especially retrospective investigations that require detailed medical data or research, the hospital may wish to establish a long retention period. Moreover, if the medical research involves experimental or innovative patient care procedures, the hospital may wish to establish retention policies of at least 75 years. The patients' medical records enable the hospital to notify patients if follow-up warnings of any type are necessary. In addition, the records will assist the hospital in defending suits arising from experimental treatments.

The American Hospital Association (AHA) and the American Medical Record Association (AMRA) have adopted a policy on record retention that recommends that the original or reproduced record be kept for a period of 10 years. Certain parts of the record should be kept permanently. After 10 years, the policy recommends that the complete record may be destroyed, unless prohibited by statute, regulation, ordinance, or law, provided that the institution retain the information specifically set out in the policy and retain the record for longer than 10 years at the request of specified individuals. Figure 31-1 shows the AHA and AMRA retention policy.

A major consideration for a hospital in establishing a retention policy is its capability for storing a large number of records. Available space, expansion rates, the durability of the paper and folders used, the cost of microfilming and computerizing records, and storage and safety requirements all affect the hospital's ability to retain records.

Microfilming

The statutes and regulations of several states authorize microfilming or other photographic reproduction of records.[16] Hospitals in these states can remedy storage problems by microfilming records and destroying the originals. Where state law or regulations do not specifically authorize microfilming, hospitals may microfilm their records and destroy the original record in accordance with law or regulations governing record destruction. Although microfilming alleviates storage problems, it may raise other administrative burdens if the records are not readily available for review. Moreover, the hospital will incur additional reading and printing equipment costs. Also, appropriate safeguards must be taken if outside sources are involved in microfilming the records.

Computerized Records

Some states also specifically authorize retention of medical records on a computer.[17] Increasingly, hospitals are beginning to consider retaining records in computerized formats. Storing records on optical disks allows hospitals to store their records as permanently as paper records in a fraction of the space and with a retrieval time measured in seconds instead of the hours or even days that it can take to find a paper chart.[18] Hospital licensing regulations in about half of the states recognize computerized medical records in some way.

In states whose regulations do not explicitly allow for computerized records, other medical record retention requirements can limit the use of computerized record storage. However, if hospitals are able legally to store records in computer formats, the hospital must ensure that the records are confidential, secure from unauthorized access, legible, durable, accessible, and accurate.

Destruction of the Record

The statutes and regulations in some states specify the method by which a record may be destroyed after the retention period has concluded or after the record has been copied onto microfilm or computer or converted to other machine-readable form. Other states require the hospital to prepare a permanent abstract of the record before destroying it.[19] Although the statutes may recommend that records be destroyed by shredding or burning, the Environmental Protection Agency has recommended shredding or recycling as the preferred methods of disposing of records.[20]

If the hospital delivers the records to a commercial organization for destruction, it should enter into a written contract with the organization that sets forth the method of destruction, establishes safeguards against breach of confidentiality, includes indemnification provisions to protect the hospital from loss due to unauthorized disclosure, and requires the contractor to certify that records delivered to it have been properly destroyed.

Figure 31-1. AHA and AMRA Policy on Medical Records Retention

Technical Advisory Bulletin

Preservation of Medical Records in Health Care Institutions

This technical advisory bulletin is intended to provide specific advice to the membership of the American Hospital Association, as approved by the Council on Patient Services.

The primary purpose of the medical record is to document the course of the patient's illness and the treatment he receives. Although the medical record is kept for the benefit of the patient, the physician, and the health care institution, it is the property of the health care institution with other interests recognized by law.

The length of time medical records should be retained will vary depending on the purposes for which the record is being kept. In formulating a record retention policy, a health care institution must be guided by its own clinical, scientific, and audit needs, and the possibility of future patient litigation.

In some jurisdictions a health care institution is not required by law to preserve its records for any given length of time. The appropriate period of retention may be affected by the statute of limitations for bringing a legal action for an injury or breach of contract. In most states the period of the applicable statute of limitations would be less than 10 years. Moreover, in many states the statute of limitations requires that an action for personal injuries sustained by a minor must be exercised within a few years after he attains his majority.

It is deemed unnecessary for a health care institution to preserve medical records that duplicate other official records that will be kept permanently. Thus, keeping records for the sole purpose of proving birth or age, residence, citizenship, or family relationship serves no useful purpose. Inasmuch as a hospital or other health care institution is seldom requested to produce medical records older than 10 years for clinical, scientific, legal, or audit purposes, it is ordinarily sufficient to retain the medical records 10 years after the most recent patient care usage in the absence of legal considerations.

Accordingly, it is recommended that complete patient medical records in health care institutions usually be retained, either in the original or reproduced form, for 10 years after the most recent patient care usage. After 10 years, such records may be destroyed unless destruction is specifically prohibited by statute, ordinance, regulation, or law, provided that the institution:

1. Retains basic information such as dates of admission and discharge, names of responsible physicians, records of disgnoses and operations, surgical procedure reports, pathology reports, and discharge resumes for all records so destroyed.

2. Retains complete medical records of minors for the period of minority plus the applicable period of statute of limitations as prescribed by statute in the state in which the health care institution is located.

3. Retains complete medical records of patients under mental disability in like manner as those of patients under disability of minority.

4. Retains complete patient medical records for longer periods when requested in writing by one of the following:

   - An attending or consultant physician of the patient

   - The patient or someone acting legally in his behalf

   - Legal counsel for a party having an interest affected by the patient medical records

If the adoption of a record retention policy as suggested by this document would reduce the previous period of retention by a health care institution, it is recommended that any new policy be developed with the full knowledge and participation of the medical staff, legal counsel for the institution, and any past or present liability insurance carrier affording coverage during any time in which the affected records were made. It is also recommended that written notice of the new policy of retention be given to state and local medical societies and bar associations and by announcement in any other media suggested by the institution's legal counsel; and, further, that the lesser period of retention either be restricted to subsequently completed patient medical records or that general application be deferred for a resonable length of time until requests for deferred destruction may be received.

This document was prepared by the American Hospital Association's Committee on Medical Records and the American Medical Record Association's Planning and Bylaws Committee as a first step toward promoting uniformity in state laws and regulations relating to statues of limitation for the retention of medical records. It is hoped that the various states will adopt legislation on regulations to implement its provisions.

The document was approved by the AHA House of Delegates February 6, 1974, and by the AMRA House of Delegates October 22, 1973, to become the AHA S80 leaflet, which replaced the Resolution on Preservation of Medical Records of Hospital Inpatients adopted by both organizations in 1960. The S80 leaflet was superseded by the statement S003 in 1975. In accordance with a new classification system for documents, it was reclassified as a technical advisory bulletin in 1980 by the Council on Patient Services.

If the hospital destroys its own records, it also must establish procedures to protect the confidentiality of the information and ensure that records are completely destroyed. The hospital employee responsible for record destruction should certify that the records have been properly destroyed.

Whether the records are destroyed commercially or by hospital staff, the hospital should retain certificates of destruction permanently as evidence of its record disposal.

With the assistance of the risk management department, the hospital should create and apply uniformly a medical records policy governing destruction of records. If the hospital fails to apply the policy uniformly or destroys records contrary to the policy, a court may allow a jury in a negligence suit to infer from the unavailability of the records that the hospital acted improperly in treating the plaintiff.

Special Types of Medical Record Information

Certain types of medical information may be difficult to retain in the medical record in its original form either because of the volume of paper required to record the information or because of the nature of the item itself.

Radiology Films, EKG Tracings, Fetal Monitor Strips

Radiology films, EKG tracings, and fetal monitor strips are among the types of medical information that pose special record retention problems. For example, one patient might have a number of EKG tracings. A maternity patient could have hours of fetal monitoring strips containing important documentation of the events of the birth. It would be impractical to retain all of this information in the patient's record. X rays, as well as the newer scanning technologies such as computed tomography scans, mammograms, and ultrasound, produce medical information in a pictorial rather than written form that may be difficult or impossible to include in the record. Although the physicians' reports and interpretations of the tests will certainly be part of the record and therefore will be retained according to hospital policy, it is less clear how the original films, strips, and scans should be retained.

If federal, state, or local statutory or regulatory provisions require hospitals to treat that type of medical record information in a particular manner, hospitals should follow the applicable requirements. For example, Medicare conditions of participation for hospitals require films, scans, and other image records to be maintained for at least five years.[21] In addition, some states require original X rays to be retained for a specified number of years. Other states require the hospital to retain all graphic data pertaining to hospital patients.[22] In the absence of specific legal guidance, institutions should develop a policy that meets the administrative and risk management objectives of the facility as well as the practical considerations involved in dealing with those items. Many institutions retain in the record any radiologic scans small enough to fit easily. Other items that cannot fit easily into the record are retained separately in the department that conducted the test, either indefinitely or at least as long as the facility retains its medical records. After the retention period has expired, institutions may find that it is prohibitively expensive to microfilm EKG tracings or fetal monitor strips. For certain technologies, such as scans, microfilming may not be possible because the microfilm may not be legible. Therefore, many institutions place these original items in long-term storage.

Dialysis Records

Patients who receive dialysis treatment for end-stage renal disease usually receive treatment several times per week on an outpatient basis for long periods of time. Those patients generate voluminous medical records. Medicare regulations require dialysis providers to retain patient records for the longest period of the following: the length of any applicable state statute or statute of limitations; or, in the absence of a state statute, for five years from the date of discharge; or, in the case of a minor, three years after the patient comes of age under state law. Medicare regulations also require that records be maintained in a manner that allows for prompt retrieval.[23] Generally, dialysis patient records should be retained for as long as the facility retains other medical records, so long as that policy meets the Medicare requirement. It may not be cost-efficient to microfilm dialysis patient records because of their volume, so many facilities store them in original form on-site for a reasonable period of time and off-site for the remainder of the retention period. Off-site storage should be acceptable as long as the records are easily retrievable.

Medical Record Entries

The medical record is often the most important document available to a hospital in defending a negligence action and ordinarily is admissible as evidence of what transpired in the care of the patient. Without a legible, complete medical record, the hospital may be unable to defend itself successfully against allegations of improper care. Therefore, hospitals must take great care to ensure that entries made in medical records are thorough and proper.

Legible and Complete Medical Records
Medical record entries should be made in clear and concise language that can be understood by all professional staff attending the patient. An ambiguous or illegible record often is worse than no record, because it documents a failure of the hospital and professional staff to communicate clearly and thus may impair the ability of the staff to provide proper treatment to the patient. In addition, an illegible record entry introduced into evidence in a court action against the hospital may create suspicion in the minds of the jury that the entry was improper and may thereby weaken the hospital's defense.

A person making entries should place his or her signature and position or title after each entry. Anyone who reads the medical record must be able to determine who participated in the patient's care should the need arise to consult on a treatment question or to reconstruct the hospitalization. Including appropriate titles also helps a reader evaluate the contents of the record entry.

The medical record should contain a complete account of the treatment given the patient.[24] A record is complete if it contains sufficient information to show clearly what treatment the patient received, why it was given, and, if some routine procedure was not given, the reason it was not. If a hospital can demonstrate by testimony about its policy, procedures, and routine practices that it regularly keeps complete and accurate records, the absence of certain notations may be used in the hospital's defense.[25] Otherwise, the failure to maintain a complete record may lead to a finding that the hospital was negligent in its treatment of the patient.[26]

The hospital's efforts to increase efficiency should never prevent its staff from keeping records that are sufficiently detailed to show the type and quality of care rendered. When careful observations are essential in particularly sensitive cases, all staff must document their contacts with patients. In some hospitals, especially tertiary care facilities, the elements of a patient's record will be kept in various departments throughout the hospital. Unless the complete record is maintained in one location, hospitals should have a cross-indexing system, so that all patient information is accessible when needed.

Accurate and Timely Completion of Medical Records
An inaccurate record not only may be detrimental to patient care and in violation of licensing statutes[27] and accreditation standards,[28] but also may allow a plaintiff in a professional negligence action to destroy the credibility of the entire record. In *Hiatt v. Groce*,[29] a Kansas court found that the clear discrepancy between what the medical record stated and what actually happened to the patient could justify the jury's finding that, if the medical record was erroneous in one respect, it could be erroneous in other respects as well and could be considered generally invalid.

Medical records must not only be accurate, but also must be completed in a timely manner. Entries should be made when the treatment they describe is given or the observations to be documented are made. Regulations governing participation in federal reimbursement programs require that hospital records be completed within 30 days following the patient's discharge.[30] Joint Commission accreditation standards require the hospital's medical staff regulations to state the time limit after discharge for completion of the record.[31] The bylaws or regulations of hospital medical staffs should require staff members to complete their patients' records within a specified time and should provide an automatic suspension of clinical privileges of members who fail to comply.

Incomplete medical records can be disastrous to a hospital's or physician's defense in a professional negligence action. Entries made in a record weeks after the patient's discharge have less credibility than those made during or immediately after the patient's hospitalization. If an entry is made after a lawsuit is threatened or filed, it may appear to have been made for purposes of establishing a defense rather than for documenting the actual treatment rendered.

It generally is the responsibility of the individual practitioner and the hospital's medical staff organization to ensure that patient records are completed within a reasonable time after the patient's discharge from the hospital.[32] The medical records department customarily is delegated responsibility for making sure that records are completed within the time specified by the hospital and for collating them into the permanent medical records. This department, with input from risk management staff, should establish procedures for notifying attending physicians when records are incomplete and for follow-up when a physician fails to respond.[33]

The final responsibility for completeness of the record rests with the patient's attending physician and the medical staff through enforcement of its bylaws and regulations. A hospital that fails to have and enforce proper medical record completion policies subjects itself and its medical staff to liability for breach of its duty to monitor a patient's treatment and for any ensuing injuries.[34]

Persons Making Entries

As the number and types of people making entries in patient medical records increase, so does the potential for increased liability. Unnecessary or improper entries can give rise to negligence liability exposure, problems involving unlicensed persons practicing nursing or medicine, and poor patient relations. In order to diminish that exposure, hospitals should have policies governing who may enter information in a record. Such policies should be carefully developed so that hospitals do not compromise patient care as they attempt to reduce liability exposure.

Given the broad legal and accrediting requirements in most states concerning the types of professionals who may write entries in the medical record,[35] any person providing care to a patient should be permitted to document that care in the patient's medical record, regardless of the person's position in the hospital. Hospitals should define the level of record documentation expected of practitioners working in the institution. To the extent that the hospital permits nurse midwives, podiatrists, dentists, clinical psychologists, physicians' assistants, social workers, and other nonphysician practitioners to provide treatment, it should require them to document their treatment in accordance with hospital medical records policy.

The entries of certain individuals require a physician's countersignature. The purpose of countersignatures is to require a professional to review and, if appropriate, indicate approval of action taken by another practitioner. Usually, the person countersigning a record entry is more experienced or has received a higher level of training than the person who made the original entry. In any case, the person required to countersign should have the authority to evaluate the entry. Countersignatures should not be viewed as needless paperwork, but rather as a means for carrying out delegated responsibility.

In most hospitals, licensed house staff may make entries in the patient charts, but attending physicians are required to countersign some or all such entries. Under Joint

Commission accreditation standards, hospitals may permit house staff to write orders in patient charts, but the patient's attending physician must document active participation in and supervision of the patient's care.[36] Each hospital should determine the extent to which countersignatures are required beyond the minimum regulatory requirements. What is important is that the medical record show clear evidence of the attending physician's supervision of house staff engaged in patient care.[37]

When undergraduate medical students and unlicensed house staff make record entries that show the application of medical judgment, medical diagnosis, the prescription of treatment, or any other act defined by applicable state law to be the practice of medicine, those entries should be countersigned by a licensed physician, who may be an attending or a resident physician. In most states, it is a violation of the medical licensure act for anyone to practice medicine without a license, unless he or she is practicing under the direct, proximate supervision of a physician licensed to practice in the state. Therefore, without evidence of such supervision, the student or unlicensed resident might be held to have violated state law. The rules governing a physician's countersignature of medical record entries made by other authorized personnel should be set forth in the hospital medical staff rules and regulations.[38]

Similarly, the entries of undergraduate nursing students should be countersigned by a licensed professional nurse, if such entries document the practice of professional nursing as defined by the state's nursing licensure act. Without evidence of proper supervision, a nursing student who practices professional nursing could be held in violation of the state's nursing licensure act, unless the act specifically authorizes nursing students to practice nursing in the course of their studies toward a registered nurse (RN) degree.[39] The nursing licensure acts of some states also authorize graduate nurses who have applied for a license to practice professional nursing for a limited time without a license.[40] Graduate, unlicensed nurses in those states may make entries in medical records without countersignature by a licensed nurse. However, in states that have no specific allowances for practice by such graduates, their entries should be properly countersigned. Moreover, hospitals may establish rules governing nursing student record entries that are more stringent than state law.

Although state and federal law generally is silent with regard to the entries of other students in the hospital, hospitals generally should require licensed professionals to countersign the record entries of students. The patient's medical record should show careful monitoring of students' scope of practice and competence.

In many hospitals, social workers participate in the care of patients and request that they be allowed to make entries in their patients' charts. Generally, there is no prohibition against entries by members of an institution's social services department, so long as the information placed in the record is relevant to the patient's treatment. Entries by social services staff should be limited to relevant factual observations or to data and judgments that such staff are competent to make; highly subjective remarks, if essential to the record, must be carefully worded and clearly relevant to the patient's care. Social workers should be discouraged from keeping other records of their observations and judgments that are not included in the medical record. These additional records may not enjoy the same confidentiality as do medical records.

Authentication of Records

The requirement that the physician or other medical practitioner sign records, or a portion of them, ensures authenticity. Most state regulations require a signature or other authentication for the record; authentication is the key element in system reliability and security. The Joint Commission requires that all entries in the record be dated and authenticated and that a method be established to identify the authors of entries. The Joint Commission further provides that entries can be authenticated by written signature, identifiable initials, or computer key.[41]

The Medicare conditions of participation require that records be authenticated by the person who is responsible for ordering, providing, or evaluating the service furnished.

The physician must authenticate each entry that he or she makes; a single signature on the face sheet of the record will not suffice to authenticate the entire record.[42]

Most states require a medical staff member to authenticate *and* sign entries in the medical record, thereby necessitating a written signature. However, a growing number of state regulations provide that entries may be either authenticated or signed, thus permitting authentication by a variety of means, including written signature, identifiable initials, computer key, rubber stamp, or mechanical means.

Several states expressly provide in their hospital regulations for authentication by means of computer keys or rubber-stamp signatures. However, all states that permit this type of authentication require that use of the authenticating devices be limited to the properly authorized individuals. With regard to rubber-stamp signatures, these states have adopted controls identical or very similar to those set forth in the Joint Commission's definition of authentication.

Although several states have adopted the Joint Commission definition of "authenticated" in their hospital regulations, it is not possible to state as a general rule that authentication of medical records may be accomplished by other than a written signature. Any health care institution that intends to automate its medical records information should confer with legal counsel to determine how its medical records may be authenticated in the proposed computer system. If state law requires a written signature for authentication, the institution must provide for such authentication in its automated system or obtain an amendment of the applicable, restrictive state law.

Verbal Orders

Verbal orders may be used when the physician is on the hospital unit but unable to write the order before it is carried out or when the physician is off the unit and must communicate orders by telephone. Joint Commission accreditation standards and hospital licensing regulations in most states require all physician orders to be written in the patient's medical record and authenticated.[43] In addition, Joint Commission accreditation standards state specifically that verbal orders must be transcribed in the medical record and that verbal orders associated with potential hazard to the patient must be signed by the physician within 24 hours.[44]

Regardless of laws or accrediting standards, hospitals should require all verbal orders to be transcribed within a specified time. A physician's signature on a transcribed verbal order authenticates the order and indicates that it was written correctly. Who may receive and transcribe a physician's verbal order is a matter of hospital policy and should be set forth in hospital policies or in the medical staff rules and regulations. The policies should be predicated on the concept that only personnel who are qualified to understand physicians' orders should be authorized to receive and transcribe verbal orders.

In view of the great potential for error in the transcription of verbal orders, hospitals should discourage all verbal orders except those that must be issued by telephone. Physicians should be responsible for writing their orders in the medical record, unless they are not present when the order must be given. If the physicians cannot write their orders in the record, they should authenticate their orders before leaving the unit. Nursing or house staff in most hospitals receive and transcribe telephone orders from attending physicians. Although not practicable in all cases, having a second person at the hospital on the telephone listening to the conversation reduces error and controversy concerning the order given. For especially sensitive orders, such as drug orders, hospitals should request that a second person listen to the order.

Corrections and Alterations

Because errors in medical record entries are inevitable, hospitals should establish clear procedures for making corrections. Generally, there are two kinds of errors: (1) minor errors in transcription and spelling and (2) more significant errors involving test results, physician orders, inadvertently omitted information, and similar substantive entries. As a general rule, the person who made the incorrect record entry should correct it. If the correction is a significant one, a senior person designated by hospital policy should review the correction to ensure that it complies with the institution's guidelines for record amendments. Hospital personnel should make changes that are within their scope of practice, as defined by state licensing and certification laws. A registered nurse, for example, should not amend a physician's medication order unless directed to do so by the physician or by a senior hospital official pursuant to established hospital policy. Obvious minor errors in spelling and the like do not require intervention by senior personnel. If possible, the person who made the error should correct it; however, any practitioner working with the record may correct such a minor error.

The person correcting an error in the record should cross out the incorrect entry, enter the correct information, initial the correction, and enter the time and date the correction was made (if not otherwise shown in the entry). Mistakes in the record should not be erased or obliterated, because erasures and obliterations are likely to make jurors suspicious about the original entry. A single line drawn through incorrect entries leaves no doubt as to the original information being corrected. Where a correction requires more space than is available near the original entry, the person correcting the record should enter a reference to an addendum to the record and enter the more lengthy correction in the addendum.

If the patient requests that the record be amended, hospital personnel should advise the patient's attending physician of the changes requested. If the physician considers the requested amendment inappropriate, he or she should discuss the matter with the patient. If the record is amended, the amendment should be made in an addendum to the record, and the physician should add an entry to document that the change was made at the request of the patient, who will thereafter bear the burden of explaining the change. The hospital should establish a policy governing such amendments.

After a claim has been made or a lawsuit has been threatened or filed against the hospital or a member of its staff, hospital personnel and medical staff should make no changes in the complainant's medical record without first consulting their defense counsel. Attempts to alter medical record entries in a way that might be favorable to the defendants are always inappropriate and do not necessarily help the defense, particularly if the patient has obtained a copy of the chart prior to the time that the changes are made. If the plaintiff can show that the record was altered without justification by a defendant, the plaintiff may be able to destroy the credibility of the entire record.[45]

If, after a claim has been made or a lawsuit threatened, an original record entry is found to be inaccurate or incomplete, the hospital should request that clarifications or additions to the record be placed in a properly signed and dated addendum to the record.

Deliberately altering a medical record or writing an incorrect record may subject the individual and the hospital to statutory sanctions. In some states, for example, a practitioner who makes a false entry on a medical record is subject to license revocation for unprofessional conduct.[46]

In other states, falsifying a medical record for purposes of cheating or defrauding is a crime.[47] Under federal statutes and regulations, altering or falsifying a chart for purposes of wrongfully obtaining government funds is a crime and subjects the violator to a substantial fine or imprisonment.[48]

Access to Medical Record Information

It is a generally accepted rule that the hospital owns the medical record, subject to the patient's interest in the information it contains. The medical record also is a confidential document; access to it should be limited to the patient, the patient's authorized representative and attending physician, and hospital staff members who have a legitimate interest in the record. There are many exceptions to this general rule that permit other individuals to review the medical record or that otherwise limit access by giving certain types of records a greater degree of confidentiality, such as psychiatric records or the records of alcohol and drug abuse patients. For a detailed discussion of access to medical records and confidentiality concerns, see chapter 24, "Confidentiality of Records Maintained in a Hospital Setting." Regardless of the applicable access rules, hospitals must devise effective record security procedures that will preserve and protect both the patient's confidentiality and the hospital's medical record.

Hospitals receive numerous forms of legal process, such as subpoenas or court orders, that require them to provide patient record information. The hospital should develop a response procedure based on a careful review of federal and state requirements. For a detailed discussion of response to legal process, see chapter 26, "Claims and Litigation Management."

Hospitals can be held liable to their patients for improper or unauthorized disclosure of medical record information. Aside from statutory penalties established in some jurisdictions, hospitals and practitioners may be liable for defamation, invasion of privacy, betrayal of professional secrets, and breach of contract for such disclosures. For a detailed discussion of liability for improper disclosure, see chapter 24.

Record Security

It is essential that hospitals establish effective procedures for safeguarding medical records, not only to protect patient confidentiality, but also to prevent intentional alteration or falsification of records by hospital staff or by individuals who wish to file a personal injury claim against a practitioner or the hospital or otherwise to use the records for an unlawful purpose.[49] Some hospitals have learned, to their misfortune, that given the opportunity, patients occasionally will remove important parts of their records or alter significant information in their records to improve their chances of bringing a successful professional negligence action. Hospitals have also found that, because medical record information can be useful to many people, some will do whatever is necessary to obtain it.

To protect their medical records from such abuse, hospitals should adopt at least the following security precautions:

- Competent medical records or risk management personnel should review a record before it is examined by the patient or by the patient's representative and should notify the appropriate hospital manager if the record is incomplete or otherwise defective, or if the record reveals a problem that could give rise to negligence liability in the hospital or its staff.
- An original medical record should not be permitted to be taken from the hospital's premises except pursuant to legal process or a defined hospital procedure allowing inpatients going to another facility for testing to take their medical record, if the patient is to return the same day and if the record is accompanied by a responsible hospital employee.
- Neither the patient, the patient's representative, nor any other person who is not an authorized hospital employee or staff member should ever be allowed to examine a medical record alone. The hospital should provide accommodations for people to inspect records in its medical records department or other location where proper surveillance is possible.

Maintenance of Legal Files

The hospital attorney, the risk management department, and the medical records department should cooperate to develop a legal file containing records of patients involved in litigation against the hospital. Other records, such as those of patients who have threatened to sue the institution but have not actually filed a lawsuit, can also be placed in the legal file according to hospital policy. Maintaining legal files is a simple method for handling records of a sensitive nature to (1) prevent them from being microfilmed, improperly altered, or destroyed; (2) allow medical record personnel to alert risk management when those records are requested and by whom; and (3) allow the risk management department and the hospital's attorney easy access to the records. After the hospital's risk manager and attorney have identified the records that should be placed in the legal file, the medical records department should secure the records in a locked, restricted location.[50]

If a patient who has litigation pending is readmitted to the hospital, the hospital should maintain the original record in the legal file. A copy of the record, with each page numbered, can go back to the file room for reference. The data from the patient's readmission should be entered as new original materials that will be combined with the rest of the original record at the conclusion of the hospitalization.

☐ Business Records

A hospital's business records may contain a number of different kinds of documents, among them incident reports and records of hospital and medical staff committees.

Incident Reports

Hospitals generally generate incident reports[51] about any event that is not consistent with the routine operation of the hospital or with the routine care of a particular patient, including actual accidents or situations that may result in an accident. In risk management programs, incident reports alert the hospital and its insurer to particular situations that could lead to liability. They also provide the institution with information that will enable it to monitor unusual occurrences.

Although incident reports may be an essential part of a claims and risk management program, they also can provide a great deal of information for parties in litigation. If the incident described in the report is the event that the plaintiff alleges caused the injury, the plaintiff will do everything legally possible to obtain the report for use as evidence. If the report contains admissions of negligent conduct by hospital employees, the plaintiff is likely to find it easier to build a case against the institution.[52] Although incident reports can be protected from discovery in legal proceedings in some instances, it is clearly the trend that incident reports will be discoverable. Therefore, hospitals should take the following precautions to protect their reports:

- Treat incident reports as confidential documents, clearly marked as such.
- Strictly limit the number of copies made and the distribution of the reports in the institution.
- Do not place a copy of the report in the patient's medical record or in a file in the patient care unit. Copies may be retained with other quality assurance records, however.
- Limit the content of the report to facts, not conclusions or assignment of blame. Analyses of the cause of an incident should be placed in a separate document.
- Address the report and any separate analysis of an incident to the hospital's attorney or claims manager, by name.
- Train hospital personnel to complete incident reports with the same care used in completing a medical record.
- Treat incident reports as quality assurance records and subject them to the same stringent policies as are applied to other quality assurance records.

Hospital and Medical Staff Committee Records

Hospitals are required by a variety of authorities to establish and maintain programs to monitor and improve the quality of the patient care they provide.[53] Included in those quality assurance programs are certain committees of the medical staff, each of which may collect data and generate records concerning the performance of individual physicians practicing in the hospital or the treatment provided to particular patients in the hospital. Counsel representing plaintiffs in professional negligence actions against practitioners and hospitals have shown an increasing interest in the proceedings, records, and reports of those committees as a source of important evidence. Peer review committees have the responsibility of monitoring and evaluating the quality of care provided by a particular hospital. Typically, a hospital will have at least the following committees: (1) executive committee, (2) credentials committee, (3) medical audit committee, (4) tissue committee, and (5) utilization review committee.[54] Each generates documents and information that could be quite damaging to a doctor charged with malpractice.

The potential value of such records to the plaintiff in a negligence action is clear, and the demand for access to them has created a substantial body of statutory and common law. A hospital should be familiar with the applicable statutory provisions and relevant court decisions in its state before it establishes procedures for creating and maintaining hospital and medical staff committee records.

Authorities do not agree on whether hospital and medical staff committee records should be discoverable. Some courts hold that, if quality assurance programs are to work properly, they must be conducted confidentially, and that the records of such are not discoverable. Other courts give greater weight to the plaintiff's need for information vital to his or her case than to policy considerations in favor of confidential committee proceedings.

In response to the decisions declaring those records to be discoverable, many state legislatures have enacted statutes protecting the records from discovery, although the extent of protection varies. Some statutes provide that such records generally are not subject to subpoena, discovery, or disclosure; other statutes state specifically that such committee records, proceedings, and reports are not discoverable, or describe such material as confidential or privileged. A common exception to nondiscovery statutes allows physicians to discover records of staff privilege committees when contesting the termination, suspension, or limitation of their staff privileges. Nondiscovery statutes typically also provide that the statute is not to be construed as protecting from discovery information, documents, and records that are otherwise available from original sources. Further, people who testify before committees are not immune from discovery, but they may not be asked about their testimony before the committee.[55] Although most statutes provide protection only to medical staff committee activities and records, a few statutes are broad enough to include other hospital review committees.[56]

Because state statutes and court decisions concerning protection of peer review and quality assurance activities from discovery vary considerably, hospitals should carefully review and thoroughly understand the applicable law. Institutions should organize and operate peer review and quality assurance activities in a manner designed to obtain the greatest possible protection under applicable law. Although arguments may be made in support of the discoverability of committee records, hospitals generally can operate with greater flexibility and efficiency and with less risk if peer review and quality assurance records carry some degree of protection.

Once the hospital has developed its policies concerning committee records, all hospital and medical staff personnel involved in committee activities should be educated as to the importance of following policies meticulously. Peer review and quality assurance activities should be identified as such and documented in a manner that reinforces their official peer review status and thereby will likely qualify them for maximum protection under state law.

All peer review committee minutes and reports should be carefully prepared and should demonstrate that the hospital performed an objective, considered review. In most states, committee minutes should document actions taken on the matters discussed and not the details of the actual discussion or personal comments made by committee members. The hospital should limit distribution of and access to committee minutes and reports to as few individuals and files as possible.

In all matters relating to developing policies governing the creation and use of peer review and quality assurance materials, hospitals should consult with their legal counsel, especially in states in which rules of discoverability are ambiguous or in which courts have narrowly construed protection statutes. Hospitals should instruct their legal counsel to advise them of changes in applicable law as they occur and to review those policies at least annually.

Retention Guidelines for Selected Business Records

Certain hospital business records will require special retention guidelines.

Policy and Procedure Manuals

Policy and procedure manuals can provide critical evidence in constructing the defense for a hospital in a lawsuit. A case could easily turn on whether the hospital had a particular policy in place at the time a certain incident occurred and whether the hospital in fact followed its policy. Therefore, hospitals should retain a master set of those manuals and keep a historical record so that someone reviewing the manuals can identify exactly what policy was in place at a particular time. That will require the hospital to date the original manual and keep a careful record of all revisions and their respective effective dates.

Indexes, Registers, and Logs

Hospitals generate enormous amounts of information through indexes, registers, daily logs, and worksheets. Those materials permit patient information and other health care information to be located and classified for patient care management and research purposes, quality of care and utilization review, administrative and financial purposes, and compliance with state regulations or licensure requirements.[57] In litigation, those records can provide crucial information for the hospital's defense. Although most states have no legal guidelines establishing retention periods for such information, hospitals should consider developing policies for the storage and retention of those records. Hospitals should retain such materials for as long as any state or local statute or regulation may require. Some institutions maintain at least the master patient indexes in original or microfilm form as permanent files. Institutions may retain other materials for as long as they retain medical records. Furthermore, because such documents contain patient-identifying information, hospitals should be certain that these secondary sources of confidential information are treated with the same degree of care as other patient information.

Equipment Purchase and Maintenance Records

A hospital could be found liable if patients are injured as a result of improperly selected or maintained equipment. If a hospital is required to defend a suit arising from an equipment defect, the records of the equipment purchase and periodic maintenance history may be useful in defending its case. The Joint Commission requires hospitals to conduct an extensive preventive maintenance program and to document the various aspects of the program.[58] The Joint Commission also requires equipment maintenance records for the pathology and medical laboratory service to be maintained for the life of each instrument used.[59] In addition, the Joint Commission requires hospitals to have a multidisciplinary safety committee to adopt, implement, and monitor a comprehensive, hospitalwide safety program. Hospitals should retain those records for as long as any state statute, regulation, or accreditation standard may require. Hospitals also may adopt a policy of retaining such records for the period of the statute of limitations applicable to professional negligence actions, so long as that period exceeds the requirements of any statute, regulation, or accreditation standard.

Corporate Records, Minutes, and Other Governance Documents
The hospital should retain original corporate documents and all amendments and updates permanently in its archives.

Billing Records
Medicare requires billing materials and related attachments, including charge slips, daily patient census, and other business and accounting records referring to specific claims to be retained in original or microfilmed form for five years after the month that the cost report is filed with the intermediary, unless state law requires a longer retention period.[60] Billing records are likely to contain patient information that should be protected in the same manner as all other patient information. In addition, the American Medical Record Association recommends that the billing records be retained in a locked storeroom accessible only to the billing manager and the health information manager.[61]

Personnel Records
Personnel records must be maintained pursuant to federal and state law and regulation. See chapter 30 for a detailed discussion of those issues.

References

1. This chapter focuses on medical records kept by hospitals or under hospital sponsorship according to the legal requirements governing hospitals. In certain instances, specialized programs under hospital sponsorship also may be subject to legal requirements governing those specific programs. These additional medical records requirements should be reviewed separately.

2. This section was adapted from *Medical Records and the Law* by W. H. Roach, Jr., S. N. Chernoff, and C. L. Esley, with permission of Aspen Publishers, Inc., ©1985, pp. 1–28.

3. Waters, K., and Murphy, G. *Medical Records in Health Information*. Germantown, MD: Aspen Publishers, 1979, pp. 39–95.

4. Fulton, D. K. Legal problems arising in the automation of medical records. *Topics in Health Record Management* 8(2):73–79, Dec. 1987; Wynstra, N. Computerized medical records: legal problems and implications. *Topics in Health Record Management* 2(2):75–84, Dec.1981 .

5. Waters and Murphy, p. 257.

6. *See, e.g.*, Foley v. Flushing Hospital and Medical Center, 34 N.Y.2d 863, 359 N.Y.S.2d 113 (1974).

7. *See, e.g.*, N.Y. Pub. Health Law sec. 4165 (McKinney 1985); Tenn. Code Ann. §68-11-302 (1987).

8. *See, e.g.*, Ill. Hosp. Licensing Requirements tit. 77 Ill. Admin. Code §250.1510 (1985).

9. Joint Commission on Accreditation of Healthcare Organizations. *Accreditation Manual for Hospitals*. Chicago: JCAHO, 1989, p. 87.

10. *Id.* at 89–93.

11. *See, e.g.*, N.M. Stat. Ann. §14-6-2 (1978).

12. *See, e.g.*, Ill. Ann. Stat. ch. 111-1/2, §157-11 (Smith-Hurd 1977).

13. *See, e.g.*, Miss. Code Ann. §41-9-69 (1981).

14. 42 C.F.R. §482.24(b)(1) (1988); 42 C.F.R. §482.25(d)(2).

15. H.I.M.-10 §§480, 480.1.

16. *See, e.g.*, Cal. Evid. Code §§1550 (1966); Mass. Gen. Laws Ann. ch. 111, §70 (1985 and West Supp. 1988); N.J. Stat. Ann. §26:8-5 (1987 and Supp. 1988); Va. Code §8.01-391 (1984).

17. *See, e.g.*, Ind. Code Ann. §34-3-15.5-1 *et seq.* (West 1983).

18. Gardner, E. Automated medical chart becoming a priority. *Modern Healthcare* 18(36):29–37, Sept. 2, 1988; Roach, W. H., Jr. The case for and against optical disk storage. *Topics in Health Record Management* 9(3):79–83, Mar. 1989.

19. *See, e.g.*, Miss. Code Ann. §41-9-75 (1981).

20. 40 C.F.R. §246 (1988).

21. 42 C.F.R. §482.25(d)(2).

22. *See, e.g.,* Tenn. Code Ann. §68-11-302 (1987).

23. 42 C.F.R. §405.2139 (1988).

24. *See, e.g.,* N.J. Stat. Ann. §26.8-5 (1987 and Supp. 1988); Tenn. Code Ann. §68-11-303 (1987); Ill. Hosp. Licensing Requirements tit. 77 Ill. Admin. Code §250.1510 (1985); Joint Commission on Accreditation of Healthcare Organizations, p. 94.

25. Smith v. Roger's Memorial Hospital, 382 A.2d 1025 (App. D.C.), *cert. denied.* 439 U.S. 847 (1978).

26. Collins v. Westlake Community Hospital, 57 Ill.2d 388, 312 N.E.2d 614 (1974).

27. *See, e.g.,* Miss. Code Ann. §41-9-63 (1981).

28. Joint Commission on Accreditation of Healthcare Organizations, p. 95.

29. 215 Kan. 14, 523 P.2d 320, 326 (1974).

30. 42 C.F.R. §482.24(c)(viii) (1988).

31. Joint Commission on Accreditation of Healthcare Organizations, p. 96.

32. *Id.*

33. Skurka, M. F. *Organization of Medical Record Departments in Hospitals.* 2d ed. Chicago: American Hospital Publishing, 1988, p. 54.

34. Bost v. Riley, 44 N.C. App. 638, 262 S.E.2d 391, *appeal denied,* 300 N.C. 194, 269 S.E.2d 621 (1980).

35. Joint Commission on Accreditation of Healthcare Organizations, p. 95.

36. *Id..*

37. Joint Commission on Accreditation of Healthcare Organizations, p. 95.

38. *Id.*

39. *See, e.g.,* Ill. Ann. Stat. ch. 111, §3504 (Smith-Hurd Supp. 1988).

40. *Id.*

41. Joint Commission on Accreditation of Healthcare Organizations, p. 95.

42. 42 C.F.R. §482.24(c)(1988).

43. Joint Commission on Accreditation of Healthcare Organizations, pp. 91, 95. Ill. Hosp. Licensing Requirements tit. 77 Ill. Admin. Code §§250.330 and 250.1510 (1985).

44. Joint Commission on Accreditation of Healthcare Organizations, p. 91, 95.

45. Pisel v. Stamford Hospital, 180 Conn. 314, 430 A.2d 1 (1980).

46. *See, e.g.,* Ky. Rev. Stat. §311.595 (1983).

47. *See, e.g.,* Tenn. Code Ann. §39-3-944 (1982).

48. 42 U.S.C. §1320a-7a (Supp. 1988); 42 U.S.C. §1320a-7b (Supp. 1988).

49. This section was adapted from *Medical Records and the Law* by W. H. Roach, Jr., S. N. Chernoff, and C. L. Esley, with permission of Aspen Publishers, Inc., © 1985, p. 71.

50. Crane, E. J., and Reckard, J. M. Hospital liability and risk management and the medical record. *Topics in Health Record Management* 2(1):49–59, Sept. 1981.

51. This section was adapted from *Medical Records and the Law* by W. H. Roach, Jr., S. N. Chernoff, and C. L. Esley, with permission of Aspen Publishers, Inc., © 1985, pp. 137–139.

52. Roach, W. H., Jr. Hospital incident reports. *Topics in Health Record Management* 2(2):85–90, Dec. 1981.

53. This section was adapted from *Medical Records and the Law* by W. H. Roach, Jr., S. N. Chernoff, and C. L. Esley, with permission of Aspen Publishers, Inc., © 1985, pp. 126–36.

54. Holbrook, R., and Dunn, L. Medical malpractice litigation: the discoverability and use of hospital quality assurance committee records. *Washburn Law Journal* 16:54, Fall 1976.

55. Ca. Evid. Code §1157 (Supp. 1989). *See also* West Covina Hosp. v. Superior Court, 153 Cal. App.3d 134, 200 Cal. Rptr. 162 (1984).

56. Tenn. Code Ann. §63-6-219(a) (1986 and Supp. 1988).

57. Skurka, p. 63.

58. Joint Commission on Accreditation of Healthcare Organizations, pp. 150, 154, 156, 208–10.

58. Joint Commission on Accreditation of Healthcare Organizations, p. 156.

60. H.I.M.-10, §480, 480.1.

61. *Confidentiality of Patient Health Information: Position Statement of the American Medical Record Association.* Chicago: American Medical Record Association, 1985.

Bibliography

Confidentiality of Patient Health Information: Position Statement of the American Medical Record Association. Chicago: American Medical Record Association, 1985.

Crane, E. J., and Reckard, J. M. Hospital liability and risk management and the medical record. *Topics in Health Record Management* 2(1):49–59, Sept. 1981.

Fulton, D. K. Legal problems arising in the automation of medical records. *Topics in Health Record Management* 8(2):73–79, Dec. 1987.

Gardner, E. Automated medical chart becoming a priority. *Modern Healthcare* 18(36):29–37, Sept. 2, 1988.

Holbrook, R., and Dunn, L. Medical malpractice litigation: the discoverability and use of hospital quality assurance committee records. *Washburn Law Journal* 16:54, Fall 1976.

Joint Commission on Accreditation of Healthcare Organizations. *Accreditation Manual for Hospitals.* Chicago: JCAHO, 1989.

Micheletti, J. A., and Shlala, T. J. Risk prevention: a market for health record services. *Journal of American Medical Record Association* 58:20–25, Feb. 1987.

Roach, W. H., Jr., Chernoff, S. N., and Esley, C. L. *Medical Records and the Law.* Rockville, MD: Aspen Publishers, 1985.

Roach, W. H., Jr. Hospital incident reports. *Topics in Health Record Management* 2(2):85–90, Dec. 1981.

Roach, W. H., Jr. The case for and against optical disk storage. *Topics in Health Record Management* 9(3):79–83, Mar. 1989.

Rowland, H. S., and Rowland, B. L. *Hospital Legal Forms, Checklists and Guidelines.* Rockville, MD: Aspen Publishers, 1988.

Skurka, M. F. *Organization of Medical Record Departments in Hospitals.* 2nd ed. Chicago: American Hospital Publishing, 1988.

Smith, J. W. *Hospital Liability.* New York City: Law Journal Seminars Press, 1988.

Waters, K., and Murphy, G. F. *Medical Records in Health Information.* Germantown, MD: Aspen Publishers, 1979.

Wynstra, N. Computerized medical records: legal problems and implications. *Topics in Health Record Management* 2(2):75–84, Dec. 1981.

Appendix A

JCAHO Risk Management Standards for 1990

The following standards are from the *Accreditation Manual for Hospitals, 1990 edition.* Copyright 1989 by the Joint Commission on Accreditation of Healthcare Organizations, Chicago. Reprinted with permission.

"Governing Body" Chapter

GB.1.19 The governing body provides for resources and support systems for the quality assurance functions and risk management functions related to patient care and safety.

"Management and Administrative Services" Chapter

MA.1.8 The chief executive officer, through the management and administrative staff, provides support for:

    MA.1.8.1 The medical staff in the following activities:

        MA.1.8.1.1 the identification of general areas of potential risk in the clinical aspects of patient care and safety;

        MA.1.8.1.2 the development of criteria for identifying specific cases with potential risk in the clinical aspects of patient care and safety, and evaluation of these cases;

        MA.1.8.1.3 the correction of problems in the clinical aspects of patient care and safety identified by risk management activities; and

        MA.1.8.1.4 the design of programs to reduce risk in the clinical aspects of patient care and safety.

    MA.1.8.2 The establishment and maintenance of operational linkages between the risk management functions related to the clinical aspects of patient care and safety and the quality assurance functions.

    MA.1.8.3 In quality assurance functions, access to existing information from risk management activities that may be useful in identifying clinical problems and/or opportunities to improve the quality of patient care.

"Quality Assurance" Chapter

QA.1   There is an ongoing quality assurance program designed to objectively and systematically monitor and evaluate the quality and appropriateness of patient care, pursue opportunities to improve patient care, and resolve identified problems.

QA.1.1   The governing body strives to assure quality patient care by requiring and supporting the establishment and maintenance of an effective hospitalwide quality assurance program.

QA.1.2   Clinical and administrative staffs monitor and evaluate the quality and appropriateness of patient care and clinical performance, resolve identified problems, and report information to the governing body that the governing body needs to assist it in fulfilling its responsibility for the quality of patient care.

QA.1.3   There is a written plan for the quality assurance program that describes the program's objectives, organization, scope, and mechanisms for overseeing the effectiveness of monitoring, evaluation, and problem-solving activities.

QA.1.4   There are operational linkages between the risk management functions related to the clinical aspects of patient care and safety and quality assurance functions.

QA.1.5   Existing information from risk management activities that may be useful in identifying clinical problems and/or opportunities to improve the quality of patient care is accessible to the quality assurance function.

QA.2.3   The following hospitalwide functions are performed:

QA.2.3.3   Review of accidents, injuries, patient safety, and safety hazards ("Plant, Technology, and Safety Management," Standard PL.1., Required Characteristics PL.1.4.2, PL.1.4.3, and PL.1.7).

"Medical Staff" Chapter

MS.1.2.3.1.3   Each applicant for medical staff membership completes an application that asks for information specified in the medical staff bylaws.

MS.1.2.3.1.3.1   Information related to the following is provided:

MS.1.2.3.1.3.1.1   Previously successful or currently pending challenges to any licensure or registration (states or district, Drug Enforcement Administration), or the voluntary relinquishment of such licensure or registration; and

MS.1.2.3.1.3.1.2   Voluntary or involuntary termination of medical staff membership or voluntary or involuntary limitation, reduction, or loss of clinical privileges at another hospital.

MS.1.2.3.1.3.3   Medical staff bylaws and rules and regulations specify the circumstances in which an individual is to report involvement in a professional liability action.

MS.1.2.3.1.3.3.1   At a minimum, final judgments or settlements involving the individual are reported.

MS.4.2   The following requirements pertinent to clinical privileges are observed:

MS.4.2.2   Professional criteria specified in the medical staff bylaws and uniformly applied to all applicants for delineated clinical privileges constitute the basis for granting clinical privileges.

MS.4.2.2.2 The criteria include, at the least, evidence of current licensure, relevant training and/or experience, current competence, and health status.

MS.4.2.2.3 Medical staff bylaws and rules and regulations specify the circumstances in which an individual is to report involvement in a professional liability action.

MS.4.2.2.3.1 At a minimum, final judgment or settlements involving the individual are reported.

MS.4.2.6 The granting of delineated clinical privileges is also based on information regarding:

MS.4.2.6.1 previously successful or currently pending challenges to any licensure or registration (state or district, Drug Enforcement Administration), or the voluntary relinquishment of such licensure or registration; and

MS.4.2.6.2 voluntary or involuntary termination of medical staff membership, or voluntary or involuntary limitation, reduction, or loss of clinical privileges at another hospital.

MS.5.3 Reappointment and/or the renewal or revision of clinical privileges is based on a reappraisal of the individual at the time of reappointment and/or the renewal or revision of clinical privileges.

MS.5.3.1 The reappraisal includes information concerning

MS.5.3.1.1 the individual's current licensure;

MS.5.3.1.2 the individual's health status;

MS.5.3.1.3 the individual's professional performance;

MS.5.3.1.4 the individual's judgment;

MS.5.3.1.5 the individual's clinical and/or technical skills, as indicated in part by the results of quality assurance activities;

MS.5.3.1.6 previously successful or currently pending challenges to any licensure or registration (state or district, Drug Enforcement Administration), or the voluntary relinquishment of such licensure or registration;

MS.5.3.1.7 voluntary or involuntary termination of medical staff membership, or voluntary or involuntary limitation, reduction, or loss of clinical privileges at another hospital; and

MS.5.3.1.8 other reasonable indicators of continuing qualifications.

MS.5.3.2 Medical staff bylaws and rules and regulations specify the circumstances in which an individual is to report involvement in a professional liability action.

MS.5.3.2.1 At a minimum, final judgments or settlements involving the individual are reported.

MS.6.1.7 Risk Management Activities

MS.6.1.7.1 The medical staff actively participates, as appropriate, in the following risk management activities related to the clinical aspects of patient care and safety:

MS.6.1.7.1.1 the identification of general areas of potential risk in the clinical aspects of patient care and safety;

MS.6.1.7.1.2 the development of criteria for identifying specific cases with potential risk in the clinical aspects of patient care and safety, and evaluation of these cases;

MS.6.1.7.1.3 the correction of problems in the clinical aspects of patient care and safety identified by risk management activities; and

MS.6.1.7.1.4 the design of programs to reduce risk in the clinical aspects of patient care and safety.

MS.6.1.8 Other Review Functions

MS.6.1.8.1 The medical staff participates in other review functions, including infection control, internal and external disaster plans, hospital safety, and utilization review.

☐ Glossary Definition

Risk Management—The standards pertaining to risk management in this *Manual* address only those risk management functions relating to clinical and administrative activities designed to identify, evaluate, and reduce the risk of patient injury associated with care. The full scope of risk management functions encompasses activities in health care organizations that are intended to conserve financial resources from loss. Those functions include a broad range of administrative activities intended to reduce losses associated with patient, employee, or visitor injuries; property loss or damages; and other sources of potential organizational liability. Many of these activities are beyond the scope of Joint Commission standards.

Appendix B

Health Care Quality Improvement Act of 1986

TITLE IV—ENCOURAGING GOOD FAITH PROFESSIONAL REVIEW ACTIVITIES

SEC. 401. SHORT TITLE.

This title may be cited as the "Health Care Quality Improvement Act of 1986."

SEC. 402. FINDINGS.

The Congress finds the following:

(1) The increasing occurrence of medical malpractice and the need to improve the quality of medical care have become nationwide problems that warrant greater efforts than those that can be undertaken by any individual State.

(2) There is a national need to restrict the ability of incompetent physicians to move from State to State without disclosure or discovery of the physician's previous damaging or incompetent performance.

(3) This nationwide problem can be remedied through effective professional peer review.

(4) The threat of private money damage liability under Federal laws, including treble damage liability under Federal antitrust law, unreasonably discourages physicians from participating in effective professional peer review.

(5) There is an overriding national need to provide incentive and protection for physicians engaging in effective professional peer review.

PART A—PROMOTION OF PROFESSIONAL REVIEW ACTIVITIES

SEC. 411. PROFESSIONAL REVIEW.

(a) IN GENERAL.—

(1) LIMITATION ON DAMAGES FOR PROFESSIONAL REVIEW ACTIONS.— If a professional review action (as defined in section 431[9]) of a professional review body meets all the standards specified in section 412(a), except as provided in subsection (b)—

(A) the professional review body,

(B) any person acting as a member or staff to the body,

(C) any person under a contract or other formal agreement with the body, and

(D) any person who participates with or assists the body with respect to the action, shall not be liable in damages under any law of the United States or of any State (or political subdivision thereof) with respect to the action. The preceding sentence shall not apply to damages under any law of the United States or any State relating to the civil rights of any person or persons, including the Civil Rights Act of 1964, 42 U.S.C. 2000e, *et seq.* and the Civil Rights Acts, 42 U.S.C. 1981, *et seq.* Nothing in this paragraph shall prevent the United States or any Attorney General of a State from bringing an action, including an action under section 4C of the Clayton Act, 15 U.S.C. 15C, where such an action is otherwise authorized.

(2) PROTECTION FOR THOSE PROVIDING INFORMATION TO PROFESSIONAL REVIEW BODIES.—Notwithstanding any other provision of law, no person (whether as a witness or otherwise) providing information to a professional review body regarding the competence or professional conduct of a physician shall be held, by reason of having provided such information, to be liable in damages under any law of the United States or of any State (or political subdivision thereof) unless such information is false and the person providing it knew that such information was false.

(b) EXCEPTION.—If the Secretary has reason to believe that a health care entity has failed to report information in accordance with section 423(a), the Secretary shall conduct an investigation. If, after providing notice of noncompliance, an opportunity to correct the noncompliance, and an opportunity for a hearing, the Secretary determines that a health care entity has failed substantially to report information in accordance with section 423(a), the Secretary shall publish the name of the entity in the *Federal Register*. The protections of subsection (a)(1) shall not apply to an entity the name of which is published in the *Federal Register* under the previous sentence with respect to professional review actions of the entity commenced during the 3-year period beginning 30 days after the date of publication of the name.

(c) TREATMENT UNDER STATE LAWS.—

(1) PROFESSIONAL REVIEW ACTIONS TAKEN ON OR AFTER OCTOBER 14, 1989.—Except as provided in paragraph (2), subsection (a) shall apply to State laws in a State only for professional review actions commenced on or after October 14, 1989.

(2) EXCEPTIONS.—

(A) STATE EARLY OPT-IN.—Subsection (a) shall apply to State laws in a State for actions commenced before October 14, 1989, if the State by legislation elects such treatment.

(B) STATE OPT-OUT.—Subsection (a) shall not apply to State laws in a State for actions commenced on or after October 14, 1989, if the State by legislation elects such treatment.

(C) EFFECTIVE DATE OF ELECTION.—An election under State law is not effective, for purposes of subparagraphs (A) and (B), for actions commenced before the effective date of the State law, which may not be earlier than the date of the enactment of that law.

SEC. 412. STANDARDS FOR PROFESSIONAL REVIEW ACTIONS.

(a) IN GENERAL.—For purposes of the protection set forth in section 411(a), a professional review action must be taken—

(1) in the reasonable belief that the action was in the furtherance of quality health care,

(2) after a reasonable effort to obtain the facts of the matter,

(3) after adequate notice and hearing procedures are afforded to the physician involved or after such other procedures as are fair to the physician under the circumstances, and

(4) in the reasonable belief that the action was warranted by the facts known after such reasonable effort to obtain facts and after meeting the requirement of paragraph (3). A professional review action shall be presumed to have met the preceding standards necessary for the protection set out in section 411(a) unless the presumption is rebutted by a preponderance of the evidence.

(b) ADEQUATE NOTICE AND HEARING.—A health care entity is deemed to have met the adequate notice and hearing requirement of subsection (a)(3) with respect to a physician if the following conditions are met (or are waived voluntarily by the physician):

(1) NOTICE OF PROPOSED ACTION.—The physician has been given notice stating—

(A) (i) that a professional review action has been proposed to be taken against the physician,

(ii) reasons for the proposed action,

(B) (i) that the physician has the right to request a hearing on the proposed action,

(ii) any time limit (of not less than 30 days) within which to request such a hearing, and

(C) a summary of the rights in the hearing under paragraph (3).

(2) NOTICE OF HEARING.—If a hearing is requested on a timely basis under paragraph (1)(B), the physician involved must be given notice stating—

(A) the place, time, and date, of the hearing, which date shall not be less than 30 days after the date of the notice, and

(B) a list of the witnesses (if any) expected to testify at the hearing on behalf of the professional review body.

(3) CONDUCT OF HEARING AND NOTICE.—If a hearing is requested on a timely basis under paragraph (1)(B)—

(A) subject to subparagraph (B), the hearing shall be held (as determined by the health care entity)—

(i) before an arbitrator mutually acceptable to the physician and the health care entity,

(ii) before a hearing officer who is appointed by the entity and who is not in direct economic competition with the physician involved, or

(iii) before a panel of individuals who are appointed by the entity and are not in direct economic competition with the physician involved;

(B) the right to the hearing may be forfeited if the physician fails, without good cause, to appear;

(C) in the hearing the physician involved has the right—

(i) to representation by an attorney or other person of the physician's choice,

(ii) to have a record made of the proceedings, copies of which may be obtained by the physician upon payment of any reasonable charges associated with the preparation thereof,

(iii) to call, examine, and cross-examine witnesses,

(iv) to present evidence determined to be relevant by the hearing officer, regardless of its admissibility in a court of law, and

(v) to submit a written statement at the close of the hearing; and

(D) upon completion of the hearing, the physician involved has the right—

(i) to receive the written recommendation of the arbitrator, officer, or panel, including a statement of the basis for the recommendations, and

(ii) to receive a written decision of the health care entity, including a statement of the basis for the decision.

A professional review body's failure to meet the conditions described in this subsection shall not, in itself, constitute failure to meet the standards of subsection (a)(3).

(c) ADEQUATE PROCEDURES IN INVESTIGATIONS OR HEALTH EMERGENCIES.—For purposes of section 411(a), nothing in this section shall be construed as—

(1) requiring the procedures referred to in subsection (a)(3)—

(A) where there is no adverse professional review action taken, or

(B) in the case of a suspension or restriction of clinical privileges, for a period of not longer than 14 days, during which an investigation is being conducted to determine the need for a professional review action; or

(2) precluding an immediate suspension or restriction of clinical privileges, subject to subsequent notice and hearing or other adequate procedures, where the failure to take such an action may result in an imminent danger to the health of any individual.

SEC. 413. PAYMENT OF REASONABLE ATTORNEYS' FEES AND COSTS IN DEFENSE OF SUIT.

In any suit brought against a defendant, to the extent that a defendant has met the standards set forth under section 412(a) and the defendant substantially prevails, the court shall, at the conclusion of the action, award to a substantially prevailing party defending against any such claim the cost of the suit attributable to such claim, including a reasonable attorney's fee, if the claim, or the claimant's conduct during the litigation of the claim, was frivolous, unreasonable, without foundation, or in bad faith. For the purposes of this section, a defendant shall not be considered to have substantially prevailed when the plaintiff obtains an award for damages or permanent injunctive or declaratory relief.

SEC. 414. GUIDELINES OF THE SECRETARY.

The Secretary may establish, after notice and opportunity for comment, such voluntary guidelines as may assist the professional review bodies in meeting the standards described in section 412(a).

SEC. 415. CONSTRUCTION.

(a) IN GENERAL.—Except as specifically provided in this part, nothing in this part shall be construed as changing the liabilities or immunities under law.

(b) SCOPE OF CLINICAL PRIVILEGES.—Nothing in this part shall be construed as requiring health care entities to provide clinical privileges to any or all classes of physicians or other licensed health care practitioners.

(c) TREATMENT OF NURSES AND OTHER PRACTITIONERS.—Nothing in this part shall be construed as affecting, or modifying any provision of Federal or State law, with respect to activities of professional review bodies regarding nurses, other licensed health care practitioners, or other health professionals who are not physicians.

(d) TREATMENT OF PATIENT MALPRACTICE CLAIMS.—Nothing in this title shall be construed as affecting in any manner the rights and remedies afforded patients under any provision of Federal or State law to seek redress for any harm or injury suffered as a result of negligent treatment or care by any physician, health care practitioner, or health care entity, or as limiting any defenses or immunities available to any physician, health care practitioner, or health care entity.

SEC. 416. EFFECTIVE DATE.

This part shall apply to professional review actions commenced on or after the date of the enactment of this Act.

PART B—REPORTING OF INFORMATION

SEC. 421. REQUIRING REPORTS ON MEDICAL MALPRACTICE PAYMENTS.

(a) IN GENERAL.—Each entity (including an insurance company) which makes payment under a policy of insurance, self-insurance, or otherwise in settlement (or partial settlement) of, or in satisfaction of a judgment in, a medical malpractice action or claim shall report, in accordance with section 424, information respecting the payment and circumstances thereof.

(b) INFORMATION TO BE REPORTED.—The information to be reported under subsection (a) includes—

(1) the name of any physician or licensed health care practitioner for whose benefit the payment is made,

(2) the amount of the payment,

(3) the name (if known) of any hospital with which the physician or practitioner is affiliated or associated,

(4) a description of the acts or omissions and injuries or illnesses upon which the action or claim was based, and

(5) such other information as the Secretary determines is required for appropriate interpretation of information reported under this section.

(c) SANCTIONS FOR FAILURE TO REPORT.—Any entity that fails to report information on a payment required to be reported under this section shall be subject to a civil money penalty of not more than $10,000 for each such payment involved. Such penalty shall be imposed and collected in the same manner as civil money penalties under subsection (a) of section 1128A of the Social Security Act are imposed and collected under that section.

(d) REPORT ON TREATMENT OF SMALL PAYMENTS.—The Secretary shall study and report to Congress, not later than two years after the date of the enactment of this Act, on whether information respecting small payments should continue to be required to be reported under subsection (a) and whether information respecting all claims made concerning a medical malpractice action should be required to be reported under such subsection.

SEC. 422. REPORTING OF SANCTIONS TAKEN BY BOARDS
OF MEDICAL EXAMINERS.

(a) IN GENERAL.—

(1) ACTIONS SUBJECT TO REPORTING.—Each Board of Medical Examiners—

(A) which revokes or suspends (or otherwise restricts) a physician's license or censures, reprimands, or places on probation a physician, for reasons relating to the physician's professional competence or professional conduct, or

(B) to which a physician's license is surrendered, shall report, in accordance with section 424, the information described in paragraph (2).

(2) INFORMATION TO BE REPORTED.—The information to be reported under paragraph (1) is—

(A) the name of the physician involved,

(B) a description of the acts or omissions or other reasons (if known) for the revocation, suspension, or surrender of license, and

(C) such other information respecting the circumstances of the action or surrender as the Secretary deems appropriate.

(b) FAILURE TO REPORT.—If, after notice of noncompliance and providing opportunity to correct noncompliance, the Secretary determines that a Board of Medical Examiners has failed to report information in accordance with subsection (a), the Secretary shall designate another qualified entity for the reporting of information under section 423.

SEC. 423. REPORTING OF CERTAIN PROFESSIONAL REVIEW ACTIONS TAKEN BY HEALTH CARE ENTITIES.

(a) REPORTING BY HEALTH CARE ENTITIES.—

(1) ON PHYSICIANS.—Each health care entity which—

(A) takes a professional review action that adversely affects the clinical privileges of a physician for a period longer than 30 days;

(B) accepts the surrender of clinical privileges of a physician—

(i) while the physician is under an investigation by the entity relating to possible incompetence or improper professional conduct, or

(ii) in return for not conducting such an investigation or proceeding; or

(C) in the case of such an entity which is a professional society, takes a professional review action which adversely affects the membership of a physician in the society, shall report to the Board of Medical Examiners, in accordance with section 424(a), the information described in paragraph (3).

(2) PERMISSIVE REPORTING ON OTHER LICENSED HEALTH CARE PRACTITIONERS.—A health care entity may report to the Board of Medical Examiners, in accordance with section 424(a), the information described in paragraph (3) in the case of a licensed health care practitioner who is not a physician, if the entity would be required to report such information under paragraph (1) with respect to the practitioner if the practitioner were a physician.

(3) INFORMATION TO BE REPORTED.—The information to be reported under this subsection is—

(A) the name of the physician or practitioner involved,

(B) a description of the acts or omissions or other reasons for the action or, if known, for the surrender, and

(C) such other information respecting the circumstances of the action or surrender as the Secretary deems appropriate.

(b) REPORTING BY BOARD OF MEDICAL EXAMINERS.—Each Board of Medical Examiners shall report, in accordance with section 424, the information reported to it under subsection (a) and known instances of a health care entity's failure to report information under subsection (a)(1).

(c) SANCTIONS.—

(1) HEALTH CARE ENTITIES.—A health care entity that fails substantially to meet the requirement of subsection (a)(1) shall lose the protections of section 411(a)(1) if the Secretary publishes the name of the entity under section 411(b).

(2) BOARD OF MEDICAL EXAMINERS.—If, after notice of noncompliance and providing an opportunity to correct noncompliance, the Secretary determines that a Board of Medical Examiners has failed to report information in accordance with subsection (b), the Secretary shall designate another qualified entity for the reporting of information under subsection (b).

(d) REFERENCES TO BOARD OF MEDICAL EXAMINERS.—Any reference in this part to a Board of Medical Examiners includes, in the case of a Board in a State that fails to meet the reporting requirements of section 422(a) or subsection (b), a reference to such other qualified entity as the Secretary designates.

SEC. 424. FORM OF REPORTING.

(a) TIMING AND FORM.—The information required to be reported under sections 421, 422(a), and 423 shall be reported regularly (but not less often than monthly) and in such form and manner as the Secretary prescribes. Such information shall first be required to be reported on a date (not later than one year after the date of the enactment of this Act) specified by the Secretary.

(b) TO WHOM REPORTED.—The information required to be reported under sections 421, 422(a), and 423(b) shall be reported to the Secretary, or, in the Secretary's discretion, to an appropriate private or public agency which has made suitable arrangements with the Secretary with respect to receipt, storage, protection of confidentiality, and dissemination of the information under this part.

(c) REPORTING TO STATE LICENSING BOARDS.—

(1) MALPRACTICE PAYMENTS.—Information required to be reported under section 421 shall also be reported to the appropriate State licensing board (or boards) in the State in which the medical malpractice claim arose.

(2) REPORTING TO OTHER LICENSING BOARDS.—Information required to be reported under section 423(b) shall also be reported to the appropriate State licensing board in the State in which the health care entity is located if it is not otherwise reported to such board under subsection (b).

SEC. 425. DUTY OF HOSPITALS TO OBTAIN INFORMATION.

(a) IN GENERAL.—It is the duty of each hospital to request from the Secretary (or the agency designated under section 424[b]), on and after the date information is first required to be reported under section 424[a]—

(1) at the time a physician or licensed health care practitioner applies to be on the medical staff (courtesy or otherwise) of, or for clinical privileges at, the hospital, information reported under this part concerning any physician or practitioner, and

(2) once every 2 years information reported under this part concerning any physician or such practitioner who is on the medical staff (courtesy or otherwise) of, or has been granted clinical privileges at, the hospital.

A hospital may request such information at other times.

(b) FAILURE TO OBTAIN INFORMATION.—With respect to a medical malpractice action, a hospital which does not request information respecting a physician or practitioner as required under subsection (a) is presumed to have knowledge of any information reported under this part to the Secretary with respect to the physician or practitioner.

(c) RELIANCE ON INFORMATION PROVIDED.—Each hospital may rely upon information provided to the hospital under this title and shall not be held liable for such reliance in the absence of the hospital's knowledge that the information provided was false.

SEC. 426. DISCLOSURE AND CORRECTION OF INFORMATION.

With respect to the information reported to the Secretary (or the agency designated under section 424[b]) under this part respecting a physician or other licensed health care practitioner, the Secretary shall, by regulation, provide for—

(1) disclosure of the information, upon request, to the physician or practitioner, and

(2) procedures in the case of disputed accuracy of the information.

SEC. 427. MISCELLANEOUS PROVISIONS.

(a) PROVIDING LICENSING BOARDS AND OTHER HEALTH CARE ENTITIES WITH ACCESS TO INFORMATION.—The Secretary (or the agency designated under section 424[b]) shall, upon request, provide information reported under this part with respect to a physician or other licensed health care practitioner to State licensing boards, to hospitals, and to other health care entities (including health maintenance organizations) that have entered (or may be entering) into an employment or affiliation relationship with the physician or practitioner or to which the physician or practitioner has applied for clinical privileges or appointment to the medical staff.

(b) CONFIDENTIALITY OF INFORMATION.—

(1) IN GENERAL.—Information reported under this part is considered confidential and shall not be disclosed (other than to the physician or practitioner involved) except with respect to professional review activity, with respect to medical malpractice actions, or in accordance with regulations of the Secretary promulgated pursuant

to subsection (a). Nothing in this subsection shall prevent the disclosure of such information by a party which is otherwise authorized, under applicable State law, to make such disclosure.

(2) PENALTY FOR VIOLATIONS.—Any person who violates paragraph (1) shall be subject to a civil money penalty of not more than $10,000 for each such violation involved. Such penalty shall be imposed and collected in the same manner as civil money penalties under subsection (a) of section 1128A of the Social Security Act are imposed and collected under that section.

(3) USE OF INFORMATION.—Subject to paragraph (1), information provided under section 425 and subsection (a) is intended to be used solely with respect to activities in the furtherance of the quality of health care.

(c) RELIEF FROM LIABILITY FOR REPORTING.—No person or entity shall be held liable in any civil action with respect to any report made under this part without knowledge of the falsity of the information contained in the report.

(d) INTERPRETATION OF INFORMATION.—In interpreting information reported under this part, a payment in settlement of a medical malpractice action or claim shall not be construed as creating a presumption that medical malpractice has occurred.

PART C—DEFINITIONS AND REPORTS

SEC. 431. DEFINITIONS.

In this title:

(1) The term "adversely affecting" includes reducing, restricting, suspending, revoking, denying, or failing to renew clinical privileges or membership in a health care entity.

(2) The term "Board of Medical Examiners" includes a body comparable to such a Board (as determined by the State) with responsibility for the licensing of physicians and also includes a subdivision of such a Board or body.

(3) The term "clinical privileges" includes privileges, membership on the medical staff, and the other circumstances pertaining to the furnishing of medical care under which a physician or other licensed health care practitioner is permitted to furnish such care by a health care entity.

(4) (A) The term "health care entity" means—

(i) a hospital that is licensed to provide health care services by the State in which it is located,

(ii) an entity (including a health maintenance organization or group medical practice) that provides health care services and that follows a formal peer review process for the purpose of furthering quality health care (as determined under regulations of the Secretary), and

(iii) subject to subparagraph (B), a professional society (or committee thereof) of physicians or other licensed health care practitioners that follows a formal peer review process for the purpose of furthering quality health care (as determined under regulations of the Secretary).

(B) The term "health care entity" does not include a professional society (or committee thereof) if, within the previous 5 years, the society has been found by the Federal Trade Commission or any court to have engaged in any anti-competitive practice which had the effect of restricting the practice of licensed health care practitioners.

(5) The term "hospital" means an entity described in paragraphs (1) and (7) of section 1861(e) of the Social Security Act.

(6) The terms "licensed health care practitioner" and "practitioner" mean, with respect to a State, an individual (other than a physician) who is licensed or otherwise authorized by the State to provide health care services.

(7) The term "medical malpractice action or claim" means a written claim or demand for payment based on a health care provider's furnishing (or failure to furnish) health care services, and includes the filing of a cause of action, based on the law of tort, brought in any court of any State or the United States seeking monetary damages.

(8) The term "physician" means a doctor of medicine or osteopathy or a doctor of dental surgery or medical dentistry legally authorized to practice medicine and surgery or dentistry by a State (or any individual who, without authority holds himself or herself out to be so authorized).

(9) The term "professional review action" means an action or recommendation of a professional review body which is taken or made in the conduct of professional review activity, which is based on the competence or professional conduct of an individual physician (which conduct affects or could affect adversely the health or welfare of a patient or patients), and which affects (or may affect) adversely the clinical privileges, or membership in a professional society, of the physician. Such term includes a formal decision of a professional review body not to take an action or make a recommendation described in the previous sentence and also includes professional review activities relating to a professional review action. In this title, an action is not considered to be based on the competence or professional conduct of a physician if the action is primarily based on—

(A) the physician's association, or lack of association, with a professional society or association,

(B) the physician's fees or the physician's advertising or engaging in other competitive acts intended to solicit or retain business,

(C) the physician's participation in prepaid group health plans, salaried employment, or any other manner of delivering health services whether on a fee-for-service or other basis,

(D) a physician's association with, supervision of, delegation of authority to, support for, training of, or participation in a private group practice with, a member or members of a particular class of health care practitioner or professional, or

(E) any other matter that does not relate to the competence or professional conduct of a physician.

(10) The term "professional review activity" means an activity of a health care entity with respect to an individual physician—

(A) to determine whether the physician may have clinical privileges with respect to, or membership in, the entity,

(B) to determine the scope or conditions of such privileges or membership, or

(C) to change or modify such privileges or membership.

(11) The term "professional review body" means a health care entity and the governing body or any committee of a health care entity which conducts professional review activity, and includes any committee of the medical staff of such an entity when assisting the governing body in a professional review activity.

(12) The term "Secretary" means the Secretary of Health and Human Services.

(13) The term "State" means the 50 States, the District of Columbia, Puerto Rico, the Virgin Islands, Guam, American Samoa, and the Northern Mariana Islands.

(14) The term "State licensing board" means, with respect to a physician or health care provider in a State, the agency of the State which is primarily responsible for the licensing of the physician or provider to furnish health care services.

SEC. 432. REPORTS AND MEMORANDA OF UNDERSTANDING.

(a) ANNUAL REPORTS TO CONGRESS.—The Secretary shall report to Congress, annually during the three years after the date of the enactment of this Act, on the implementation of this title.

(b) MEMORANDA OF UNDERSTANDING.—The Secretary of Health and Human Services shall seek to enter into memoranda of understanding with the Secretary of Defense and the Administrator of Veterans' Affairs to apply the provisions of part B of this title to hospitals and other facilities and health care providers under the jurisdiction of the Secretary or Administrator, respectively. The Secretary shall report to Congress, not later than two years after the date of the enactment of this Act, on any such memoranda and on the cooperation among such officials in establishing such memoranda.

(c) MEMORANDUM OF UNDERSTANDING WITH DRUG ENFORCEMENT ADMINISTRATION.—The Secretary of Health and Human Services shall seek to enter into a memorandum of understanding with the Administrator of Drug Enforcement relating to providing for the reporting by the Administrator to the Secretary of information respecting physicians and other practitioners whose registration to dispense controlled substances has been suspended or revoked under section 304 of the Controlled Substances Act. The Secretary shall report to Congress, not later than two years after the date of the enactment of this Act, on any such memorandum and on the cooperation between the Secretary and the Administrator in establishing such a memorandum.

Appendix C
National Practitioner Data Bank Regulations

DEPARTMENT OF HEALTH AND HUMAN SERVICES
Public Health Service
45 CFR Part 60

National Practitioner Data Bank for Adverse Information on Physicians and Other Health Care Practitioners

AGENCY: Public Health Service, HHS.
ACTION: Final regulations.

SUMMARY: This rule sets forth criteria and procedures for information to be collected in and released from a National Practitioner Data Bank, in accordance with the requirements of title IV, part B, of the Health Care Quality Improvement Act of 1986. These regulations govern the reporting and release of information concerning: (1) Payments made for the benefit of physicians, dentists, and other health care practitioners as a result of medical malpractice actions and claims; and (2) certain adverse actions taken regarding the licenses and clinical privileges of physicians and dentists.

EFFECTIVE DATE: These regulations will be effective on the date on which the National Practitioner Data Bank is operational. The Secretary will publish this date in an announcement in the *Federal Register.*

A separate announcement will be published in the *Federal Register* when the Department obtains Office of Management and Budget approval for section 60.6(b) which contains information collection requirements.

FOR FURTHER INFORMATION CONTACT: Daniel D. Cowell, M.S., Director, Division of Quality Assurance and Liability Management, Bureau of Health Professions, Health Resources and Services Administration, Room 8-15, Parklawn Building, 5600 Fishers Lane, Rockville, Maryland 20857; telephone number: 301/443-2300.

SUPPLEMENTARY INFORMATION: On March 21, 1988, the Secretary published a Notice of Proposed Rulemaking (NPRM) to implement the Health Care Quality Improvement Act of 1986 (the Act), title IV of Public Law 99-660, through the establishment of a National Practitioner Data Bank (the Data Bank). The Department received more than

140 comments which were postmarked on or before May 20, the end of the comment period, from health professionals' organizations, hospitals, health maintenance organizations, State licensing boards, other units of State government, insurers, health care consultants, attorneys, physicians, and others.

The Secretary would like to thank the respondents for the quality and the thoroughness of their comments. As a result of the comments, many modifications have been made to the NPRM. The comments and the Department's response to the comments are discussed below. For clarity, the comments and responses are arranged according to the section numbers and titles of the NPRM to which they pertain. We note that a new section 60.6 has been added to the final regulations, which results in renumbering the sections following new section 60.6.

As the Secretary indicated in the March 21, 1988 NPRM, the Act does not require the application of these provisions to Federal health care entities, physicians, dentists, and other health care providers. However, the intent of the law appears clear that coverage be as broad as possible, and hence that Federal providers be included to the extent feasible. Accordingly, the Secretary has signed Memoranda of Understanding with the Department of Defense and the Drug Enforcement Administration of the Department of Justice, and is pursuing the execution of such a memorandum with the Department of Veterans Affairs. Also, the Secretary is developing a policy and procedure regarding the manner in which health care providers in the Department of Health and Human Services will participate in the Data Bank.

Subpart A—General Provisions

Section 60.1 The National Practitioner Data Bank

The Department has revised the title of "The National Data Bank," to "The National Practitioner Data Bank" to more precisely represent the purpose of the Data Bank. Accordingly, references to the Data Bank have been so revised throughout these regulations.

Section 60.3 Definitions

Several respondents indicated that the reference to "failing to renew State licensure" in the definition of "adversely affecting" was incorrect, since "adversely affecting" is used in the body of the regulations only in connection with professional review actions concerning clinical privileges and membership in a professional society.

The Department agrees with the comments and has deleted the phrase "failing to renew State licensure" from this definition.

A large number of respondents indicated that the definition of "adversely affecting" was overbroad in its incorporation of actions by specialty boards. "Adversely affecting," as proposed, referenced specialty boards for consistency with the proposed definition of "health care entity," which included specialty boards. These respondents similarly felt that including "specialty board" within "health care entity" was an overexpansion of the Act.

In response, the Department has deleted the reference to "specialty board" both from the term "adversely affecting" and from "health care entity." A more detailed explanation of the comments and the basis for these revisions is contained in the discussion below of the term "health care entity."

A board of dental examiners stated that the definition of "dentist" was inaccurate. The board indicated that D.M.D. means "doctor of dental medicine," not "doctor of medical dentistry," as proposed. It was also indicated that some dentists, generally foreign graduates, may hold a degree other than doctor of dental surgery or doctor of dental medicine which qualifies them to hold licenses and practice in a State.

In response, the Department has deleted the abbreviations for degrees and retained the statutory references for the credentials of a dentist. For consistency, the Department has made the same revisions in the definition of "physician." The definition of "dentist" was also expanded to include dentists with degrees equivalent to doctor of dental surgery or doctor of dental medicine who otherwise meet the statutory criteria.

Numerous attorneys, associations, and medical boards found the definition of "health care entity" to be unclear and questioned whether various organizations, such as Individual Practice Associations and Preferred Provider Organizations, would fall within the term.

In clarification, the Department's intent is that an entity apply the criteria of paragraph (b) of the definition of "health care entity" to itself in order to make a factual determination of whether the definition would encompass it. Specifically, these criteria are that an entity: (1) Provides health care services; and (2) engages in professional review activity through a formal peer review process for the purpose of furthering quality health care. The Department prefers to define this term broadly, rather than to attempt to focus on the myriad of health care organizations, practice arrangements, and professional societies, so as to ensure that the regulations include all the entities within the scope of the statute. In keeping with this intent, the Department has revised the description of "group medical practice" in the definition of "health care entity" to delete the specific criteria of shared facilities, personnel, medical records, and responsibilities, and incomes set by contract. The modification generalizes the definition to indicate that a health care entity includes any group or prepaid medical practice which meets the criteria of paragraph (b).

As previously mentioned, the Department has further revised "health care entity" to delete the reference to "specialty board" based on numerous comments that the proposal was overly broad. In addition, respondents pointed out that membership in a specialty board is voluntary, and that curtailment of this membership does not necessarily reflect lack of competence. The comments generally indicated that equating "specialty board" with "professional society" within the definition of "health care entity" was not within the intent of the Act.

Several respondents questioned the definition of licensed "health care practitioner" as it refers to "an individual who is licensed or otherwise authorized by a State to provide health care services." The Department used "otherwise authorized" to include disciplines for which States grant authority to provide health care services by mechanisms other than licensure, such as registration and certification. All health care practitioners authorized by a State to provide health care services by whatever formal mechanism the State employs are included within this definition. The Act similarly uses "otherwise authorized" to define "licensed health care practitioner."

Some respondents requested the Department to include a list of health care practitioners subject to these regulations. To include such a list in the regulations would be unfeasible since regulatory amendments would then be necessary each time the list would require revisions. However, the Department does intend to make available to members of the public, upon request, a list by State of those practitioners who are the subject of these regulations.

Numerous respondents found the definition of "medical malpractice action or claim" to be in need of clarification. Several comments questioned whether this term was limited to claims or actions filed in court or included administrative claims. Other respondents questioned the meaning of "other adjudicative body" as used in this term in reference to where a medical malpractice action or claim may be filed.

In response to these comments, the Department has adopted some of the suggested revisions to clarify the definition as follows:

"Medical malpractice action or claim" means a written complaint or claim demanding payment based on a physician's, dentist's, or other health care practitioner's provision of or failure to provide health care services, and includes the filing of a cause of action based on the law of tort, brought in any State or Federal court or other adjudicative body.

This definition, as did that in the NPRM, includes the filing of medical malpractice claims on an administrative level, as well as judicial claims and actions. The revised definition more closely tracks the language of the Act.

"Other adjudicative body," as used in this definition, is intended to specify medical malpractice actions which are brought before arbitration boards and other dispute resolution mechanisms prior to or instead of a formal court action.

Two associations opposed the definition of "professional review action." One stated that including within the term "a formal decision not to take an action or to make a recommendation" was inappropriate, since this phrase is relevant to the immunity provisions of part A of the Act but not the reporting provisions of part B. The other association found that the definition implied that a decision to not take an action should be reported.

The Department agrees with these comments. Since these regulations implement only the reporting provisions of part B of the Act and not the immunity provisions of part A, the Secretary has revised the definition of "professional review action" to delete the above-referenced phrase. However, the Secretary points out that "a formal decision not to take an action or to make a recommendation" which would result in the voluntary surrender of clinical privileges would be reported under section 60.9(a)(i) and (ii). The Department has similarly deleted the reference to "professional review activities related to a professional review action" as being unnecessary in the implementation of the reporting requirements of part B.

Numerous respondents requested clarification of the meaning of "professional competence or conduct" as used in the definition of "professional review action." They inquired whether revocation or suspension of privileges related to nonclinical factors would be reportable, such as failure to attend staff meetings or to complete medical records or billing forms. Another respondent questioned whether it would include criminal activities committed by the professional outside the employment setting.

In response, the Department has revised the form of the definition of "professional review action" to stress that it encompasses only professional competence or conduct which affects or could affect adversely the health or welfare of a patient. Hence, "professional review action" does not include an action taken against a physician, dentist, or other health care practitioner based on a technical or administrative failing unrelated to the health or welfare of patients. With respect to criminal activities, it would obviously be necessary to analyze the criminal action to make a determination whether the health or welfare of a patient was or could be adversely affected by the situation. In short, the Department believes that "professional review action" is best defined in generic terms which allows each health care entity to make its own factual determinations.

Several respondents found the definition of "professional review activity" to be unclear. They felt, for example, that a health care entity could have many reasons unrelated to professional competence for making an initial determination not to grant clinical privileges. For example, it may have a sufficient number of anesthesiologists currently on its staff and not need the services of another. Another comment stated that many hospitals routinely grant initial privileges on a probationary basis.

The Department clarifies that, as used in the Act as well as in the NPRM, the definition of "professional review activity" is not descriptive of the reasons for modification or curtailment of clinical privileges or membership but relates only to various types of actions that may or may not lead to modification or curtailment of clinical privileges and membership. This definition's significance is in how it relates to the definition of "professional review action." It is only "professional review actions," not "professional review activities," which are reportable under Part B of the Act. The definition of "professional review action" encompasses only professional review activities which are related to the professional competence or conduct of a physician, dentist, or other health care practitioner and which could adversely affect the health or welfare of a patient. In fact, paragraph (d)(5) specifically excludes from the definition of "professional review action" matters that do not relate to the competence or professional conduct of a physician, dentist, or other health care practitioner. Thus, it is clear that although the definition of "professional review activities" does not by its own terms exclude such actions as refusing privileges to an anesthesiologist because a health care entity already has enough such practitioners, such actions would not be reportable under section 60.9.

Subpart B—Reporting of Information

Section 60.4 How Information Must Be Reported

To improve the clarity of the structure of these regulations, the Secretary has moved the portion of proposed section 60.4 that related to errors and omissions in reports to a new section 60.6.

Section 60.5 When Information Must Be Reported

There were approximately 40 comments on this section. Most of them addressed the timing of reports. Some respondents found the time periods outlined in the NPRM too stringent; others, particularly insurers, proposed alternate report submission schemes or the submission of reports in batches; still others asked for clarification of the events which trigger the time periods.

With the few exceptions noted below, the Department has decided to retain the language of the NPRM in the final rule. In this decision, the Department was guided both by the language of the Act which specifies that reports shall be made "not less often than monthly," and by the importance of maintaining current information for the protection of the public.

Several respondents questioned why section 60.5(c), as proposed, required health care entities to report adverse actions within 20 days, whereas other reports were required within a 30-day timeframe. The rationale for the 20-day period is that the reporting of adverse actions is a two-step process, with the health care entity making a report to the Board of Medical Examiners, and the Board then submitting this report to the Data Bank, both of which actions are to be accomplished within a single 30-day timeframe.

Several respondents opposed section 60.5(c) on the basis that the 10-day timeframe for reports by Boards of Medical Examiners to the Data Bank placed an undue burden on Boards whose resources are limited.

The Department is sympathetic to the difficulties of meeting a 10-day deadline and, in response, has revised section 60.5(c) to shorten the time for health care entities to file reports with Boards of Medical Examiners from 20 to 15 days and increase the time for Boards to file their reports from 10 to 15 days. Nevertheless, we stress that this particular type of reporting simply requires Boards of Medical Examiners to pass through information which they have received from the health care entity in the form that they received it and does not require the preparation of a new document or Board action on the contents of the report.

With respect to inquiries concerning the triggering event of the applicable time period for reporting, the Department views the events as follows:

(1) For malpractice payments (section 60.7)—the date of the check in payment of the medical malpractice action or claim.

(2) For licensure and adverse actions (section 60.8 and section 60.9)—the date of formal approval of the adverse action by the Board's or entity's authorized official.

The Department will be issuing guidelines to explain these points further, as well as other regulatory provisions in need of greater discussion, and provide examples.

The Secretary emphasizes that individuals and entities will not be held responsible for reporting any information under these regulations or the Act until the Data Bank has been established and the Secretary has announced the date of the beginning of its operation in the *Federal Register*. The reporting requirements are not retroactive from November 14, 1987, the statutory date on which the Data Bank was to have been in operation.

Section 60.6 Reporting Errors, Omissions, and Revisions (New)

As stated earlier, the Department reorganized these regulations, moving the provision concerning errors and omissions from section 60.4. One medical association had commented on the lack of any reference to time in reporting an omission or error. Several respondents expressed concern about the accuracy of the information in the Data Bank.

The Secretary is sensitive to the importance of accuracy of the information in the Data Bank, for the protection of the users of the information, the subjects of the reports, and the public. In response to the comments on the proposed section 60.4, the Department has added "as soon as possible" to indicate the urgency of correcting reports on file.

The Secretary has added the requirement that individuals and entities who file reports must update them when they learn of revisions, such as the reinstatement of a license or the reversal or modification of a professional review action. The procedures for reporting revisions will be the same as those which applied to the reporting of the original event.

To increase the accuracy of the information in the Data Bank, all reports which are filed will be held for 30 days after receipt prior to release to any parties other than to the subjects of the reports. This period will provide opportunity for disputes, corrections, or revisions to be filed prior to release of the information. In addition, the Data Bank will maintain a record of all inquiries made to it and any information provided as a result of an inquiry. It will then issue corrections or supplementary reports to all who have received erroneous or incomplete information.

Section 60.7 (Proposed section 60.6) Reporting Medical Malpractice Payments

More than 50 respondents commented on proposed section 60.6 (section 60.7 below). The majority of comments expressed concern over the burden of reporting all payments, regardless of size. About one-fourth of the respondents suggested setting a floor for the size of medical malpractice payments below which reporting would not be required. For example, several respondents recommended that payments below $30,000 not be reported.

The Department cannot accept these comments due to the statutory requirement that medical malpractice payments of any size be reported. However, as stated in the NPRM, the Secretary will be filing a report with Congress on whether information on small payments should continue to be collected. These comments will be considered when making this report.

Numerous comments were made regarding the interpretation of malpractice payments. Respondents pointed out that nuisance or frivolous claims are frequently settled by small payments which do not reflect on the professional competence or conduct of the physician, dentist, or other health care practitioner in issue.

The Secretary agrees with these comments and therefore has revised section 60.7 to include a new paragraph (d) entitled "Interpretation of information." This paragraph reiterates section 427(d) of the Act, which states that a payment in settlement of a medical malpractice action or claim shall not be construed as creating a presumption that medical malpractice has occurred.

Several associations requested that the "acts or omissions" which must be reported under section 60.7 be described as "alleged" acts or omissions. These respondents stated that if a payment were made in a settlement, then "alleged" should be used as a modifier because the acts or omissions may never have occurred. They also felt that to add "alleged" would be consistent with the statutory provision of section 427(d) of the Act, that a payment in settlement of a medical malpractice claim shall not be construed as creating a presumption that medical malpractice has occurred.

The Department has not accepted these comments. The Secretary believes that section 60.7, as proposed, is closer to the statutory intent and language. For example, section 421(b)(4) of the Act requires a report on a payment on a medical malpractice claim or action to contain "a description of the acts or omissions and injuries or illnesses upon which the action or claim was based." The Department has, however, revised section

60.7(a) so that it reflects the language of the Act. Further, as mentioned above, the Department has included a new paragraph (d) in section 60.7 to set forth the interpretation of medical malpractice payments contained in section 427(d).

Several respondents suggested that information in the Data Bank be "purged" after a periodic interval of, perhaps, 5 years.

The Department has not accepted these comments because the deletion of reports from the Data Bank would be inconsistent with the statutory purpose of protecting the public. However, the Secretary wishes to make every effort to maintain the accuracy of the information and thus, as discussed earlier, has added new section 60.6 to require the filing of updated information. The Department acknowledges that data retained over very long periods of time can lose practical utility. For that reason, the Department will assess the desirability of indefinite retention of information in the Data Bank.

An association of insurers requested clarification of section 60.7(a) to emphasize that reportable payments are those for medical malpractice claims or actions and for the benefit of a physician, dentist, or other health care practitioner. This respondent was concerned that a suit could include multiple defendants and multiple allegations, such as libel or slander.

The Department has accepted this comment and has revised section 60.7(a) accordingly.

Numerous health care entities inquired whether the waiver of an outstanding bill to settle a medical malpractice claim or action would be required to be reported under section 60.7.

Both the Act and these regulations require the reporting of payments in response to medical malpractice claims or actions. The Department interprets "payment" as meaning an exchange of money; therefore, the waiver of a debt as described above would not be a reportable event. The Department has revised section 60.7(a) to clarify this point.

Several insurers and professional organizations opposed the requirements of section 60.7(b)(1), subitems (iii), (vii), and (viii) to report the home address, the license number, and the Drug Enforcement Administration registration number of the subject of the report. They indicated that this information is neither routinely collected nor readily known.

In response, the Department has modified section 60.7(b)(1)(viii) to allow for the reporting of the Drug Enforcement Administration registration number, if known. Since an individual's home address could be a useful identifier, it has been retained but has been modified to be required only if it is known. The reporting data of section 60.8 and section 60.9 for licensure and adverse actions have been similarly revised. The Department has retained the requirement of the license number, since it is an important provider identifier.

The Department is requiring the reporting of additional information to distinguish more precisely among individual physicians, dentists, and other health care practitioners on whom information is reported to the Data Bank. The additional personal identifiers to be reported are: Date of birth; name of each professional school attended and year of graduation; the field of licensure and the name of the State or Territory in which the license is held. The reporting requirements in section 60.8 and section 60.9 for licensure and adverse actions have been similarly revised.

As previously mentioned, the Secretary is sensitive to the importance of accuracy of the information in the Data Bank. The combination of identifiers required to be reported to the Bank will help prevent errors in distinguishing among more than one practitioner with the same name.

To correct the references to the Privacy Act in the proposed rule at sections 60.6(b)(1)(v), 60.7(b)(5), and 60.8(a)(3)(v), the Secretary has removed from those sections the phrase, "* * * and released in accordance with applicable provisions of the Privacy Act (5 U.S.C. 552a)* * *" and has inserted in its place the phrase, "In accordance with section 7 of the Privacy Act of 1974."

Numerous respondents expressed concern over section 60.7(b)(3)(viii), which stated that the Secretary would require other information from time to time, as announced in the *Federal Register*. They opposed this provision as omitting the rulemaking requirements of the Administrative Procedure Act.

The Secretary never intended these additional data requirements to be imposed without public notice and comment. This section, and the parallel provisions of section 60.8 and section 60.9, have been revised to clarify that any such additional requirements would be proposed in the *Federal Register* for public comment.

Many insurers sought clarification on how payments should be reported when they are made on a periodic basis or on behalf of more than one individual.

In response, the Department interprets section 60.7 as requiring reporting only at the time of the first payment of periodic payment terms. The accompanying report would indicate the expectation of periodic payments. In the case of a payment on behalf of multiple individuals, the insurer would report the total payment, list the details concerning each health care provider, and indicate that the payment was made on behalf of all the listed providers. The Department will be issuing guidelines with illustrative examples to advise individuals and entities in the filing of all required reports.

Several respondents expressed a need for a uniform system of classification of medical malpractice claims to assist in reporting.

The Department recognizes this need and has added new section 60.7(b)(3)(vii). This requirement is similar to proposed section 60.7(b)(8) which requires the reporting of the classification of licensure actions in accordance with a reporting code to be adopted by the Secretary. The Department is consulting with liability insurers and others to develop a system to classify acts or omissions upon which a medical malpractice claim or action is based. A classification for each category of reportable actions, such as malpractice claims and licensure actions, will be developed with an opportunity for public comment in accordance with the review procedures of the Paperwork Reduction Act of 1980.

The Secretary notes that the procedures for the imposition of sanctions for failure to report malpractice payments, as referenced in section 60.7(c), were proposed in the *Federal Register* on March 21, 1988. Final regulations for the latter will be published separately in the *Federal Register* by the Office of the Inspector General (OIG), Department of Health and Human Services, shortly after the publication of these Title IV regulations. The OIG regulations will be codified at 42 CFR part 1003.

Section 60.8 (Proposed section 60.7) Reporting Licensure Actions Taken by Boards of Medical Examiners

The majority of comments on proposed section section 60.7 (section 60.8 below) criticized this section for requiring licensure actions which are unrelated to professional conduct or competence to be reported. As proposed, section 60.8(a)(1) and (3) required a Board of Medical Examiners to report actions which revoke or suspend a physician's or dentist's license or under which such license is surrendered. Only section 60.8(a)(2), which requires the reporting of an action to censure, reprimand or place on probation a physician or dentist, conditioned the clause with "reasons relating to the physician's or dentist's professional competence or professional conduct." Insurers, associations, and boards pointed out that a license may be surrendered simply due to retirement or relocation. Also, licensure actions may be taken for reasons related to licensees' fees, or advertising, which do not relate to professional competence or conduct.

The Department has accepted these comments. Since the purpose of the Data Bank is to improve the quality of medical care by restricting the ability of certain physicians and dentists to continue to change practice locations without the disclosure or discovery of their previous incompetent performance or misconduct, the Secretary intends to collect only data relating to professional competence or conduct. The regulations have been revised accordingly.

Several associations found section 60.8(b)(11) to be unclear. This section requires a report to contain a classification of the action per State reporting code.

In response, the Department has revised this section to delete the reference to "State," and to note that the code will be one adopted by the Secretary. The Department intends to develop a code or codes for reporting licensure actions to the Data Bank and to distribute this code to reporting agencies and entities. To the extent feasible, the reporting scheme which is most commonly used by Boards will be incorporated.

The Department notes that section 60.8(b)(3) and (8) have been revised, as explained in the preamble discussion of section 60.7, entitled "Reporting medical malpractice payments."

Section 60.9 (Proposed section 60.8) Reporting Adverse Actions on Clinical Privileges

The Department received nearly 50 comments on proposed section 60.8 (section 60.9 below). The vast majority addressed section 60.9(c), concerning sanctions for noncompliance with reporting requirements. The comments generally requested clarification of some provisions but also contained many helpful suggestions. As noted in preceding discussion pertaining to section 60.7(c), final regulations regarding sanctions for failure to comply with these reporting requirements will be published shortly and codified at 42 CFR part 1003.

Numerous respondents expressed dismay over their interpretation of section 60.9 as requiring the reporting of voluntary decisions to limit clinical privileges, such as a family practitioner's decision to stop accepting obstetrical or minor surgical cases, when these decisions are not motivated by investigations or threats of investigation of clinical competence or professional conduct.

The Department shares the view of these respondents that the Data Bank should contain only information which reflects adversely on a practitioner's professional competence or conduct. However, section 60.9, as proposed, achieves this purpose. A "professional review action," as referenced in section 60.9(a)(1)(i), requires, by definition, both a formal peer review process and a relationship to professional competence or conduct. The same is true of section 60.9(a)(1)(iii) for professional review actions by professional societies. Thus, a physician's or dentist's voluntary reduction in clinical privileges for reasons of personal preference is not a reportable event.

Another respondent objected to section 60.9(a)(1)(ii) as lacking clarity. This section requires the reporting of the "surrender of clinical privileges" by a physician or a dentist in situations where the physician or dentist is under investigation for possible incompetence or improper professional conduct, or where the physician or dentist surrenders clinical privileges in return for not conducting such investigation. The respondent was concerned that the reporting of the surrender of clinical privileges would not include a partial surrender of such privileges.

The Department has accepted this comment and revised section 60.9(a)(1)(ii) accordingly, to clarify that the restriction of clinical privileges in those situations would be reported.

A dental association commented on section 60.9(a)(1)(iii) concerning professional review actions by professional societies. The association suggested the deletion of "which adversely affects the membership of a physician or dentist" as being redundant with "professional review action."

The Department has accepted this comment and revised this provision accordingly.

A medical board supported section 60.9 but suggested that the regulations should require the reporting of a loss of clinical privileges of any length, not just of 30 days or more. This respondent suggested that suspensions of 29 days might become a common mechanism for avoiding the reporting requirement.

The Secretary appreciates this concern. However, the provision has been retained as proposed, since the 30-day time period is explicit in the Act.

An association felt that "appropriate" as modifying "Board of Medical Examiners" in section 60.9(a)(1) was unclear.

In response, the Department has revised this provision to require a health care entity to report to the "Board of Medical Examiners" *in the State in which the health care entity is located* (emphasis added).

Most of the comments on section 60.9 addressed paragraph (c), which describes the Department's procedures for imposing sanctions for noncompliance with reporting requirements of this section. With regard to requests for hearings, several respondents asked what constituted "substantive and relevant" issues, and how the Department would determine whether the statement of factual issues submitted was "frivolous or inconsequential." Some respondents questioned whether it was appropriate for the Department to deny hearing requests, given the substantial nature of the sanction. Finally, many comments opposed the provision of this subsection which requires that hearings be held in the Washington, DC, area. These respondents stated that the requirement will limit the opportunity for adequate representation during proceedings and recommended that there be regional hearings instead.

In response, the Department emphasizes that the intent of the proposal is to assure that the hearing process is administered as efficiently and cost-effectively as possible for the health care entities and the Department, and concludes that it is consistent with both due process and legislative requirements.

A determination of what constitutes a factual issue in dispute is directly tied to the reporting requirements in section 60.9. An example of a factual issue in dispute would be a case where a health care entity alleges facts which, if true, would undercut the Department's determination that the health care entity has not met the requirements of the reporting provision. Such a case would involve a material, factual issue in dispute that would be appropriate for resolution through a hearing.

The proposed procedure for determining whether a hearing must be conducted is essentially an administrative "summary judgment" proceeding. It is a well-settled principle that an agency has the authority to deny a hearing when it appears from the request that no substantial issue of fact is in dispute. *Weinberger v. Hynson, Westcott & Dunning,* 412 U.S. 609 (1973); *United States v. Storer Broadcasting Co.,* 352 U.S. 192, 202-205 (1956); *Pineapple Growers Association of Hawaii v. F.D.A.,* 673 F.2d 1083 (9th Cir. 1982).

Section 411(b) of the Act, which requires the Secretary to provide an opportunity for a hearing, does not constitute a bar to such summary judgment. When it is apparent from a request that there are no substantive issues in dispute, no purpose could be served by holding a public hearing. In upholding a similar summary judgment provision promulgated by the Food and Drug Administration, the U.S. Court of Appeals for the Eighth Circuit articulated the rationale for the provision as follows:

* * * The hearing is solely for the purpose of receiving evidence "relevant and material to the issues raised by such objections." Certainly, then the objections, in order to be effective and necessitate the hearing requested, must be legally adequate so that, if true, the order complained of could not prevail. The objections must raise "issues." The issues must be material to the question involved; that is, the legality of the order attacked. They may not be frivolous or inconsequential. Where the objections stated and the issues raised thereby are, even if true, legally insufficient, their effect is a nullity and no objections have been stated. Congress did not intend the governmental agencies created by it to perform useless or unfruitful tasks. If it is perfectly clear that the petitioner's appeal for a hearing contains nothing material and the objections stated do not abrogate the legality of the order attacked, no hearing is required by law. *Dyestuffs and Chemicals, Inc. v. Flemming,* 271 F.2d 281 (8th Cir. 1959), *cert. denied* 362 U.S. 911 (1960).

With regard to the recommendation for regional hearings, the Secretary continues to believe that the location of hearings for most cases must be limited to the Washington, DC, metropolitan area due to constraints in departmental resources.

Several respondents noted that section 60.9(c)(1) as proposed, concerning sanctions for health care entities, omitted the statutory language of "substantially" as used to modify "failed to report information in accordance with section 60.9."

The Department acknowledges this oversight and has revised this provision accordingly.

Another respondent pointed out that section 60.9(c)(1) as proposed also omitted the statutory requirement that the Secretary must give a health care entity an opportunity to correct noncompliance before imposing a sanction.

The Secretary accepts this comment and has revised the provision accordingly.

Subpart C—Disclosure of Information by the National Practitioner Data Bank

Section 60.10 (Proposed section 60.9) Information Which Hospitals Must Request From the National Practitioner Data Bank

Several respondents opposed the requirement that hospitals "obtain" information, suggesting that it be replaced by "request." They asserted that hospitals could only be held responsible for making requests from the Data Bank and should not be held responsible if they fail to receive it due to a deficiency on the part of the Data Bank.

The Secretary accepts these comments and has revised section 60.10 accordingly.

Another respondent opposed as burdensome the requirement that a hospital request information from the Data Bank every 2 years for its medical staff and those who have clinical privileges.

The Department is unable to accept this comment since this requirement is mandated by the Act.

A dental association pointed out that dentists had not been included in the requirement of section 60.10(a)(2) that a hospital query the Data Bank every 2 years concerning its staff.

The Department has corrected this oversight by revising section 60.10(a)(2) accordingly.

Several associations requested that section 60.10 be revised to include "authorized agents" of hospitals as entities who may query the Data Bank. These respondents pointed out that many hospitals rely on centralized medical staff application and reappointment programs operated by local medical societies.

The Secretary has accepted these comments and has revised section 60.10(a) accordingly. However, it should be noted that section 60.11(a) already specifically provides that "authorized agents" of persons or entities may request and obtain information from the Data Bank. The Secretary has nevertheless made the requested changes for additional clarity.

Section 60.11 (Proposed section 60.10) Requesting Information From the National Practitioner Data Bank

The Department received over 80 comments on this section.

Several respondents suggested that the regulations provide for timely responses by the Data Bank to requests for information.

The Secretary emphasizes that all efforts will be made by the Department and the contractor who will be operating the Data Bank to insure that requests for information are fulfilled on a timely basis. However, at this time it is not feasible to incorporate a response time in these regulations because the Data Bank has not been established. It is the intent of the Secretary to establish a timeframe for the Data Bank to respond to requests after it is in operation. This information will be available to the public at that time.

Several insurers and an educational institution requested access to information in the Data Bank.

The Secretary cannot expand access to the Data Bank beyond what the Act authorizes. It should be noted that individuals are permitted to obtain information about themselves and may share this information with a potential employer or insurer. In addition, information requested in a form that does not identify any health care entity or health care practitioner will be available to anyone making such a request.

Numerous respondents questioned what information would be given in response to authorized requests concerning physicians, dentists, or other health care practitioners.

Persons and entities who make such requests will be given the substantive content of all reports on the subject individual which are contained in the Data Bank.

The majority of the respondents expressed concern over verification of the identity of individuals and entities who request information from the Data Bank. Some suggested procedures involving identification codes for verification of requestors.

The Secretary shares these concerns about maintaining the confidentiality of the information in the Data Bank and will take measures necessary to insure the proper release of this information. Since the Data Bank has not been established at this time, it is impossible to detail the precise procedures which will be used for the verification of the identity of requestors. At the time of operation of the Data Bank, the Department intends to provide this information to the public in the form of guidelines.

The Department notes that it will be maintaining a list of all requests for information on each individual in the Data Bank. Upon request, the subject individual may receive a copy of the list of requestors.

Several comments stated that section 60.11(a)(3), as proposed, was confusing and that Boards of Medical Examiners and State licensing boards should be separated from health care entities.

The Department has accepted these comments and revised section 60.11(a) accordingly.

The majority of comments received on this section expressed great concern over section 60.11(a)(5), which provides for access by attorneys to information in the Data Bank. Many respondents requested its deletion. Others requested that it be narrowed as much as possible. Some comments indicated that attorney access is contrary to the intent and purpose of the Act—that of promoting effective professional peer review and furthering quality health care. Most respondents felt that attorney access threatened the confidentiality of the Data Bank records.

In response, the Secretary stresses that section 60.11(a)(5) implements section 427(b)(1) of the Act as narrowly as possible. Access by attorneys cannot be eliminated without an amendment to the Act. The Department points out that attorney access to the Data Bank is extremely limited. To clarify, a plaintiff's attorney (or a person representing himself or herself in a medical malpractice action) may request information from the Data Bank on a health care provider if, and only if, he or she meets these tests:

(1) The attorney or individual has filed a medical malpractice action or claim in a State or Federal court or other adjudicative body against a hospital and requests information regarding a specific physician, dentist or other health care practitioner also named in the action or claim; *and*

(2) The attorney or individual produces evidence that the hospital failed to request information from the Data Bank on the physician, dentist or other health care practitioner, as required by these regulations.

The information so obtained may be used solely with respect to the action or claim against the hospital. In short, the applicability of section 60.11(a)(5) is limited to judicial cases filed against a hospital where the hospital failed to make a request from the Data Bank, as required under section 60.10. In this instance, the hospital is then presumed, under section 425(b) of the Act, to have knowledge of the information contained in the Data Bank. Thus, if the attorney who filed the action against the hospital could not obtain the information at issue from the Data Bank, the parties and the court would not know what information must be imputed to the defendant hospital and could not effectively litigate the case.

Several comments questioned the purpose of providing access in section 60.11(a)(5) to an individual "acting on his own behalf" and suggested clarification of the provision.

In response, the Department intended simply to allow access to pro se litigants, as well as attorneys, for purposes of section 60.11(a)(5). This section has been revised for greater clarity.

One respondent requested access for the defendant's attorney, as well as the plaintiff's, in section 60.11(a)(5).

In response, no revision is necessary for this purpose because the defendant physician, dentist, or other health care practitioner can always obtain information about himself, or the hospital can obtain the information which it should have requested under section 60.10.

Numerous respondents requested clarification of what "evidence" of a hospital's failure to request information would be required to obtain information from the Data Bank. Many comments suggested that a court order to this effect would be appropriate.

The Secretary agrees that evidence of an objective, factual nature should be required to obtain access under section 60.11(a)(5). Due to the variety of possible forums for these medical malpractice actions—State courts, Federal courts, county courts, etc., and their accompanying varying procedural rules—the Department prefers to retain the general requirement of "evidence" in this provision. This would permit an attorney to present a court order, a deposition, a response to an interrogatory, an admission, or other evidence of the failure of a hospital to request information. The Department will be providing guidance of this nature in guidelines for the Data Bank.

A few respondents indicated concern about possible breaches of confidentiality under section 60.11(a)(7), the release of information for research purposes. Others requested clarification. This regulation explicitly states that information released for research purposes will be released only in a form which will not allow the identification of an individual health care entity, physician, dentist or health care practitioner.

The Department has deleted the word "patient" from this provision. Its inclusion may have given the mistaken impression that the Bank would collect information that would allow the identification of patients. This is not the case. The Department wishes to emphasize that no information that would allow patient identification will be contained in the Data Bank.

The Department wants to take this opportunity to notify the public that it plans to request additional information regarding reported adverse actions to support important medical liability and malpractice research. In the Department's publication, "Report of the Task Force on Medical Liability and Malpractice," August 1987, the Task Force found a significant need for additional data (part IV: Research Issues). The type of information that the Department plans to request will be specified through the rulemaking process with an opportunity for public comment.

It should be noted that giving researchers access to Data Bank information does not imply that the Data Bank will act as a research service, but its data, without identifiers, will be available to researchers who request it. As in other requests for data information, appropriate user fees will be charged according to section 60.12.

Section 60.12 (Proposed section 60.11) Fees Applicable to Requests for Information

The Department received 15 comments on section 60.12. Most of these stressed the importance of keeping fees at a "reasonable" level or requested that funds be waived or reduced for various classes of users. Several respondents noted the limited financial resources of State Boards. One association suggested that fees for statutorily required requests, such as those by hospitals under section 60.10, be at a lower scale than "optional" requests.

In response, the Department recognizes these concerns. Although section 60.12 has not been revised, the Secretary wishes to assure the public that, as the regulation states, fees will be based on the costs of processing requests and providing information. It should be noted, however, that the President's Budget for Fiscal Year 1990 proposes appropriation language that would require fees for the disclosure of information from the Data Bank to be calculated so that the full costs of operating the Data Bank can be recovered.

The Department will endeavor to keep costs associated with operating the Data Bank, and the consequent costs of querying it, as low as possible.

*Section 60.13 (Proposed section 60.12) Confidentiality of National
Practitioner Data Bank Information*

Several respondents requested clarification of the confidentiality provisions in section 60.13. One State board suggested a revision to clarify the point that information from the Data Bank may only be used for the purpose for which it was provided, whether the information was received directly from the Data Bank or received indirectly from the requesting party. A group of insurers suggested that this section be revised to forbid the requesting party from disclosing the information received from the Data Bank.

In response, the Department has revised section 60.13 to emphasize that the confidentiality restrictions apply to parties who receive information from the Data Bank indirectly, as well as directly. However, it has not accepted the suggestion to forbid further disclosure of information from a requesting party because this is contrary to the intent of the Act. An individual or entity who receives information from the Data Bank is permitted to disclose it further in the course of carrying out the activity for which it was sought. For example, a hospital may request information from the Data Bank on a physician who is applying for a staff position and may share this information with the officials who make the employment review and decision on this physician's application. Nevertheless, the confidentiality limitations of the Act apply both to the initial hospital staff who receive the information and to the specific department staff who subsequently review it. They may each only use and disclose the information with respect to the employment decision.

*Section 60.14 (Proposed section 60.13) How to Dispute the Accuracy of the National Practitioner
Data Bank Information*

Numerous respondents opposed the procedures for disputing the accuracy of information in the Data Bank. Some found them to be vague. Several comments suggested withholding information from parties who make requests pending resolution of a dispute.

In response, the Secretary has made some revisions to clarify the procedures for disputing information. Section 60.14 now explicitly states that the Secretary will routinely mail copies of reports to the subject individual. In order to determine the accuracy of Data Bank information in an expeditious manner, section 60.14(b) now provides a 60-day time period within which to challenge a report.

The Department has not accepted the suggestion that information in dispute be withheld from requestors pending the resolution of the dispute. The Secretary believes that labeling the report as "disputed" provides sufficient notice that the report is in question. The Secretary further believes that the potential threat to the public of withholding valuable information which may well be accurate is not outweighed by a possible detriment to the subject physician, dentist, or other health care practitioner.

Several respondents were disturbed by the statement that, in resolving a dispute, the Secretary would review "related information which is available, including, but not limited to, that available from malpractice insurers, test examination results, State administrative procedures and judicial decisions, and the Health Care Financing Administration." These respondents felt that the Secretary's review should be limited to the statements on file by the reporting and disputing parties, since they would have no further opportunity to challenge this information.

The Secretary has accepted these comments and revised section 60.14 accordingly.

Numerous comments indicated that the Secretary should not continue to label reports as "disputed" if the Secretary determines that the information is accurate. The comments stated that in such a case this label would be misleading.

The Secretary has accepted this comment and has revised section 60.14(c)(2)(i) to indicate that when the information is determined to be accurate, it will simply contain a statement by the subject individual describing the basis for challenge and an explanation of the Secretary's decision.

The Secretary wishes to point out that section 5 of the Medicare and Medicaid Patient and Program Protection Act of 1987 (Pub. L. 100-93), enacted August 18, 1987, requires that States have in effect a system of reporting information to the Secretary with respect to formal proceedings concluded against health care practitioners or entities by authorities responsible for the licensing of health care practitioners or entities. This Act requires the Secretary to provide for the maximum appropriate coordination in implementing section 5 and the Health Care Quality Improvement Act. Proposed regulations implementing section 5 are being developed. When issued, those regulations will complement these final regulations.

The Department will be republishing in the *Federal Register* for public comment the notice of a new system of records for the Data Bank, with proposed routine uses. Although a Privacy Act systems of records notice had been published on September 14, 1987 (52 FR 34721), legislative amendments necessitate the republication of this notice.

Regulatory Flexibility Act and Executive Order 12291

The Secretary certifies that these regulations do not have a significant economic impact on a substantial number of small entities, and therefore do not require a regulatory flexibility analysis under the Regulatory Flexibility Act of 1980.

Regulatory Flexibility Act

Consistent with the Regulatory Flexibility Act of 1980 (Pub. L. 96-354, 5 U.S.C. 604[a]), the Department prepares and publishes an initial regulatory flexibility analysis for proposed regulations unless the Secretary certifies that the regulation would not have a significant economic impact on a substantial number of small business entities. The analysis is intended to explain what effect the regulatory action by the agency would have on small businesses and other small entities and to develop lower cost or burden alternatives. As indicated above, these final regulations would not have a significant economic impact. While some of the penalties and fees the Department could impose as a result of these regulations might have an impact on small entities, the Department does not anticipate that a substantial number of these small entities would be significantly affected by this rulemaking. Therefore, the Secretary certifies that these final regulations would not have a significant economic impact on a substantial number of small entities.

Executive Order 12291

Executive Order 12291 requires the Department to prepare and publish an initial regulatory impact analysis for any proposed major rule. A major rule is defined as any regulation that is likely to: (1) Have an annual effect on the economy of $100 million or more; (2) cause a major increase in costs or prices for consumers, individual industries, government agencies, or geographic regions; or (3) result in significant adverse effects on competition, employment, investment, productivity, innovation, or on the ability of United States-based enterprises to compete with foreign-based enterprises in domestic or export markets.

The Department has determined that these regulations do not meet the criteria for a major rule as defined by section 1(b) of Executive Order 12291. This final regulation establishes procedures for the reporting and releasing of information from the Data Bank. As such, the regulations would have little direct effect on the economy or on Federal or State expenditures. Consequently, the Department has concluded that an initial regulatory impact analysis is not required.

Paperwork Reduction Act of 1980

Section 60.4 of this regulation requires that information to be reported under sections 60.7, 60.8 and 60.9 shall be provided in the form and manner prescribed by the Secretary. Section 60.11(b) provides that requests for information from the Data Bank, including those required under section 60.10, shall be made in the form and manner prescribed by the Secretary. The actual forms to be used for reporting information to or requesting information from the Data Bank will be submitted to the Office of Management and Budget for review and public comment in accordance with the Paperwork Reduction Act of 1980 as soon as they are available.

Sections 60.6(a), 60.7, 60.8, 60.9, 60.10, and 60.14 contain information collection requirements which have been approved by the Office of Management and Budget (OMB) under section 3504(h) of the Paperwork Reduction Act of 1980 and assigned control number 0915-0126.

Section 60.6(b) contains information collection requirements which are subject to OMB review. We have submitted an information request to OMB for approval under section 3504(h) of the Paperwork Reduction Act of 1980. These requirements will not be effective until the Department obtains OMB approval, at which time a notice will be published in the *Federal Register* to notify the public of such action.

List of Subjects in 45 CFR Part 60

Health professions, Malpractice, Insurance companies.

Accordingly, the Department of Health and Human Services adds a new part 60 to title 45 of the Code of Federal Regulations, as set forth below.

Dated: September 7, 1989.

James O. Mason,
Assistant Secretary for Health.

Approved October 11, 1989.

Louis W. Sullivan, Secretary.

PART 60—NATIONAL PRACTITIONER DATA BANK FOR ADVERSE INFORMATION ON PHYSICIANS AND OTHER HEALTH CARE PRACTITIONERS

Subpart A—General Provisions

Sec.

60.1   The National Practitioner Data Bank.
60.2   Applicability of these regulations.
60.3   Definitions.

Subpart B—Reporting of Information

60.4   How information must be reported.
60.5   When information must be reported.
60.6   Reporting errors, omissions, and revisions.
60.7   Reporting medical malpractice payments.
60.8   Reporting licensure actions taken by Boards of Medical Examiners.
60.9   Reporting adverse actions on clinical privileges.

Subpart C—Disclosure of Information by the National Practitioner Data Bank

60.10   Information which hospitals must request from the National Practitioner Data Bank.
60.11   Requesting information from the National Practitioner Data Bank.
60.12   Fees applicable to requests for information.

60.13 Confidentiality of National Practitioner Data Bank information.

60.14 How to dispute the accuracy of National Practitioner Data Bank information.

Authority: Secs. 401-432 of the Health Care Quality Improvement Act of 1986, Pub. L. 99-660, 100 Stat. 3784-3794, as amended by section 402 of Pub. L. 100-177, 101 Stat. 1007-1008 (42 U.S.C. 11101-11152).

Subpart A—General Provisions

Section 60.1 The National Practitioner Data Bank.

The Health Care Quality Improvement Act of 1986 (the Act), title IV of Pub. L. 99-660, as amended, authorizes the Secretary to establish (either directly or by contract) a National Practitioner Data Bank to collect and release certain information relating to the professional competence and conduct of physicians, dentists and other health care practitioners. These regulations set forth the reporting and disclosure requirements for the National Practitioner Data Bank.

Section 60.2 Applicability of These Regulations.

These regulations establish reporting requirements applicable to hospitals; health care entities; Boards of Medical Examiners; professional societies of physicians, dentists or other health care practitioners which take adverse licensure or professional review actions; and individuals and entities (including insurance companies) making payments as a result of medical malpractice actions or claims. They also establish procedures to enable individuals or entities to obtain information from the National Practitioner Data Bank or to dispute the accuracy of National Practitioner Data Bank information.

Section 60.3 Definitions.

Act means the Health Care Quality Improvement Act of 1986, title IV of Pub. L. 99-660, as amended.

Adversely affecting means reducing, restricting, suspending, revoking, or denying clinical privileges or membership in a health care entity.

Board of Medical Examiners, or "Board," means a body or subdivision of such body which is designated by a State for the purpose of licensing, monitoring and disciplining physicians or dentists. This term includes a Board of Osteopathic Examiners or its subdivision, a Board of Dentistry or its subdivision, or an equivalent body as determined by the State. Where the Secretary, pursuant to section 423(c)(2) of the Act, has designated an alternate entity to carry out the reporting activities of section 60.9 due to a Board's failure to comply with section 60.8, the term "Board of Medical Examiners" or "Board" refers to this alternate entity.

Clinical privileges means the authorization by a health care entity to a physician, dentist or other health care practitioner for the provision of health care services, including privileges and membership on the medical staff.

Dentist means a doctor of dental surgery, doctor of dental medicine, or the equivalent who is legally authorized to practice dentistry by a State (or who, without authority, holds himself or herself out to be so authorized).

Formal peer review process means the conduct of professional review activities through formally adopted written procedures which provide for adequate notice and an opportunity for a hearing.

Health care entity means:

(a) A hospital;

(b) An entity that provides health care services, and engages in professional review activity through a formal peer review process for the purpose of furthering quality health care, or a committee of that entity; or

(c) A professional society or a committee or agent thereof, including those at the national, State, or local level, of physicians, dentists, or other health care practitioners that engages in professional review activity through a formal peer review process, for the purpose of furthering quality health care. For purposes of paragraph (b) of this definition, an entity includes: a health maintenance organization which is licensed by a State or determined to be qualified as such by the Department of Health and Human Services; and any group or prepaid medical or dental practice which meets the criteria of paragraph (b).

Health care practitioners means an individual other than a physician or dentist, who is licensed or otherwise authorized by a State to provide health care services.

Hospital means an entity described in paragraphs (1) and (7) of section 1861(e) of the Social Security Act.

Medical malpractice action or claim means a written complaint or claim demanding payment based on a physician's, dentist's or other health care practitioner's provision of or failure to provide health care services, and includes the filing of a cause of action based on the law of tort, brought in any State or Federal Court or other adjudicative body.

Physician means a doctor of medicine or osteopathy legally authorized to practice medicine or surgery by a State (or who, without authority, holds himself or herself out to be so authorized).

Professional review action means an action or recommendation of a health care entity:

(a) Taken in the course of professional review activity;

(b) Based on the professional competence or professional conduct of an individual physician, dentist or other health care practitioner which affects or could affect adversely the health or welfare of a patient or patients; and

(c) Which adversely affects or may adversely affect the clinical privileges or membership in a professional society of the physician, dentist or other health care practitioner.

(d) This term excludes actions which are primarily based on:

(1) The physician's, dentist's or other health care practitioner's association, or lack of association, with a professional society or association;

(2) The physician's, dentist's or other health care practitioner's fees or the physician's, dentist's or other health care practitioner's advertising or engaging in other competitive acts intended to solicit or retain business;

(3) The physician's, dentist's or other health care practitioner's participation in prepaid group health plans, salaried employment, or any other manner of delivering health services whether on a fee-for-service or other basis;

(4) A physician's, dentist's or other health care practitioner's association with, supervision of, delegation of authority to, support for, training of, or participation in a private group practice with, a member or members of a particular class of health care practitioner or professional; or

(5) Any other matter that does not relate to the competence or professional conduct of a physician, dentist or other health care practitioner.

Professional review activity means an activity of a health care entity with respect to an individual physician, dentist or other health care practitioner:

(a) To determine whether the physician, dentist or other health care practitioner may have clinical privileges with respect to, or membership in, the entity;

(b) To determine the scope or conditions of such privileges or membership; or

(c) To change or modify such privileges or membership.

Secretary means the Secretary of Health and Human Services and any other officer or employee of the Department of Health and Human Services to whom the authority involved had been delegated.

State means the fifty States, the District of Columbia, Puerto Rico, the Virgin Islands, Guam, American Samoa, and the Northern Mariana Islands.

Subpart B—Reporting of Information

Section 60.4 How Information Must Be Reported.

Information must be reported to the Data Bank or to a Board of Medical Examiners as required under sections 60.7, 60.8, and 60.9 in such form and manner as the Secretary may prescribe.

Section 60.5 When Information Must Be Reported.

Information required under sections 60.7, 60.8, and 60.9 must be submitted to the Data Bank within 30 days following the action to be reported, beginning with actions occurring on or after the effective date of these regulations or the date of the establishment of the Data Bank, whichever is later, as follows:

(a) *Malpractice Payments (section 60.7).* Persons or entities must submit information to the Data Bank within 30 days from the date that a payment, as described in section 60.7, is made. If required under section 60.7, this information must be submitted simultaneously to the appropriate State licensing board.

(b) *Licensure Actions (section 60.8).* The Board must submit information within 30 days from the date the licensure action was taken.

(c) *Adverse Actions (section 60.9).* A health care entity must report an adverse action to the Board within 15 days from the date the adverse action was taken. The Board must submit the information received from a health care entity within 15 days from the date on which it received this information. If required under section 60.9, this information must be submitted by the Board simultaneously to the appropriate State licensing board in the State in which the health care entity is located, if the Board is not such licensing Board.

Section 60.6 Reporting Errors, Omissions, and Revisions.

(a) Persons and entities are responsible for the accuracy of information which they report to the Data Bank. If errors or omissions are found after information has been reported, the person or entity which reported it must send an addition or correction to the Data Bank or, in the case of reports made under section 60.9, to the Board of Medical Examiners, as soon as possible.

(b) An individual or entity which reports information on licensure or clinical privileges under sections 60.8 or 60.9 must also report any revision of the action originally reported. Revisions include reversal of a professional review action or reinstatement of a license. Revisions are subject to the same time constraints and procedures of sections 60.5, 60.8, and 60.9, as applicable to the original action which was reported.

Section 60.7 Reporting Medical Malpractice Payments.

(a) *Who must report.* Each person or entity, including an insurance company, which makes a payment under an insurance policy, self-insurance, or otherwise, for the benefit of a physician, dentist or other health care practitioner in settlement of or in satisfaction in whole or in part of a claim or a judgment against such physician, dentist or other health care practitioner for medical malpractice, must report information as set forth in paragraph (b) to the Data Bank and to the appropriate State licensing board(s) in the State in which the act or omission upon which the medical malpractice claim was based. For purposes of this section, the waiver of an outstanding debt is not construed as a "payment" and is not required to be reported.

(b) *What information must be reported.* Persons or entities described in paragraph (a) must report the following information:

(1) With respect to the physician, dentist or other health care practitioner for whose benefit the payment is made—

(i) Name,

(ii) Work address,

(iii) Home address, if known,

(iv) Social Security number, if known, and if obtained in accordance with section 7 of the Privacy Act of 1974,

(v) Date of birth,

(vi) Name of each professional school attended and year of graduation,

(vii) For each professional license: the license number, the field of licensure, and the name of the State or Territory in which the license is held,

(viii) Drug Enforcement Administration registration number, if known,

(ix) Name of each hospital with which he or she is affiliated, if known;

(2) With respect to the reporting person or entity—

(i) Name and address of the person or entity making the payment,

(ii) Name, title, and telephone number of the responsible official submitting the report on behalf of the entity, and

(iii) Relationship of the reporting person or entity to the physician, dentist, or other health care practitioner for whose benefit the payment is made;

(3) With respect the judgment or settlement resulting in the payment—

(i) Where an action or claim has been filed with an adjudicative body and the case number,

(ii) Date or dates on which the act(s) or omission(s) which gave rise to the action or claim occurred,

(iii) Date of judgment or settlement,

(iv) Amount paid, date of payment, and whether payment is for a judgment or a settlement,

(v) Description and amount of judgment or settlement and any conditions attached thereto, including terms of payment,

(vi) A description of the acts or omissions and injuries or illnesses upon which the action or claim was based,

(vii) Classification of the acts or omissions in accordance with a reporting code adopted by the Secretary, and

(viii) Other information as required by the Secretary from time to time after publication in the *Federal Register* and after an opportunity for public comment.

(c) *Sanctions.* Any person or entity that fails to report information on a payment required to be reported under this section is subject to a civil money penalty of up to $10,000 for each such payment involved. This penalty will be imposed pursuant to procedures at 42 CFR part 1003.

(d) *Interpretation of information.* A payment in settlement of a medical malpractice action or claim shall not be construed as creating a presumption that medical malpractice has occurred.

Section 60.8 Reporting Licensure Actions Taken by Boards of Medical Examiners.

(a) *What actions must be reported.* Each Board of Medical Examiners must report to the Data Bank any action based on reasons relating to a physician's or dentist's professional competence or professional conduct—

(1) Which revokes or suspends (or otherwise restricts) a physician's or dentist's license,

(2) Which censures, reprimands, or places on probation a physician or dentist, or

(3) Under which a physician's or dentist's license is surrendered.

(b) *Information that must be reported.* The Board must report the following information for each action:

(1) The physician's or dentist's name,

(2) The physician's or dentist's work address,

(3) The physician's or dentist's home address, if known,

(4) The physician's or dentist's Social Security number, if known, and if obtained in accordance with section 7 of the Privacy Act of 1974,

(5) The physician's or dentist's date of birth,

(6) Name of each professional school attended by the physician or dentist and year of graduation,

(7) For each professional license, the physician's or dentist's license number, the field of licensure and the name of the State or Territory in which the license is held,

(8) The physician's or dentist's Drug Enforcement Administration registration number, if known,

(9) A description of the acts or omissions or other reasons for the action taken,

(10) A description of the Board action, the date the action was taken, and its effective date,

(11) Classification of the action in accordance with a reporting code adopted by the Secretary, and

(12) Other information as required by the Secretary from time to time after publication in the *Federal Register* and after an opportunity for public comment.

(c) *Sanctions.* If, after notice of noncompliance and providing opportunity to correct noncompliance, the Secretary determines that a Board has failed to submit a report as required by this section, the Secretary will designate another qualified entity for the reporting of information under section 60.9.

Section 60.9 Reporting Adverse Actions on Clinical Privileges.

(a) *Reporting to the Board of Medical Examiners.* — (1) *Actions that must be reported and to whom the report must be made.* Each health care entity must report to the Board of Medical Examiners in the State in which the health care entity is located the following actions:

(i) Any professional review action that adversely affects the clinical privileges of a physician or dentist for a period longer than 30 days;

(ii) Acceptance of the surrender of clinical privileges or any restriction of such privileges by a physician or dentist—

(A) While the physician or dentist is under investigation by the health care entity relating to possible incompetence or improper professional conduct, or

(B) In return for not conducting such an investigation or proceeding; or

(iii) In the case of a health care entity which is a professional society, when it takes a professional review action.

(2) *Voluntary reporting on other health care practitioners.* A health care entity may report to the Board of Medical Examiners information as described in paragraph (a)(3) of this section concerning actions described in paragraph (a)(1) in this section with respect to other health care practitioners.

(3) *What information must be reported.* The health care entity must report the following information concerning actions described in paragraph (a)(1) of this section with respect to the physician or dentist:

(i) Name,

(ii) Work address,

(iii) Home address, if known,

(iv) Social Security number, if known, and if obtained in accordance with section 7 of the Privacy Act of 1974,

(v) Date of birth,

(vi) Name of each professional school attended and year of graduation,

(vii) For each professional license: the license number, the field of licensure, and the name of the State or Territory in which the license is held,

(viii) Drug Enforcement Administration registration number, if known,

(ix) A description of the acts or omissions or other reasons for privilege loss, or, if known, for surrender,

(x) Action taken, date the action was taken, and effective date of the action, and

(xi) Other information as required by the Secretary from time to time after publication in the *Federal Register* and after an opportunity for public comment.

(b) *Reporting by the Board of Medical Examiners to the National Practitioner Data Bank.* Each Board must report, in accordance with sections 60.4 and 60.5, the information reported to it by a health care entity and any known instances of a health care entity's failure to report information as required under paragraph (a)(1) of this section. In addition, each Board must simultaneously report this information to the appropriate State licensing board in the State in which the health care entity is located, if the Board is not such licensing board.

(c) *Sanctions*—(1) *Health care entities.* If the Secretary has reason to believe that a health care entity has substantially failed to report information in accordance with section 60.9, the Secretary will conduct an investigation. If the investigation shows that the health care entity has not complied with section 60.9, the Secretary will provide the entity with a written notice describing the noncompliance, giving the health care entity an opportunity to correct the noncompliance, and stating that the entity may request, within 30 days after receipt of such notice, a hearing with respect to the noncompliance. The request for a hearing must contain a statement of the material factual issues in dispute to demonstrate that there is cause for a hearing. These issues must be both substantive and relevant. The hearing will be held in the Washington, DC, metropolitan area. The Secretary will deny a hearing if:

(i) The request for a hearing is untimely,

(ii) The health care entity does not provide a statement of material factual issues in dispute, or

(iii) The statement of factual issues in dispute is frivolous or inconsequential.

In the event that the Secretary denies a hearing, the Secretary will send a written denial to the health care entity setting forth the reasons for denial. If a hearing is denied, or if as a result of the hearing the entity is found to be in noncompliance, the Secretary will publish the name of the health care entity in the *Federal Register*. In such case, the immunity protections provided under section 411(a) of the Act will not apply to the health care entity for professional review activities that occur during the 3-year period beginning 30 days after the date of publication of the entity's name in the *Federal Register*.

(2) *Board of Medical Examiners.* If, after notice of noncompliance and providing opportunity to correct noncompliance, the Secretary determines that a Board has failed to report information in accordance with paragraph (b) of this section, the Secretary will designate another qualified entity for the reporting of this information.

Subpart C—Disclosure of Information by the National Practitioner Data Bank

Section 60.10 Information which Hospitals Must Request from the National Practitioner Data Bank.

(a) *When information must be requested.* Each hospital, either directly or through an authorized agent, must request information from the Data Bank concerning a physician, dentist or other health care practitioner as follows:

(1) At the time a physician, dentist or other health care practitioner applies for a position on its medical staff (courtesy or otherwise), or for clinical privileges at the hospital; and

(2) Every 2 years concerning any physician, dentist or other health care practitioner who is on its medical staff (courtesy or otherwise), or has clinical privileges at the hospital.

(b) *Failure to request information.* Any hospital which does not request the information as required in paragraph (a) of this section is presumed to have knowledge of any information reported to the Data Bank concerning this physician, dentist or other health care practitioner.

(c) *Reliance on the obtained information.* Each hospital may rely upon the information provided by the Data Bank to the hospital. A hospital shall not be held liable for this reliance unless the hospital has knowledge that the information provided was false.

Section 60.11 Requesting Information from the National Practitioner Data Bank.

(a) *Who may request information and what information may be available.* Information in the Data Bank will be available, upon request, to the persons or entities, or their authorized agents, as described below:

(1) A hospital that requests information concerning a physician, dentist or other health care practitioner who is on its medical staff (courtesy or otherwise) or has clinical privileges at the hospital,

(2) A physician, dentist, or other health care practitioner who requests information concerning himself or herself,

(3) Boards of Medical Examiners or other State licensing boards,

(4) Health care entities which have entered or may be entering employment or affiliation relationships with a physician, dentist or other health care practitioner [who] has applied for clinical privileges or appointment to the medical staff,

(5) An attorney, or individual representing himself or herself, who has filed a medical malpractice action or claim in a State or Federal court or other adjudicative body against a hospital, and who requests information regarding a specific physician, dentist, or other health care practitioner who is also named in the action or claim. Provided, that this information will be disclosed only upon the submission of evidence that the hospital failed to request information from the Data Bank as required by section 60.10(a), and may be used solely with respect to litigation resulting from the action or claim against the hospital.

(6) A health care entity with respect to professional review activity, and

(7) A person or entity who requests information in a form which does not permit the identification of any particular health care entity, physician, dentist, or other health care practitioner.

(b) *Procedures for obtaining National Practitioner Data Bank information.* Persons and entities may obtain information from the Data Bank by submitting a request in such form and manner as the Secretary may prescribe. These requests are subject to fees as described in section 60.12.

Section 60.12 Fees Applicable to Requests for Information.

(a) *Policy on fees.* The fees described in this section apply to all requests for information from the Data Bank, other than those of individuals for information concerning themselves. These fees are authorized by section 427(b)(4) of the Health Care Quality Improvement Act of 1986 (42 U.S.C. 11137). They reflect the costs of processing requests for disclosure and of providing such information. The actual fees will be announced by the Secretary in periodic notices in the *Federal Register.*

(b) *Criteria for determining the fee.* The amount of each fee will be determined based on the following criteria:

(1) Use of electronic data processing equipment to obtain information—the actual cost for the service, including computer search time, runs, printouts, and time of computer programmers and operators, or other employees,

(2) Photocopying or other forms of reproduction, such as magnetic tapes—actual cost of the operator's time, plus the cost of the machine time and the materials used,

(3) Postage—actual cost, and

(4) Sending information by special methods requested by the applicant, such as express mail or electronic transfer—the actual cost of the special service.

(c) *Assessing and collecting fees.* (1) A request for information from the Data Bank will be regarded as also an agreement to pay the associated fee.

(2) Normally, a bill will be sent along with or following the delivery of the requested information. However, in order to avoid sending numerous small bills to frequent requesters, the charges may be aggregated for certain periods. For example, such a requester may receive a bill monthly or quarterly.

(3) In the event that a requester has failed to pay previous bills, the requester will be required to pay the fee before a request for information is processed.

(4) Fees must be paid by check or money order made payable to "U.S. Department of Health and Human Services" or to the unit stated in the billing and must be sent to the billing unit. Payment must be received within 30 days of the billing date or the applicant will be charged interest and a late fee on the amount overdue.

Section 60.13 Confidentiality of National Practitioner Data Bank Information.

(a) *Limitations on disclosure.* Information reported to the Data Bank is considered confidential and shall not be disclosed outside the Department of Health and Human Services, except as specified in sections 60.10, 60.11, and 60.14. Persons and entities which receive information from the Data Bank either directly or from another party must use it solely with respect to the purpose for which it was provided. Nothing in this paragraph shall prevent the disclosure of information by a party which is authorized under applicable State law to make such disclosure.

(b) *Penalty for violations.* Any person who violates paragraph (a) shall be subject to a civil money penalty of up to $10,000 for each violation. This penalty will be imposed pursuant to procedures at 42 CFR part 1003.

Section 60.14 How to Dispute the Accuracy of National Practitioner Data Bank Information.

(a) *Who may dispute National Practitioner Data Bank information.* Any physician, dentist or other health care practitioner may dispute the accuracy of information in the Data Bank concerning himself or herself. The Secretary will routinely mail a copy of any report filed in the Data Bank to the subject individual.

(b) *Procedures for filing a dispute.* A physician, dentist or other health care practitioner has 60 days from the date on which the Secretary mails the report in question to him or her in which to dispute the accuracy of the report. The procedures for disputing a report are:

(1) Informing the Secretary and the reporting entity, in writing, of the disagreement, and the basis for it,

(2) Requesting simultaneously that the disputed information be entered into a "disputed" status and be reported to inquirers as being in a "disputed" status, and

(3) Attempting to enter into discussion with the reporting entity to resolve the dispute.

(c) *Procedures for revising disputed information.* (1) If the reporting entity revises the information originally submitted to the Data Bank, the Secretary will notify all entities to whom reports have been sent that the original information has been revised.

(2) If the reporting entity does not revise the reported information, the Secretary will, upon request, review the written information submitted by both parties (the physician, dentist or other health care practitioner), and the reporting entity. After review, the Secretary will either—

(i) If the Secretary concludes that the information is accurate, include a brief statement by the physician, dentist or other health care practitioner describing the disagreement concerning the information, and an explanation of the basis for the decision that it is accurate, or

(ii) If the Secretary concludes that the information was incorrect, send corrected information to previous inquirers.

Resources

As the practice of risk management has grown over the years, so has the number of resources available in that field. This section presents a selected listing of organizations, periodicals, books, and audiovisual materials related to health care risk management. *Listings are supplied for information only and do not constitute an endorsement by the American Hospital Association, the American Society for Healthcare Risk Management, or American Hospital Publishing, Inc.*

☐ Organizations

Following is a list of organizations that can supply risk managers with information on particular aspects of health care delivery, health law, insurance, and risk management. Besides the organizations listed here, many other groups, such as the state health department, state hospital association, and local or regional risk management society, can provide information. The 31 local groups that are affiliated with the American Society for Healthcare Risk Management (ASHRM) are listed under the general ASHRM entry. Risk managers who live in a state that does not have an affiliated chapter should contact their state hospital association for information on local health care risk management groups.

Many insurance companies provide consulting services. For referrals to consultants, risk managers can contact their state bar association or the American Association of Health Care Consultants (listed below). The state insurance commissioner can also be a valuable source of information and assistance.

There are many risk management organizations that are not related to health care but may prove valuable to the new risk manager. The best source of information on such organizations is the Risk and Insurance Management Society (listed below), which has local chapters throughout the country.

American Academy of Hospital
Attorneys
840 N. Lake Shore Dr.
Chicago, IL 60611
312/280-6601

American Academy of Pediatrics
141 Northwest Point Blvd.
P.O. Box 927
Elk Grove Village, IL 60009
708/228-5005

American Association of Health Care
  Consultants
11208 Waples Mill Rd., STE 109
Fairfax, VA 22030
703/691-AAHC

American Association of Nurse
  Anesthetists
216 W. Higgins Rd.
Park Ridge, IL 60068
708/692-7050

American Bar Association
750 N. Lake Shore Dr.
Chicago, IL 60611
312/988-5000

American College of Emergency
  Physicians
P.O. Box 619911
Dallas, TX 75261
214/550-0911

American College of Healthcare
  Executives
840 N. Lake Shore Dr.
Chicago, IL 60611
312/943-0544

American College of Legal Medicine
P.O. Box 3190
Maple Glen, PA 19002
215/646-6800

American College of Nurse Midwives
1522 K St., N.W., STE 1120
Washington, DC 20005
202/347-5445

American College of Obstetricians and
  Gynecologists
600 Maryland Ave., S.W., STE 300
Washington, DC 20024
202/638-5577

American College of Surgeons
55 E. Erie St.
Chicago, IL 60611
312/664-4050

American Health Care Association
1201 L St., N.W.
Washington, DC 20005
202/842-4444

American Hospital Association
840 N. Lake Shore Dr.
Chicago, IL 60611
312/280-6000

American Medical Association
535 N. Dearborn St.
Chicago, IL 60610
312/645-5000

American Medical Peer Review
  Association
810 First St., N.E., STE 410
Washington, DC 20002
202/371-5610

American Medical Record Association
919 N. Michigan Ave.
Chicago, IL 60611
312/787-2672

American Nurses' Association
2420 Pershing Rd.
Kansas City, MO 64108
816/474-5720

American Society for Healthcare Risk
  Management
840 N. Lake Shore Dr.
Chicago, IL 60611
312/280-6430

Association for Hospital Risk Management of New York, Inc.

California Society for Hospital Risk Management

Colorado Hospital Associated Risk Managers

Connecticut Society for Hospital Risk Management

Delaware Valley Health Care Risk Management Association

Florida Society for Healthcare Risk Management

Georgia Society for Healthcare Risk Managers

Greater Houston Society for Healthcare Risk Management

Hawaii Association for Hospital Risk Management

Healthcare Risk Management Council of New Orleans

Healthcare Risk Management Society of Metropolitan Chicago

Illinois Society of Healthcare Risk Management

Indiana Society for Hospital Risk Management

Maryland Society for Healthcare Risk Management

Massachusetts Society for Hospital Risk Management, Inc.

Michigan Society of Hospital Risk Management

Missouri Association of Hospital Risk Managers

New Hampshire/Vermont Society for Health Care Risk Management, Inc.

North Carolina Chapter of ASHRM

North Texas Society for Healthcare Risk Management

Ohio Society of Hospital Risk Managers

Oregon Health Care Risk Management Society

Pennsylvania Association of Health Care Risk Management

Risk Management Division, Hospital Council of the National Capital Area, Inc.

Society for Health Care Risk Management of New Jersey

South Carolina Society for Hospital Risk Managers and Quality Assurance Professionals

Southern California Association of Healthcare Risk Managers

Tennessee Society for Healthcare Risk Management

Virginia Chapter of the American Society for Healthcare Risk Management

Washington Health Care Risk Management Society

Wisconsin Society of Healthcare Risk Management

American Society of Anesthesiologists
515 Busse Highway
Park Ridge, IL 60068
708/825-5586

American Society of Law & Medicine
765 Commonwealth Ave.
Boston, MA 02215
617/262-4990

American Society of Post-Anesthesia
   Nurses
2315 Westwood Ave., STE 100
P.O. Box 11083
Richmond, VA 23230
804/359-3557

American Tort Reform Association
1250 Connecticut Ave., N.W., STE 700
Washington, DC 20036
202/637-6490

Anesthesia Patient Safety Foundation
515 Busse Highway
Park Ridge, IL 60068
708/825-5586

Association of Operating Room Nurses
10170 E. Mississippi Ave.
Denver, CO 80231
303/755-6300

Council of Medical Specialty Societies
P.O. Box 70
Lake Forest, IL 60045
708/295-3456

Emergency Nurses Association
230 E. Ohio St., STE 600
Chicago, IL 60611
312/649-0297

Healthcare Financial Management
Association
Two Westbrook Corporate Center,
STE 700
Westchester, IL 60154
708/531-9600

Insurance Institute of America
720 Providence Rd.
Malvern, PA 19355-0770
215/644-2100

Insurance Services Office
175 Water St.
New York, NY 10038
212/487-5000

International Healthcare Safety
Professional Certification Board
5010A Nicholson Lane
Rockville, MD 20852
301/984-8969

Joint Commission on Accreditation of
Healthcare Organizations
1 Renaissance Blvd.
Oakbrook Terrace, IL 60181
708/916-5600

National Association of Insurance
Commissioners
120 W. 12th St., STE 1100
Kansas City, MO 64105
816/842-3600

National Association of Quality
Assurance Professionals
104 Wilmot Rd., STE 201
Deerfield, IL 60015-5195
708/940-8800

National Board of Medical Examiners
3930 Chestnut St.
Philadelphia, PA 19104
215/349-6400

National Fire Protection Association
Batterymarch Park
Quincy, MA 02269
617/770-3000

National Health Lawyers Association
1620 I St., N.W., STE 900
Washington, DC 20006
202/833-1100

National Society for Patient
Representatives and Consumer
Affairs
840 N. Lake Shore Dr.
Chicago, IL 60611
312/280-6424

Nurses' Association of the American
College of Obstetricians and
Gynecologists
409 12th St., S.W.
Washington, DC 20024
202/638-0026

Physician Insurers Association of
America
2 Princess Rd.
Lawrenceville, NJ 08648
609/896-4131

Risk and Insurance Management
Society
205 E. 42nd St.
New York, NY 10017
212/286-9292

☐ Materials

The following selected lists of periodicals, books, and audiovisuals were compiled with the assistance of the American Hospital Association Resource Center. Items were chosen based on their ready availability, the practical guidance they offer to the new risk manager, or their consistent popularity among practicing health care risk managers. (Some are membership publications only and may not be available by subscription.)

For information on how to obtain these materials, risk managers should contact their hospital or organization library or a university library in their area. Many libraries belong to interlibrary loan systems and can obtain these materials. Also, the American Hospital Association Resource Center, 840 N. Lake Shore Dr., Chicago, IL 60611 (telephone 312/280-6263) can obtain many of these materials for a fee. Insurance companies are a good source of excellent audiovisual materials.

Periodicals

American Journal of Law & Medicine, published quarterly by the American Society of Law & Medicine, 765 Commonwealth Ave., Boston, MA 02215, 617/262-4990

Best's Review Property/Casualty Insurance Edition, published monthly by A.M. Best Co., Oldwick, NJ 08858, 201/439-2200

Business Insurance, published weekly by Crain Communications, Inc., 740 N. Rush St., Chicago, IL 60611, 312/649-5275

The Citation—A Medicolegal Digest for Physicians, published twice monthly by the Office of the General Counsel of the American Medical Association, 535 N. Dearborn St., Chicago, IL 60610, 312/645-5000

Drug Utilization Review, published monthly by American Health Consultants, Inc., 60 Peachtree Park Dr., N.E., Atlanta, GA 30309, 404/351-4523

Emergency Department Law, published biweekly by Buraff Publications, 1350 Connecticut Ave., N.W., Washington, DC 20036, 202/452-7889

Fire News, published bimonthly by the National Fire Protection Association, Batterymarch Park, Quincy, MA 02269, 800/344-3555

Forum, published bimonthly by the Risk Management Foundation of the Harvard Medical Institutions, 840 Memorial Dr., Cambridge, MA 02139, 617/495-5100

Hazardous Materials Management, published monthly by Emergency Care Research Institute (ECRI), 5200 Butler Pike, Plymouth Meeting, PA 19462, 215/825-6000

Hospital Law Newsletter, published monthly by Aspen Publishers, Inc., 7201 McKinney Circle, Frederick, MD 21701, 301/251-8500

Hospital Litigation Reporter, published monthly by Strafford Publications, Inc., 1375 Peachtree St., N.E., STE 235, Atlanta, GA 30367, 404/881-1141

Hospital Peer Review, published monthly by American Health Consultants, Inc., 60 Peachtree Park Dr., N.E., Atlanta, GA 30309, 404/351-4523

Hospital Risk Management, published monthly by American Health Consultants, Inc., 60 Peachtree Park Dr., N.E., Atlanta, GA 30309, 404/351-4523

Hospitals, published twice monthly by American Hospital Publishing, Inc., 211 E. Chicago Ave., Chicago, IL 60611, 312/440-6800

Joint Commission Perspectives, published bimonthly by the Joint Commission on Accreditation of Healthcare Organizations, 1 Renaissance Blvd., Oakbrook Terrace, IL 60181, 708/916-5600

Journal of Legal Medicine, published quarterly by Shugar Publishing, Inc., 270 Lafayette St., New York, NY 10012, 212/966-8800

Law, Medicine & Health Care, published quarterly by the American Society of Law & Medicine, 765 Commonwealth Ave., Boston, MA 02215, 617/262-4990

Legal Aspects of Medical Practice, published monthly by Shugar Publishing, Inc., 270 Lafayette St., New York, NY 10012, 212/966-8800

Malpractice Digest, published quarterly by the Medical Services Division of St. Paul Fire and Marine Insurance Co., 385 Washington St., St. Paul, MN 55102, 612/221-7123

Medical Economics, published twice monthly by the Medical Economics Company, P.O. Box 552, Oradell, NJ 07649, 201/262-3030

Medical Liability Advisory Service, published monthly by Business Publishers, 951 Pershing Dr., Silver Spring, MD 20910, 301/587-6300

Medical Liability Monitor, published monthly by Malpractice Lifeline, Inc., P.O. Box 9011, Winnetka, IL 60093, 708/446-3100

Medical Liability Reporter, published monthly by Shepard's McGraw-Hill, P.O. Box 1235, Colorado Springs, CO 80901, 719/475-7230

Medical Malpractice Verdicts, Settlements & Experts, published monthly by Lewis Laska, 901 Church St., Nashville, TN 37203, 615/255-6288

Modern Healthcare, published weekly by Crain Communications, 740 N. Rush St., Chicago, IL 60611, 312/649-5350

National Underwriter Property & Casualty/Employee Benefits Edition, published weekly by National Underwriter Co., 420 E. 4th St., Cincinnati, OH 45202, 513/721-2140

Occupational Health & Safety, published monthly by Stevens Publishing, P.O. Box 7573, Waco, TX 76710-7573, 817/776-9000

Occurrence, published quarterly by the Chicago Hospital Risk Pooling Program, 222 S. Riverside Plaza, Chicago, IL 60606, 312/906-6169

Perspectives in Healthcare Risk Management, published quarterly by the American Society for Healthcare Risk Management, 840 N. Lake Shore Dr., Chicago, IL 60611, 312/280-6198

QRC Advisor, published monthly by Aspen Publishers, Inc., 7201 McKinney Circle, Frederick, MD 21701, 800/638-8437

Quality Assurance Quarterly, published quarterly by the Canadian Association of Quality Assurance Professionals, 1 Eva Rd., STE 409, Etobicoke, Ontario, Canada M9C 4Z5, 416/626-0102

Quality Review Bulletin, published monthly by the Joint Commission on Accreditation of Healthcare Organizations, 1 Renaissance Blvd., Oakbrook Terrace, IL 60181, 708/916-5600

Regan Report on Nursing Law, published monthly by Medica Press, 1231 Fleet National Bank Bldg., Providence, RI 02903, 401/421-4747

Risk Management, published monthly by the Risk and Insurance Management Society, 205 E. 42nd St., New York, NY 10017, 212/286-9292

Specialty Law Digest: Health Care, published monthly by Specialty Digest Publications, Inc., STE 105, 10301 University Ave., N.E., Blaine, MN 55433, 612/780-3157

Staff Privileges Report, published monthly by Little, Brown and Company, 34 Beacon St., Boston, MA 02108, 617/227-0730

Books

American College of Surgeons. *Patient Safety Manual.* 2nd ed. Chicago: ACS, 1985.

Brown, B. L. *Risk Management for Hospitals: A Practical Approach.* Rockville, MD: Aspen Publishers, 1979.

Craddick, J. W. *Medical Management Analysis.* 2 vols. Auburn, CA: J. W. Craddick, 1983.

Emergency Care Research Institute. *Hospital Risk Control.* Plymouth Meeting, PA: ECRI. (Four-binder information system sold by subscription. To subscribe, contact Pennsylvania Insurance Management Company, One PHICO Dr., P.O. Box 85, Mechanicsburg, PA 17055-0085.)

Hospital Law Manual. Rockville, MD: Aspen Publishers. Updated quarterly.

Kapp, M. *Preventing Malpractice in Long-Term Care.* New York City: Springer Publishing Co., 1987.

Kraus, G. P. *Health Care Risk Management: Organization and Claims Administration.* Owings Mills, MD: National Health Publishing Co., 1986.

Lamade, L. L., editor. *Hospital Contracts Manual.* Rockville, MD: Aspen Publishers. Updated semiannually.

MacDonald, M. G., Meyer, K. C., and Essig, B. *Health Care Law.* New York City: Matthew Bender & Co., 1985.

Modern Health Care Law. 12 vols. Blaine, MN: Specialty Digest Publications. Updated yearly.

Monagle, J. F. *Risk Management: A Guide for Health Care Professionals.* Rockville, MD: Aspen Publishers, 1985.

Orlikoff, J. E., and Vanagunas, A. *Malpractice Prevention and Liability Control for Hospitals.* 2nd ed. Chicago: American Hospital Publishing, 1988.

Personal Injury Valuation Handbooks. Solon, OH: Jury Verdict Research. Updated monthly.

Richards, E. P., and Rathbun, K. C. *Medical Risk Management: Preventive Legal Strategies for Health Care Providers.* Rockville, MD: Aspen Publishers, 1983.

Risk Management: A Self-Evaluation Guide. Columbus, OH: Ohio Hospital Association, 1981.

Roach, W. H., Chernoff, S. N., and Esley, C. L. *Medical Records and the Law.* Rockville, MD: Aspen Publishers, 1985.

Rowland, H. S., and Rowland, B. L. *Hospital Legal Forms, Checklists, and Guidelines.* Rockville, MD: Aspen Publishers. Updated periodically.

Rowland, H. S., and Rowland, B. L. *Hospital Risk Management: Forms, Checklists, and Guidelines.* Rockville, MD: Aspen Publishers, 1989.

Rozovsky, F. A. *Consent to Treatment: A Practical Guide.* 2nd ed. Boston: Little, Brown & Co., 1990 (with annual supplements).

Safety Handbook. Columbus, OH: Ohio Hospital Association, 1981.

Southwick, A. *The Law of Hospital and Health Care Administration.* 2nd ed. Ann Arbor, MI: Health Administration Press, 1988.

Troyer, G., and Salman, S. *Handbook of Health Care Risk Management.* Rockville, MD: Aspen Publishers, 1985.

Wade, R. D. *Risk Management Hospital Professional Liability Primer.* Columbus, OH: Ohio Hospital Insurance Co., 1983.

Wilson, C. R. M. *Hospital-Wide Quality Assurance.* Toronto: W. B. Saunders Canada Ltd., 1987.

Youngberg, B. J. *Essentials of Hospital Risk Management.* Rockville, MD: Aspen Publishers, 1989.

Audiovisuals

(Addresses and telephone numbers for the distributors of these audiovisual materials are given at the end of this section.)

Accountability and Liability in Nursing Practice
    1986   28 mins   VHS, ¾ U-matic
    American Journal of Nursing Co.

Completing the Incident Report
    1987   12 mins   ¾ U-matic
    Fairview Audio-Visuals

DNR Dilemma
> 1987   21 mins   Beta, VHS, ¾ U-matic
> Carle Medical Communications

How to Recognize a Medical Malpractice Case
> 1986   210 mins   Beta, VHS, ¾ U-matic
> American Law Institute

Legal Aspects of Documentation for Nurses
> 1981   49 mins Beta,   VHS, ¾ U-matic
> Emory Medical Television Network

Medical Malpractice Litigation
> 1987   7 tapes (each 1 hr.)   Beta, VHS
> American Bar Association Division of Professional Education

Minimizing Nurses' Liabilities
> 1984   60 mins   Beta, VHS, ¾ U-matic
> American Hospital Association

Nursing Quality Assurance: Defining Quality Patient Care
> 1988   28 mins   VHS, ¾ U-matic
> American Journal of Nursing Co.

Protecting Directors and Officers in an Era of Uncertain D & O Liability Insurance
> 1986   210 mins   Beta, VHS, ¾ U-matic
> American Law Institute

Resource: A Monthly Audio Digest of Current Issues in Health Care Risk Management
> Monthly   audiocassette produced by the Risk Management Foundation of the
> Harvard Medical Institutions
> Tillinghast

Risk Management: Effective Hospital Management Series
> 1980   20 mins   VHS, ¾ U-matic
> Health Communications Network

Risk Management in the O.R.
> 1985   21 mins   VHS
> Davis & Geck

Structured Settlements in Tort Liability Cases
> 1984   180 mins   Beta, VHS, ¾ U-matic
> American Law Institute

Distributor Addresses and Telephone Numbers

American Bar Association
Division of Professional Education
750 N. Lake Shore Dr.
Chicago, IL 60611
800/621-8986

American Hospital Association
840 N. Lake Shore Dr.
Chicago, IL 60611
800/AHA-2626

American Journal of Nursing Co.
Educational Services Division
555 W. 57th St.
New York, NY 10019
212/582-8820

American Law Institute
ABA Committee on Continuing
  Education
4025 Chestnut St.
Philadelphia, PA 19104
800/CLE-NEWS

Carle Medical Communications
110 W. Main St.
Urbana, IL 61801-2700
217/384-4838

Davis & Geck
1 Casper St.
Danbury, CT 06810
800/633-0004

Emory Medical Television Network
Health Sciences Center Library
Emory University
1462 Clifton Rd., N.E.
Atlanta, GA 30322
(no telephone orders accepted)

Fairview Audio-Visuals
17909 Groveland Ave.
Cleveland, OH 44111-5656
216/476-7054

Health Communications Network
Division of Television Services
Medical University of South Carolina
171 Ashely Ave.
Charleston, SC 29425
803/792-4980

Tillinghast
Financial Centre, STE 600
695 E. Main St.
Stamford, CT 06901-2138
203/326-5400

Glossary

Actual cash value (ACV) versus replacement cost: A property policy may be issued on an actual cash-value or replacement-cost basis. Replacement-cost coverage replaces the damaged property without deduction for depreciation, whereas actual cash-value coverage is based on replacement cost at time of loss minus a deduction for depreciation.

Actuary: A person who uses statistics to compute loss probabilities to establish premiums for insurance companies and self-insurance trusts.

Additional insured: A person or entity added to a policy by endorsement who or which is protected by the terms of that policy. Other insureds are the "named insured" shown on the policy declaration and "insureds" who are defined in the policy wording.

Affirmative defense: In a civil lawsuit, a denial of wrongdoing by which the defendant asserts new evidence or matters unrelated to the claim asserted by the plaintiff. Examples of affirmative defenses include stating that the plaintiff filed after the statute of limitations had run or that the plaintiff's own actions contributed to the plaintiff's injuries.

Aggregate limits: Used most frequently in liability policies. The maximum amount an insurer will pay for all covered losses in a given policy period. For example, if the occurrence limit on a professional liability policy is $100,000 and the aggregate limit is $300,000, the policy will pay $100,000 for as many as three losses during the policy period, or for as many as six losses of $50,000 each, or for 300,000 losses of $1 each.

Allied lines: A term that has been adopted to refer to the lines that are allied with property insurance. These coverages provide protection against perils traditionally written by fire insurance companies, such as sprinkler leakage, water damage, and earthquake.

Answer: The initial document filed by the defendants, in response to a complaint, in which the defendants admit or deny the allegations in the complaint.

Antitrust: An illegal trust, as defined under federal law and the laws of most states, whereby two or more persons act jointly to restrain or monopolize trade or fix prices.

Appellant: If the party against whom the verdict has gone in a lawsuit appeals the verdict to a higher court, the appealing party becomes the "appellant," and the other party becomes the "appellee."

Appellee: The party who prevails in a lawsuit becomes the "appellee" if the other party files an appeal of the verdict to a higher court.

Arbitration: An adversarial means of dispute resolution in which the parties to the dispute present their cases to an arbitrator or panel of arbitrators who decide the issue in question. Arbitration may be either binding or nonbinding on one or both parties.

Assigned risk pool: In many states, workers' compensation and automobile liability insurance is compulsory—an entity must furnish proof of coverage to operate a business. Some entities (because of poor experience or start-up entities with no insurance "track record") cannot find an insurance company willing to provide them coverage. Recognizing the need to make coverage available, most states created "assigned risk pools." Every insurance company writing these types of coverage is required to participate in these pools. Participating companies are assigned the responsibility of providing coverage.

Assured: A term used interchangeably with "insured."

Automobile liability insurance: An insurance contract that protects the insured against liability for bodily injury or property damage by the use of an owned automobile. Coverage may be written to extend this protection to others using the insured's vehicles or when vehicles of others are used by an insured.

Automobile physical damage insurance: Coverage for damages or loss to an insured's automobile resulting from collision, fire, theft, and other perils.

Bailee: A person or concern having possession of property committed in trust from the owner.

Barrier protection: The use of physical barriers to decrease the probability of person-to-person transmission of infectious organisms. Barriers may include gloves, masks, gowns, goggles, or plastic aprons as appropriate to the situation.

Binder: A preliminary, temporary agreement indicating that insurance is in place, which obligates the insurance company to pay if the loss insured against occurs before the policy is written.

Bodily injury liability: The liability that may arise from injury to or death of another person.

Boiler and machinery liability: Coverage for loss arising out of the operation of pressure, mechanical, and electrical equipment. It may cover loss suffered by the equipment itself and may include damage done to other property, as well as business-interruption losses.

Brain death: The Uniform Determination of Death has been codified in the laws of most states as follows:

> Only an individual who has sustained either (1) irreversible cessation of circulatory and respiratory functions or (2) irreversible cessation of all functions of the entire brain, including the brain stem, is dead. A determination of death must be made in accordance with accepted medical standards.

Breach: The failure, for which the law may provide a remedy, to carry out duties or obligations assumed under a contract.

Burglary and theft insurance: Protection for loss of property as a result of burglary, robbery, or larceny.

Business interruption: A kind of insurance that reimburses an insured for lost earnings resulting from an insured peril.

Capacity: The ability to act. In health care, competent persons under the laws of the state have the capacity to make health care decisions for themselves. Also, the legal ability to sue or be brought into court.

Captive insurance company: An insurance company whose stock is owned by the insured or insureds of that company, primarily to insure the exposures of its owners. Captives are established in an attempt to reduce insurance costs to the participants.

Certificate of insurance: A document that verifies that an insurance policy has been written and states the nature of the coverage in general terms. Such a certificate is often used as proof of insurance.

Chain of custody/chain of evidence: A rule of evidence in a legal proceeding requiring that custody of a piece of evidence, such as a piece of malfunctioning equipment alleged to have caused an injury, be continuously documented from the time of the incident until its introduction into evidence. The chain of custody includes identification of each custodian and each transfer of custody.

Claim: In health care, a patient's demand for payment for injury, illness, or lost or damaged property that resulted from the alleged negligence of the hospital, the physician, or the employees or agents of either.

Claims-made coverage: Provides that the insured will be covered for an occurrence that takes place (1) during the policy period, or (2) subsequent to a retroactive date stated in the policy declarations and prior to the expiration date of the policy, if the insurer is notified of the claim (in accordance with the insurer's definition of proper notification) during the term of the policy.

Claims management: A risk management function. The person who performs this function gets reports of professional and general liability claims against the institution, its employees, and agents, and manages them to conclusion.

Closed claim surveys: A method of determining trends in professional liability by keeping track of significant information from claims as they are closed. Examples of significant events to be trended include the allegation brought by the claimant, the amount of payment required to close the claim, the amount of expense incurred in managing the claim, and who was named in the claim.

Closing argument: At the end of a trial, attorneys for the plaintiff and for the defendant each give their closing argument, a summary of the case and of what their evidence has shown.

Coinsurance: A provision in an insurance policy that requires the insured to carry insurance equal to a certain specified percentage of the value of the property. It provides for the full payment, up to the amount of the policy, of all losses if the insurance carried is at least equal to the value specified. Otherwise, the loss payment would be only a percentage of the actual loss. The insured pays a lower premium if there is a coinsurance provision.

Collateral: Money, property, or other security pledged to a creditor for the repayment of a loan.

Commercial multiple peril policy: A type of package insurance policy for the commercial establishment that includes a wide range of essential coverage.

Common law: That body of law, originally established in England by the practices and usages of the community, that has been passed down by precedent or prior court decisions. It is contrasted with statutory law, which is the body of law that has been enacted by the legislature.

Competent: Legally able to make decisions for oneself. In health care, adults who have not been determined in a court of law to be unable to make decisions are presumed to be competent.

Complaint: The document, filed in a court of law, that states the complainant's cause of action and the facts upon which the action is based. The summons and complaint usually are the initial pleadings in a lawsuit.

Comprehensive policy: A term used for various insurance contracts that provide protection for a variety of the insured's exposures. A comprehensive boiler and machinery insurance policy, a comprehensive automobile liability, or a comprehensive general liability are examples of this type of contract.

Concurrent insurance: Two or more insurance policies with the same conditions that cover the same interest in identical property and are concurrent.

Conditions: In an insurance policy, the clauses in the contract that describe the obligations, rights, and privileges of the insured. For example, as a condition to the insurer's obligation to provide coverage for the claim, the insured usually is obligated to provide prompt notice to the insurer that a claim covered under the policy has been made.

Consequential loss: A loss not directly caused by damage to property, but that arises as a result of such damage, as in the case of food spoilage from refrigeration failure resulting from fire damage to the refrigerator.

Contract: An agreement by two or more parties to assume obligations, not otherwise required of them, for consideration that is enforceable in a court of law. Contracts may be written, oral, or implied by conduct.

Counterclaim: A claim that a defendant in a civil case files against the plaintiff.

Credentialing/privileging: A process undertaken by a hospital's governing board, upon the recommendation of its medical staff, to review and approve the qualifications of applicants for appointment to the medical staff and of those seeking reappointment, and defining their scope of practice and the procedures they may perform in the institution.

Cross-claim: A claim that a party in a civil case files against a coparty arising out of the transaction or occurrence that is the subject matter of the action.

Damages: Monetary compensation for an injury.

Deductible: A clause in an insurance policy that identifies the portion of loss that is the responsibility of the insured. A deductible reduces the policy premium and usually is stated in a dollar amount or as a percentage of each loss.

"Deep pocket": A colloquial term for an organization, corporation, or sometimes an individual who or which is perceived to have sufficient assets to pay a loss and so is worth bringing into a lawsuit to ensure a larger pool of money to pay damages.

Defamation: A cause of action in law for which a plaintiff may recover damages if the plaintiff proves that the defendant made false statements that injured the plaintiff's reputation. Both libel, which is a false written statement, and slander, which is a false oral statement, are defamatory.

Defendant: In a civil lawsuit, a term designating the party who denies wrongdoing or defends against the allegations made by the plaintiff; the party against whom recovery is sought.

Deposition: Testimony taken during discovery by either party of the other party or of witnesses. The testimony is taken orally under oath outside the courtroom, and a word-for-word record is made.

Depreciation: The difference between the actual cash value of property and the cost of replacing that property with material of like kind or quality.

Difference in conditions coverage: A property insurance policy that provides coverage for perils that are excluded from an insured's "named peril" or standard "all-risks" property policy. Often used as a vehicle to purchase flood and earthquake insurance, although other perils also are included.

Directed verdict: The judge's direction to the jury to bring the verdict for the party the judge specifies. The judge may grant a motion for a directed verdict only when the evidence or the law is so clearly in the favor of one of the parties that the trial should not proceed.

Directors' and officers' (D & O) liability: The liability incurred, because of breaches of duty that result in negligence, errors, or omissions, by an individual serving as an officer or director of an organization. The organization may purchase insurance to cover their officers and directors for losses and expenses of defending claims.

Discovery: Techniques used by the parties to a lawsuit to gather information that is in the jurisdiction and control of the other party. Common discovery techniques include requests for the production of documents, depositions, and interrogatories.

DRGs: Stands for diagnosis-related groups. The Health Care Financing Administration, which administers the Medicare program, has developed 467 groups of diagnoses of illnesses upon which it bases its payments to hospitals for care of Medicare patients.

Dual capacity doctrine: A doctrine recognizing that under the law of some states, a physician employed by a company to treat employment-related accidents or illnesses of that company's employees operates in a "dual capacity." That is, the physician, as a company employee, has an obligation to the employer, but also has an obligation to the employees by virtue of the physician–patient relationship. If an employee alleges malpractice against the physician for treatment of workplace-related accidents or illnesses, the physician may be sued outside the state's workers' compensation statute in the capacity of the patient's treating physician, and the employer may be held liable for the acts of its agent.

Durable power of attorney: A document through which a competent person of legal majority age grants certain powers to another to be exercised on that person's behalf. In health care, such documents are sometimes used to designate someone to make health care decisions in the event of the maker's incompetence.

Employment at will: A legal theory under which the employer may terminate an employee at will and without cause.

Endorsement: A document that modifies the original terms of the insurance policy to which it is attached.

Escrow: Money or other property held by an uninvolved party in a fiduciary capacity and released only upon the occurrence of a specified event or under conditions specified in advance of setting up the escrow arrangement.

Excess insurance: An insurance policy covering the insured only for losses in excess of a stated amount. Losses below that stated amount may be self-insured or insured in a primary policy.

Expense reserve: That portion of the amount reserved by an insurer or self-insured trust to pay the anticipated expenses, such as legal fees and costs of investigation, of defending or settling a claim.

Exposure: Defined by risk managers as a risk of loss. In insurance, an exposure is the total value of that which is insured under a policy of insurance.

Extended coverage insurance: Protection for loss or damage to the insured's property caused by windstorm, hail, smoke, explosion, riot, riot attending a strike, civil commotion, vehicle, or aircraft. It is provided in conjunction with the fire insurance policy.

Fidelity bond: A form of protection that reimburses an employer for losses caused by dishonest or fraudulent acts of its employees.

Fiduciary: One who holds another person's funds or other assets in a trust relationship.

Fire insurance: A basic property insurance policy that covers losses caused by fire, lightning, and resultant damage.

Floating: A practice in hospitals whereby nurses are temporarily assigned to work in units other than the ones to which they usually are assigned. Nurses usually float to units that are understaffed.

Fronting insurance company: An insurance carrier that has an arrangement with a reinsurer (or reinsurers) to issue an insurance contract (fronting policy) for which the obligation is then ceded back to the reinsurer(s). The fronting company usually handles claims, makes state filings, and issues certificates of insurance.

Generic occurrence screening: The screening of patient records for defined adverse clinical events. *See* Occurrence screening.

Going bare: The decision not to transfer risk of loss by purchasing insurance, but instead to pay losses as they may occur.

Governing board: Those individuals elected or appointed by the members of an organization to have ultimate responsibility to set policy for the organization and control its activities.

Hard insurance market: Period of limited availability and high prices of insurance coverage.

Health care proxy: A document through which a competent person of legal majority may designate another to make health care decisions on the person's behalf in the event of the person's incompetence. Such a document is valid only if state law authorizes it by statute.

Hold harmless: A clause frequently inserted in contracts between buyers and sellers of products or services by which party A to the contract requires party B to assume the costs of claims when both are sued by party C, who is not a party to the contract but who claims injury as a result of the product or service.

Iatrogenic illness (or disorder): Illness or disorder caused by diagnosis or treatment by a physician.

Immunity: Protection from being sued for actions for which the person or institution otherwise could be sued. In some states, peer review statutes have granted immunity to those involved in peer review.

Implied consent: Consent to health care diagnosis or treatment manifested by action or by a silence that raises the presumption that an authorization is given. For example, a patient who attends a mass immunization clinic gives implied consent to inoculations being administered at the site. Also, in a life-threatening emergency, the law implies consent to such reasonable treatment as is deemed medically necessary.

Incident: Generally accepted by most risk managers to mean any happening not consistent with the routine operation of the facility or the routine care of a particular patient.

Incident reporting: A system in health care institutions by which employees use a standardized form to report any occurrence outside the routine so that the information can be used for loss prevention and claims management activities.

Indemnify: To agree to reimburse another for an actual loss sustained. Bonds and some insurance policies provide for indemnification of the insured in consideration for the premium charged.

Indemnity: The amount paid to a claimant by an insurer or self-insured trust on behalf of the insured for a loss that the insured is legally liable to pay.

Indemnity reserve: That portion of the funds reserved by an insurer or self-insured trust to pay the amount it anticipates a claimant may recover from its insured.

Independent contractor: A corporation, person, or other entity who is engaged to do work for another, but who has control of the manner and method by which the work is performed. Unlike an employee, who is supervised by the employer as to the manner and method of the work performed, the independent contractor is responsible to the party who has engaged the work only for the final product.

Infection control: A function performed in health care institutions to monitor and control diseases resulting from infections acquired in the health care institution.

Informed consent: A patient's agreement to a particular course of treatment based upon disclosure by the physician (or other provider who has the legal duty to seek consent before providing treatment) of the relevant facts.

Inland marine insurance: A type of insurance providing coverage for movable property and fixed property used in the transportation and communication industries. Inland marine insurance can cover such property at a fixed location, while being shipped overland, or while being shipped by inland waterways. Marine insurance, another form of coverage, provides protection when property is shipped overseas.

Insurable interest: Any interest in, or relation to, property of such a nature that the occurrence of an event insured against would cause financial loss to the insured. Only one who may suffer a loss may insure against it.

Insurance: A contract in which an insurance company agrees to protect or indemnify an insured for certain losses or against certain perils.

Insurance agent: A person or agency, usually licensed under the insurance laws of a state and authorized by one or more insurance companies, to represent the company or companies in selling insurance or providing service to the insureds. An agent receives a commission from a company for selling its insurance.

Insurance broker: A person licensed to do business in a given state who represents the insurance buyer in arranging coverage with insurance companies or through insurance intermediaries.

Insurance declaration: That part of a contract of insurance identifying the named insured and describing each property or activity for which the policy will provide coverage.

Insurance exclusion: Provisions of an insurance policy stating perils, property, and circumstances that are not covered.

Insuring agreement: That part of an insurance policy or bond stating the obligations of the insurance company to pay to the insured those losses covered under the policy that the insured becomes legally obligated to pay. The insuring agreements and the exclusions, read together, describe the coverage under a policy of insurance.

Interrogatories: Written questions submitted during discovery by one party to the other party or to witnesses, to which the party or witnesses must provide written answers under oath.

JCAHO: Stands for the Joint Commission on Accreditation of Healthcare Organizations. The Joint Commission is a private not-for-profit agency founded by the American Hospital Association, the American Medical Association, and the American College of Surgeons that provides a voluntary accreditation process for health care organizations. Many third-party payers, including the Medicare program, accept Joint Commission accreditation as a qualification for reimbursement for the care of patients.

Layering insurance: An insurance program consisting of two or more insurance contracts that together achieve the desired limits for the insured. The lowest-level policy is usually referred to as primary insurance, and each policy above it is referred to as an excess layer. Thus, in order to reach the desired limit of protection, several policies may be used, one above another, in layers.

Liability: Having legal responsibility; also, a debt or obligation.

Liability limits: The amount of money for which the insurance company agrees to protect the insured under the terms of the policy. The liability limits are shown on the declaration page of the policy as separate bodily injury and property damage amounts or as a combined single limit for bodily injury and property damage.

Liquidated damages: A specified amount of money that has been determined to fully compensate a party injured by the breach of a contract. The term also is applied when a court has made a judgment in an action and has ascertained the amount of damages.

Living will: A document created by someone who wishes to specify the medical treatment to be provided or not provided in the event that the person's illness is terminal and makes him or her unable to make medical decisions at the time treatment is proposed. Many people make living wills to prevent being put on life-support systems or kept alive on life-support systems. A living will is a legal document in a state only to the extent that the state's statutes make it so.

"Long tail": A period of several years between the occurrence of an event and the filing of a claim arising from that event. Common in professional liability.

Loss adjustment costs: Costs of investigating and defending claims. They include such expenses as attorney fees, expert reviews of medical records, and billings for independent medical examinations.

Loss prevention: A risk management function. The person who performs this function identifies the risk of loss throughout the institution and implements systems to prevent or minimize the risk of loss.

Maintenance deductible: A dollar amount or a percentage of a claim that the insured must pay. Normally used by excess insurers to ensure that if primary coverage has been exhausted, the insured will continue to participate in the financial burden of the claim. For example, the insurer providing $5 million of excess coverage over a primary $1 million policy may require a maintenance deductible. Claims arising after the first $1 million in coverage has been exhausted will be subject to the maintenance deductible.

Malpractice: The failure of one providing professional services, such as a lawyer, doctor, or accountant, to exercise that degree of skill that would be exercised by the average, prudent member of that profession, with the result that the person seeking the service has suffered an injury or other loss.

Material safety data sheets (MSDS): A document prepared in accordance with Occupational Safety and Health Administration requirements containing storage, handling, physical, and health hazard information concerning a hazardous chemical.

MDA: Medical Doctor of Anesthesiology.

Medical specials: Compensatory damages specifically related to actual out-of-pocket expenses for medical treatment such as the cost of hospitalization, physician fees, prescription drugs, physical therapy, prosthetic devices, and so forth.

Negligence: Failure to use that degree of care that a reasonably prudent person would use under similar circumstances. Negligence may be constituted by acts of either omission or commission, or both.

Negligent hiring: A legal theory under which an employer may be held liable for the wrongful acts of its employee if the employer failed to discover facts about the employee that were available to the employer and would have predicted the wrongful act.

Nursing assessment: An initial evaluation by a nurse of a patient's condition, based on various clinical indications, such as patient history, vital signs, and laboratory reports. A nursing assessment is required for every patient admitted to the hospital.

Nursing care plan: A plan, made by the nurse responsible for the patient's care, that identifies nursing care goals for the particular patient, states methods to achieve the goals, and lists the benefits to the patient. The Joint Commission on Accreditation of Healthcare Organizations requires that every hospitalized patient in an accredited facility have a nursing care plan that is evaluated and restated daily.

Occurrence coverage: Provides that the insured will be covered for an event that takes place during the policy period regardless of when the claim is brought.

Occurrence screening: The screening of patient records for defined adverse clinical events, including such occurrences as adverse drug reactions, unplanned transfers to critical care units, or returns to the emergency department within a specified number of days for the same illness or injury.

Opening statements: Presentations given by attorneys representing the plaintiff and the defendant at the beginning of a trial in which the attorneys state their respective cases and the supporting evidence to be presented.

Package policy: An insurance policy with two or more different insurance coverages combined. A typical package might include property insurance, liability insurance, and crime insurance.

Patient's bill of rights: A document mandated by the Joint Commission on Accreditation of Healthcare Organizations for accredited health care facilities that describes the rights to which patients in institutions are entitled. Statutes in some states may also require that institutions develop and prominently display such documents.

Peer review: The process by which the diagnosis, care, and treatment of patients is reviewed and evaluated by those who have training and experience similar to the professional being evaluated, for purposes of employment, appointment, reappointment, privileging, or corrective action.

Peer review privilege: A doctrine whereby some states recognize either a statutory or common law prohibition against requiring the release of peer review records and discussions.

Peril: Something that destroys or causes loss—a type of loss for which an insured is protected in a policy. Perils that may be covered in a property policy include fire, lightning, and windstorm.

Plaintiff: In a lawsuit, a term designating the party who brings the action.

Pleadings: The documents filed in a lawsuit, including the summons and complaint, the answer, and any cross-claims or counterclaims, that set forth the facts and name the issues to be litigated.

Policy: A written contract of insurance.

Policy holder: The person or company protected by an insurance contract. This term is synonymous with "insured."

Potentially compensable events: Events that have the potential for becoming claims for which the claimant may be compensated.

Precedent: A court decision that becomes authority for cases or questions of law arising later that are similar to the decided case.

Prefunding: Setting money aside that is designated to pay certain obligations that will come due in the future.

Premises liability: The liability incurred by an individual or organization for injury to the public created by negligence in maintaining or operating a business premises.

Premium: The amount of money an insured pays to an insurance company to be provided coverage for specified losses under a contract of insurance.

Primary insurer: An insurer that provides coverage from "first dollar" of loss. In recent years, some primary insurers of professional liability have required that the insured pay a deductible in lieu of carrying pure "first dollar" coverage. This deductible may range from $5,000 to $250,000 per occurrence. Primary insurers handle all claims, including those within the deductible.

Prior acts coverage: Coverage that can be offered in a claims-made liability policy for claims that occurred but were not reported for a specific time before the effective date of that policy.

Privilege: Protection from being required to disclose information. The most commonly held privileges include the patient–physician privilege, the clergy–penitent privilege, and the attorney–client privilege. The laws of each state define the privileges held in that state and who may hold them.

Procedural law: That part of the law involving the rules that govern bringing and prosecuting an action in court. Procedural law includes such issues as the structure for the presentation of evidence and for determining where the lawsuit is filed, the time limits for filing legal documents, and the limits of the discovery process.

Professional liability: Losses an individual or institution may incur as a result of professional misconduct or departure from the ordinary standard of care in the performance of services.

Promissory note: A written agreement to pay a sum of money at a specified time or upon demand to a person or an entity designated in the note.

Proof of loss: A formal statement made by the insured to the insurance company regarding a claim, so that the company may determine its liability under the policy or bond.

Quality assurance: A function performed in health care institutions, and required for accreditation by the Joint Commission on Accreditation of Healthcare Organizations, to monitor the quality of care provided to patients by the hospital staff and the medical staff.

Release: A document signed by a claimant foreclosing the claimant's ability to bring future claims arising out of a specified occurrence.

Reservation of rights: Formal written notice to the insured from the insurer that investigation of a claim by the insurer does not constitute an admission that the insurer agrees to pay the loss.

Reserve: An amount of money designated on the financial records of an insurance company or self-insured program to pay an identified loss. When a claim is reported to an insurance company, the company usually will determine what its ultimate liability and its expenses will be for the loss and will establish an indemnity reserve and an expense reserve.

Respondeat superior: A legal theory that says that an employer, through supervision and control of employees, is responsible for the acts of the employees done in furtherance of the employer's business.

Retrospective rating: A method of determining the premium for an insurance policy that is based on the insured's actual loss experience. The final premium is calculated after all losses have been closed for a policy period.

Right to know laws (or ordinances): Those laws or ordinances, effective in some states and municipalities, that require employers to provide information, education, and/or treatment to employees regarding hazardous materials to which employees may be exposed during their employment.

Risk acceptance: The decision not to transfer an identified risk but instead to assume its financial consequences.

Risk analysis: The process used by the person or persons assigned risk management functions to determine the potential severity of the loss from an identified risk, the probability that the loss will happen, and alternatives for dealing with the risk.

Risk avoidance: The decision not to undertake a particular activity because the risk associated with the activity is unacceptable.

Risk financing: A management plan to develop the sources and uses of funds that an organization would need to recover from a loss.

Risk identification: The process used by the person or persons assigned risk management functions to identify situations, policies, or practices that could result in financial loss to the institution.

Risk reduction: A loss control strategy by which a risk is identified and steps are taken to minimize its financial impact or the frequency of its occurrence.

Risk retention group: An insuring vehicle formed under the Federal Liability Risk Retention Act of 1986 or the Product Liability Risk Retention Act of 1981. A risk retention group provides liability insurance coverage to its member policy holders, all of which must have exposure to similar risk. Such groups are subject to rules and regulations established by the Risk Retention Act under which they are formed, rather than state insurance licensing laws. Unlike a captive insurance company, which must be licensed in each state in which it does business, a risk retention group, if it meets the requirements of the federal statute creating risk retention groups, may do business in all states if it is licensed by one state.

Risk transfer: The procedure of shifting risk of loss to another party who agrees to accept it. Examples of risk transfer are insurance, warranties, and hold harmless agreements.

Risk treatment: The range of choices with which to handle an identified risk that are available to the person or persons assigned risk management functions.

Rules of evidence: That part of procedural law governing how the attorneys for the plaintiff and defendant may question witnesses, what questions may be asked, and how documentary evidence, such as the patient's medical record, may be introduced into evidence.

Scope of practice: In the health professions, the professional activities that a health professional is authorized to perform under the laws of the state in which the health professional is licensed.

Self-insured retention (SIR): That portion of an institution's total exposure to loss that it chooses to pay directly (out of a self-insured trust) rather than transfer to another party by the purchase of insurance.

Situs: When used as a part of a contract, the location where the contract is considered to be entered into; the contract is interpreted according to the laws of that jurisdiction.

Soft insurance market: Period of ample availability and low prices of insurance coverage.

Spread loss program: A method of retaining the risk of loss rather than transferring it through purchasing commercial insurance. Under this program, a company retains its risk and has a plan for borrowing money to pay losses over a long period if those losses exceed its ability to pay them out of its own funds.

Standard of care: In a legal proceeding, the standard against which the defendant's conduct is measured. The defendant is expected to act as an ordinary, prudent person with similar training and skill would have acted in a similar situation. If the defendant's conduct falls below this standard, the defendant may be determined to have acted negligently.

Statute of limitations: The time period, specified by statute, during which a party must file an action; after that period has expired, the party is foreclosed from filing it.

Structured settlement: A method of paying a judgment or settlement whereby an agreed-upon amount of money is invested and the payments to the claimant are paid out from the principal and earnings over a period of years. The total amount paid out exceeds the initial sum invested.

Subpoena/subpoena duces tecum: An order issued by a court or an attorney to a witness requiring the witness to appear and give testimony. A *subpoena duces tecum* requires that the witness bring specified documents or other property.

Substantive law: That part of the law that creates, defines, and regulates the rights and duties of parties in a legal action. For example, under substantive law, a patient who has been injured as a result of the negligent act or omission of a health care provider has a right to damages from the health care provider.

Summons: The document that notifies defendants that legal action has been brought against them.

Surety bond: An agreement providing for monetary compensation should there be a failure to perform certain specified acts within a stated period. For example, the surety company becomes responsible for fulfilling a contract if the contractor defaults.

"Tail" coverage: Coverage provided by a claims-made liability policy that extends the protection of the policy beyond the expiration date for claims that occurred within the original policy period. There usually is an additional charge for this extension, and the extension may be for a limited time.

Time-weighted average (TWA): An average concentration for a normal 8-hour workday or 40-hour workweek, to which nearly all workers may be repeatedly exposed, day after day, without adverse effect.

Umbrella insurance: A comprehensive insurance policy providing broader coverage and higher limits than underlying insurance policies.

Utilization review: A function performed in health care institutions to ascertain that the number of days that patients are hospitalized is appropriate for the severity of their illness and that the resources used in their care are appropriate.

Venue: The locality where a legal proceeding occurs.

Verbal order: An order given by a physician for the care of the physician's patient, usually by telephone, that is not written by the physician but is entered in the patient's record by an authorized staff member and is required to be signed by the physician within a designated length of time.

Vicarious liability: Legal responsibility for the acts of someone else. For example, the hospital may be found to be vicariously liable for the acts of its employees.

Voir dire: The process by which the attorney for the plaintiff and the attorney for the defendant examine the qualifications of prospective jurors and select a qualified panel.

With prejudice: When used in connection with a court's dismissal of a legal action, a dismissal with prejudice terminates the rights of the parties just as if final judgment had been rendered against the plaintiff. Conversely, a dismissal without prejudice allows the action to be brought again on the same cause of action.

Work product doctrine: A doctrine whereby material prepared by an attorney in anticipation of litigation may be protected from discovery. The work product doctrine applies to the notes, statements of witnesses, private memoranda, and mental impressions formed by the attorney.

Workers' compensation: A program that provides protection to workers who are injured while engaged in the business of their employer, regardless of whether the injury resulted from the fault of the employee or the employer. Statutory limits of coverage are set by each state. The employer may purchase commercial insurance, participate in a state fund, or self-insure, based on the regulations of the particular state.

Wrongful termination: A claim brought by a former employee against the employer that the termination of employment was without cause, in violation of a contract of employment, or otherwise in violation of the law.

Index

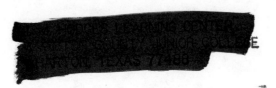

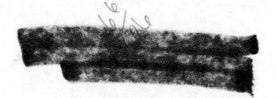